AAS
Agents and Actions Supplements
Vol. 37

Series Editors
K. Brune, Erlangen
M. J. Parnham, Bonn

Birkhäuser Verlag
Basel · Boston · Berlin

Prostaglandins in the Cardiovascular System

Edited by

H. F. Sinzinger
K. Schrör

1992

Birkhäuser Verlag
Basel · Boston · Berlin

Volume Editors' Addresses:

Prof. Dr. med. H. F. Sinzinger
Wilhelm Auerswald
Atherosclerosis Research Group
Nadlergasse 1
A–1090 Vienna
Austria

Prof. Dr. med. K. Schrör
Institut für Pharmakologie
Heinrich-Heine-Universität
Moorenstrasse 5
D–W–4000 Düsseldorf 1
FRG

Library of Congress Cataloging-in-Publication Data

Prostaglandins in the cardiovascular system / edited by
H. F. Sinzinger, K. Schrör.
(Agents and actions supplements ; vol. 37)
Includes bibliographical references and index.
ISBN 3-7643-2701-4 (acid-free paper) – ISBN 0-8176-2701-4 (acid-free paper)
1. Prostaglandins-Therapeutic use-Testing-Congresses.
2. Cardiovascular system-Diseases-Congresses. 3. Eicosanoic acid-
Derivatives-Therapeutic use-Testing-Congresses.
I. Sinzinger, H. (Helmut) II. Schrör, Karsten. III. Series: Agents and actions
supplements ; AAS 37.
[DNLM: 1. Cardiovascular System-drug effects-congresses.
2. Prostaglandins-congresses. W1 AG33A v. 37]
RC684.P76P78 1992
616.1'061 – dc20

Deutsche Bibliothek Cataloging-in-Publication Data

Prostaglandins in the cardiovascular system / ed. by H. F.
Sinzinger ; K. Schrör. – Basel ; Boston ; Berlin : Birkhäuser,
1992
(Agents and actions : Supplements ; Vol. 37)
ISBN 3-7643-2701-4 (Basel ...) Gb.
ISBN 0-8176-2701-4 (Boston) Gb.
NE: Sinzinger, Helmut F. [Hrsg.]; Agents and actions / Supplements

Printed in Germany on acid-free paper, directly from the authors' camera-ready manuscripts.

ISBN 3-7643-2701-4
ISBN 0-8176-2701-4

Contents

Preface

This volume contains the proceedings of the 5th International "Symposion on Prostaglandins in the Cardiovascular System" held in Vienna, Austria from September 22nd to 26th, 1991.

This Conference was the fifth in a series of meetings started 1982 in Bad Ischl, Austria, aiming to discuss the role of these compounds.

Eicosanoids attracted increasing scientific interest during the last few decades, especially concerning their role in the cardiovascular system. Not only the body of experimental and laboratory data is continuously enlarging, it looks also likely that despite the sometimes organizing slowness various substances are entering the stage of wider clinical use now.

The organizers are particularly grateful to Mrs Eva Unger and the staff of the Wilhelm Auerswald Atherosclerosis Research Group, Vienna for the expert technical support, both in organizing the Conference and arranging this volume. The Scientific Committee assisted greatly, especially in preparing the program, as did all the contributors, chairpersons and participants, to make this a successful event. It is a great pleasure to gratefully acknowledge the generous support by Schering AG, Berlin and Schwarz Pharma, Monheim, Germany. Last but not least the editors are thankful to Prof. Dr.K.Brune (Erlangen/Nürnberg, Germany) for the permission to edit this volume in Agents & Actions and finally Dr. C.F. Habicht and the staff of Birkhäuser (Basle, Switzerland) for expert and fast processing.

Helmut Sinzinger

Vienna, November 1991

AAS 37
Prostaglandins in the
Cardiovascular System

ROLE OF LEUKOTRIENE B_4 IN NEUTROPHIL-ENDOTHELIUM INTERACTIONS

Allan M. Lefer and Xin-liang Ma

Department of Physiology
Jefferson Medical College
Thomas Jefferson University
Philadelphia, Pennsylvania 19107
U.S.A.

Ischemia-reperfusion related tissue injury forms the basis of many important clinical disorders, including myocardial infarction, stroke, and circulatory shock. Abundant evidence exists to indicate that the process of reperfusion injury involvés components of a typical inflammatory reaction in which polymorphonuclear leukocyte (PMN) activation and infiltration play a critical role (Bulkley, 1989; Lucchesi, 1990; Weissman, 1989).

Adherence of PMNs to vascular endothelial cells (EC) is an initial step preceding PMN activation, migration and extravasation. Furthermore, the receptors on the PMN surface that are primarily responsible for this adhesive event have been identified as the CD11/CD18 glycoprotein complex (Smith, 1990). Administration of monoclonal antibodies (MAb) against the CD18 family of adhesive glycoproteins is effective in inhibiting PMN accumulation in inflammatory tissue and attenuating tissue injury (Ma et al., 1991; Vedder et al., 1990). However, recent experimental results have indicated that the importance of the CD11/CD18 complex in PMN-endothelial interaction depends upon the species and the conditions of PMN and EC activation (Carlos and Harlan, 1990).

One of the most potent and physiologically relevant chemoattractant and chemokinetic substances responsible for promoting PMN adherence to the endothelium is leukotriene B_4

(LTB_4) (Brain and Williams, 1990). LTB_4 has been identified as an important pro-inflammatory eicosanoid (Ford-Hutchinson, 1990).

We have developed a new method for assessing PMN adherence to endothelial cells (EC) using opened rings of blood vessels (Ma et al., 1991) and autologous PMNs isolated by density gradient methods and stained with a fluorescent dye according to the method of Yuan and Fleming (1990). PMNs adhering to the vascular endothelium after rinsing away loose PMNs are then corrected by epifluorescence microscopy. This system has been found to work well in both arteries and veins from rats, rabbits, cats and dogs.

Fig. 1 illustrates the concentration-response relationship for adherence of cat PMNs activated with either the chemotactic peptide formyl-methionyl-leucyl-phenylalanine (fMLP). There is an increase in PMN adherence up to a maximum concentration of 100 nM for both agonists. Moreover, the LTB_4 receptor antagonist LY 255283 almost totally blocked the LTB_4 induced PMN adherence. Although not shown, LY 255283 did not alter fMLP induced PMN adherence in this system. Thus, 100 nM LTB_4 appears to be maximal for adherence of cat PMNs to EC, a concentration which is also maximally adherent for fMLP. Therefore, we employed 100 nM LTB_4 as the PMN stimulating agonist.

Similar results were obtained with rat PMNs in rat superior mesenteric artery rings (Fig. 2). LTB_4 (100 nM) induced a 5-fold increase in PMN adherence which was blocked by 92% with the LTB_4 receptor antagonist LY 255283 (5 µg/ml), but not by the chemically related compound LY 189444 which is not a LTB_4 antagonist. Again, LY 255283 did not inhibit fMLP-induced PMN adherence to EC. Thus, LTB_4 is a very effective chemotactic agent for both rat and cat PMNs.

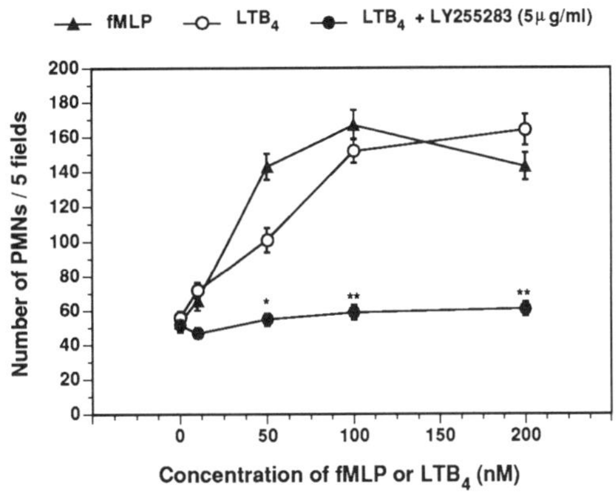

Fig. 1. Concentration-response curves of fMLP and LTB_4 on cat PMN adherence to unstimulated cat coronary EC. All values are means ± SEM for 7-9 rings from 5 or more cats. $^{*}p<0.05$; $^{**}p<0.01$ vs LTB_4 stimulation without LY 255283.

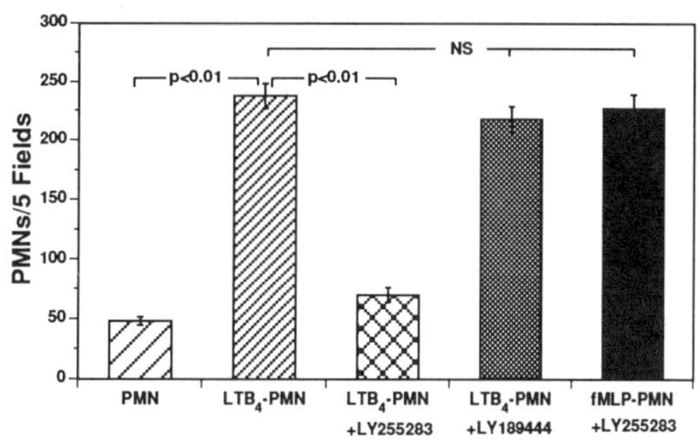

Fig. 2. Adherence of rat PMNs to rat SMA endothelial cells. Heights of bars are numbers of PMNs adhering after 20 min of activation; brackets indicate ± SEM for 7-10 experiments. LTB_4 and fMLP were present at 100 nM. LY compounds were present at concentrations of 5 μg/ml.

Further investigations were made regarding the specific adhesive proteins responsible for this PMN-EC interaction. PMN adherence to EC involves several adhesion molecules on the surface of both cell types (Tonnesen, 1989). Among those adhesion receptors found on PMNs, the CD11/CD18 glycoprotein complex appears to play a critical role in PMN-EC interaction. A number of factors, including fMLP, LTB_4, C5a, calcium ionophore and phorbol esters, may upregulate the surface expression of CD11/CD18 complex within minutes, thereby increasing PMN adherence to EC (Freyer et al., 1988). Furthermore, increased PMN adherence to EC induced by these factors is completely inhibited by MAbs against either the α-subunit of Mac-1 (i.e., CD11b) or the common β-chain of the glycoprotein complex (i.e., CD18). Moreover, the degree of PMN adherence to EC is significantly dependent upon the ligands expressed on the endothelial surface under different conditions.

Fig. 3 illustrates the relationship among adhesive proteins in mediating the LTB_4 induced PMN adherent to EC. Using a monoclonal antibody (MAbR15.7) against the common β-chain (i.e., CD18) of the adherence glycoprotein complex on PMN membranes, and one against the endothelial ligand ICAM-1 (MAbRR1/1), we were able to determine these relationships. Thus, MAbR15.7 almost totally inhibited (i.e., 87% inhibition) LTB_4-induced PMN adherence to cat coronary artery EC, whereas an isotype IGg-1 antibody (i.e., MAbR3.1) which does not bind to cat PMNs, was inactive. These findings strongly implicate the CD11/CD18 glycoprotein complex in the adherence process. Moreover, use of MAbRR1/1, a monoclonal antibody, against the endothelial ligand ICAM-1, also markedly attenuated adherence (i.e., 80% inhibition) in the same system. This strongly implicates ICAM-1 as a major endothelial ligand for PMN adherence induced by LTB_4.

The significance of PMN adherence goes far beyond the accumulation of PMNs in the vasculature. Activated and adhered

PMNs release a variety of humoral mediators including oxygen derived free radicals (i.e., superoxide) cytokines (e.g., TNF-α, IL-1β), proteases (e.g., elastase) and lipid mediators (e.g., LTD_4, PAF). Some of these mediators influence the vascular smooth muscle of the blood vessels to which the PMNs adhere. In this regard, superoxide radicals have been shown to inactivate endothelium-derived relaxing factor (EDRF) resulting in a severe vasoconstriction (Ma et al., 1991) in coronary arteries. The same phenomena occur in superior mesenteric arteries, as illustrated in Figure 4.

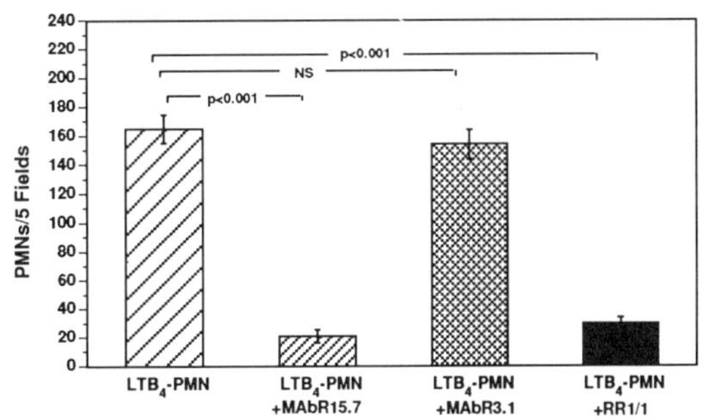

Fig. 3. LTB_4-stimulated PMN adherence to unstimulated endothelial cells and the effects of MAbs. MAbR15.7 (antibody against CD18) and MAbR3.1 (non-binding control antibody) was added before addition of 100 nM LTB_4. MAbRR1/1 (antibody against ICAM-1) was added before addition of PMN and LTB_4. Bar heights are means, brackets indicate ± SEM for 7-10 experiments.

Fig. 4 shows that 100 nM LTB_4 alone does not influence vascular tone in isolated SMA rings, nor does addition of 500,000 unactivated PMNs/ml to the bath. However, when PMNs are added to

SMA rings and then activated with 100 nM LTB_4, a marked degree of arterial contraction occurs. This contraction was almost totally inhibited when 5 µg/ml of the LTB_4 receptor antagonist, LY 255283 was added to the bath, confirming the effect of LTB_4 receptors in activating the PMNs. Additional experiments have clearly shown that the agent produced by the PMNs responsible for the arterial contraction is superoxide radicals acting against the basal release of EDRF (i.e., nitric oxide) (Ma et al., 1991).

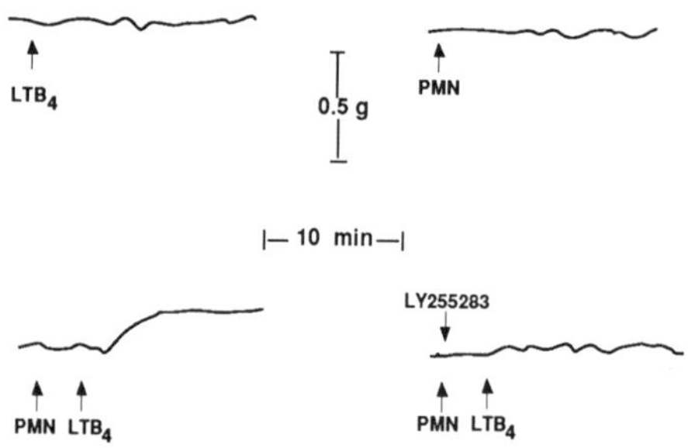

Fig. 4. Representative recordings of contractile responses of isolated rat SMA rings. PMN, polymorphonuclear leukocytes; LTB_4, leukotriene B_4.

These previous experiments show that activated PMNs can produce a significant anti-EDRF effect in isolated vessels which increases vascular tone. However, the question arises as to whether this phenomenon or a related event occurs *in vivo.* In order to answer this question, we subjected rats to splanchnic artery occlusion (SAO) and reperfusion (Karasawa et al., 1991). In this model, the celiac and superior mesenteric arteries were totally occluded for 90 minutes and then reperfused. When post-reperfusion mean arterial blood pressure fell to 45 mm Hg, usually about 90 to 120 min later, the SMA was removed, and arterial rings prepared in isolated muscle chambers. Fig. 5 illustrates representative recordings of SMA rings contracted with 10 nM U46619 (9,11-methanoepoxy-PGH_2) and challenged with acetylcholine (ACh) and A23187, two endothelium-dependent vasodilators, and acidified sodium nitrite ($NaNO_2$), an endothelium-independent vasodilator (Karasawa et al., 1991). All three vasodilators fully relaxed SMA rings isolated from sham SAO shock rats. In contrast, in SMA rings isolated from SAO shock rats, the two endothelium-dependent dilators failed to relax the SMA rings by more than 10-20%, whereas $NaNO_2$ fully relaxed these vascular rings. This provides strong evidence that SAO and reperfusion results in a significant endothelial dysfunction without impairment of vascular smooth muscle. LY 255283 given to the rats just prior to reperfusion preserved SMA vasorelaxation to ACh and A23187 by 60-70%. Thus, blockade of the effects of LTB_4 preserves the SMA vascular endothelium. This is consistent with the anti-PMN effects of LY 255283 in these same rats. Also, LY 255283 reduced intestinal myeloperoxidase (MPO) activity by half, indicating a significant inhibitory effect of the LTB_4 antagonist on PMN accumulation in the intestine following reperfusion. Since loss of EDRF promotes PMN adherence to cat mesenteric endothelium (Kubes et al., 1991). This endothelial dysfunction may be a key step in the pathophysiology of SAO reperfusion injury.

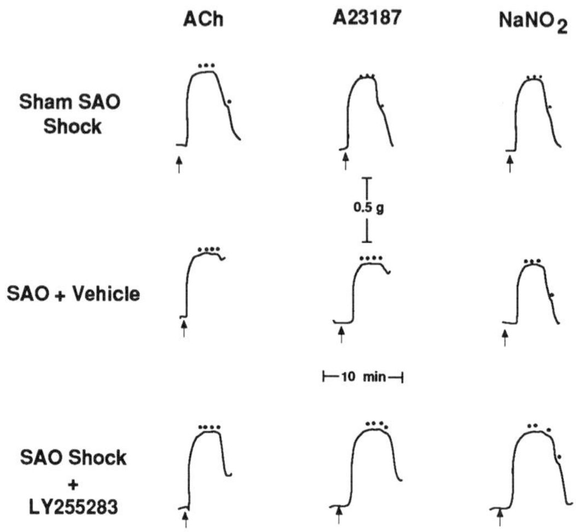

Fig. 5. Representative recordings of isolated rings of rat superior mesenteric artery (SMA) showing protective effect of LY 255283 on endothelium dysfunction after SAO and reperfusion. SMA rings were contracted with 10 nM U46619 and relaxation responses were observed for endothelium-dependent vasodilators, ACh (0.1, 1, 10, and 100 nM) and A23187 (1, 10, 100, and 1,000 nM), and for an endothelium-independent vasodilator, acidified $NaNO_2$ (0.1, 1, 10, and 100 μM). (From: Karasawa et al., 1991).

In summary, LTB_4 appears to play a key role in ischemia-reperfusion injury due to its prominent recruitment of PMNs to the ischemic site on reperfusion. LTB_4 also promotes PMN adherence to the vascular endothelium via upregulation of CD11/CD18 adhesive glycoprotein receptors on the PMN membrane and upregulation of ICAM-1 ligands on the EC membrane. Adherence leads to activation of PMNs with the subsequent release of humoral mediators including superoxide radicals (O_2^-). Superoxide radicals inactivate EDRF, resulting in vasoconstriction and enhanced PMN activation and aggregation, thus promoting a positive feedback loop which accentuates reperfusion injury. Coupled with TNF-α, O_2^- radicals erode EDRF (Kubes et al., 1991) and promote additional adherence of PMNs.

REFERENCES

Brain, S.D., and Williams, T.J. Leukotrienes and inflammation. Pharmacol. Therap. (1990) 46, 57-66.

Bulkley, G.B. Mediators of splanchnic organ injury: Overview and perspective. (1989). In: Splanchnic Ischemia and Multiple Organ Failure (A. Marston, G.B. Bulkley, R.G. Fiddian-Green and U.H. Haglund, Eds), London, Edward Arnold Publishers, pp. 183-191.

Carlos, T.M., and Harlan, J.M. (1990). Membrane proteins involved in phagocyte adherence to endothelium. Immunol. Rev. 114, 6-28.

Ford-Hutchinson, A.W. (1990). Leukotriene B_4 in inflammation. Crit. Rev. Immunol. 109, 1-12.

Freyer, D.R., Morganroth, M.L., Rogers, C.E., Arnaout, M.A., and Todd, R.F. (1988). Modulation of surface CD11/CD18 glycoproteins (Mol, LFA-1, p150,95) by human mononuclear phagocytes. Clin. Immunol. Immunopath. 46, 272-283.

Karasawa, A., Guo, J-p., Ma, X-l., Tsao, P.S., and Lefer, A.M. (1991). Protective actions of a leukotriene B_4 antagonist in splanchnic ischemia and reperfusion in rats. Am. J. Physiol. (G.I. and Liver Physiol.) 261, G191-G198.

Kubes, P., Suzuki, M., and Granger, D.N. (1991). Nitric Oxide: An endogenous modulator of leukocyte adhesion. Proc. Natl. Acad. Sci. USA 88, 4651-4655.

Lucchesi, B.R. (1990). Modulation of leukocyte-mediated myocardial reperfusion injury. Annu. Rev. Physiol.52, 561-576.

Ma, X-l., Tsao, P.S., Viehman, G.E., and Lefer, A.M. (1991). Neutrophil-mediated vasoconstriction and endothelial dysfunction in low-flow perfusion-reperfused cat coronary artery. Circ. Res. 69, 95-107.

Smith, C.W. (1990). Molecular determinants of neutrophil adhesion. Am. J. Respir. Cell. Mol. Biol. 2, 487-489.

Tonnesen, M.G. (1989). Neutrophil-endothelial cell interaction: Mechanisms of neutrophil adherence to vascular endothelium. J. Invest. Dermatol. 93, 53S-58S.

Vedder, N.B., Winn, R.K., Rice, C.L., Chi, E.Y., Arfors, K.E., and Harlan, J.M. (1990). Inhibition of leukocyte adherence by anti-CD18 monoclonal antibody attenuates reperfusion injury in the rabbit ear. Proc. Natl. Acad. Sci. USA 87, 2643-2646.

Weissman, G. (1989). The role of neutrophils in vascular injury: A summary of signal transduction mechanisms in cell/cell interactions. Springer Semin. Immunopathol. 11, 235-258.

Yuan, Y., and Fleming, B.P. (1990). A method for isolation and fluorescent labeling of rat neutrophils for intravital microvascular studies. Microvasc. Res. 40, 218-229.

AAS 37
Prostaglandins in the
Cardiovascular System

THROMBOXANE BIOSYNTHESIS AND METABOLISM IN RELATION TO CARDIOVASCULAR RISK FACTORS

Carlo Patrono, Giovanni Davì and Giovanni Ciabattoni

Departments of Pharmacology and Hematology, University of Chieti "G. D'Annunzio" School of Medicine, Chieti and Department of Pharmacology, Catholic University School of Medicine, Rome, Italy

SUMMARY: Enhanced platelet biosynthesis of thromboxane A_2 is associated with several cardiovascular risk factors, as a consequence of a direct effect on platelet biochemistry and/or some form of endothelial dysfunction. Moreover, episodic increases in thromboxane biosynthesis occur in acute coronary and cerebral ischemic syndromes. Thromboxane-dependent platelet activation represents an important mechanism that amplifies the consequences of acute vascular lesions as well as those of long-standing metabolic or hemodynamic disturbances, and results in increased risk of vascular occlusive events.

Thromboxane (TX) A_2 is a labile eicosanoid affecting contractile elements of the circulating blood (i.e., platelets), vasculature (i.e., smooth muscle cells), kidney (i.e., mesangial cells) and respiratory apparatus (i.e., bronchial smooth muscle cells). These effects are mediated through specific membrane receptors, one of which has recently been cloned and sequenced (Hirata et al., 1991). In platelets, TXA_2 represents an amplifying mechanism of activation and aggregation by virtue of its being synthesized and released in response to a variety of agonists (e.g. collagen, epinephrine, ADP, thrombin) and in turn inducing platelet aggregation.

MEASUREMENT OF TXA_2 BIOSYNTHESIS AND METABOLISM IN MAN

Measurement of TXB_2 in either plasma or urine is not a reliable index of *in vivo* platelet TXA_2 production (Patrono et al., 1986). TXB_2 undergoes two major pathways of metabolism in man, one involving ß-oxidation resulting in the formation of 2,3-dinor-TXB_2 and the other involving dehydrogenation of the hemiacetal alcohol group at C-11, resulting in the formation of a series of metabolites with a δ-lactone ring structure (e.g. 11-dehydro-TXB_2: Roberts et al., 1981). Although the former was originally described as the prevailing form of enzymatic degradation of infused TXB_2 in humans (Roberts et al., 1981), the latter has received considerable attention following the demonstration that 11-dehydro-TXB_2 has a substantially longer plasma half-life (Lawson et al., 1986) and is excreted at a higher rate (Catella and FitzGerald, 1987) than 2,3-dinor-TXB_2. Measurement of both would obviate the theoretical possibility of drug- or disease-related alterations in the metabolic disposition of TXB_2 (Ciabattoni et al., 1989).

Owing to its chemical instability, natural TXA_2 has not been isolated and characterized as a pure compound. It was not until 10 years after its discovery (Hamberg et al., 1975) that chemical synthesis of the proposed structure of TXA_2 was achieved (Bhagwat et al., 1985), thus allowing a direct comparison of the metabolism of synthetic TXA_2 and TXB_2 in the cynomolgus monkey (Patrignani et al., 1989). Similar metabolic disposition of TXA_2 and TXB_2 was demonstrated in this study, thereby suggesting that TXA_2 is likely to be hydrolyzed to TXB_2 before being converted to 11-dehydro-TXB_2 and 2,3-dinor-TXB_2. Thus, measurement of the urinary excretion of these metabolites provides a reliable indication of *in vivo* TXA_2 biosynthesis and release. Potential limitations in the interpretation of these measurements have been discussed previously (Patrono et al., 1989).

THROMBOXANE BIOSYNTHESIS AND CORONARY RISK FACTORS

AGE AND SEX: No major differences have been reported in thromboxane metabolite excretion as a function of age or sex. Fischer et al. (1986) found elevated levels of urinary 2,3-dinor-TXB_2 in neonates, on their third and fifth day of life, decreasing rapidly thereafter. Metabolite excretion was in the range of adult levels by the third year of life. No gender differences were found in the same study. Similarly, we found comparable excretion of 11-dehydro-TXB_2 in healthy subjects of both sexes who were 23 to 37 years old and those 42 to 73 years old (Davì et al., 1990). In the US Physicians' Health Study (1989), the reduction in the risk of myocardial infarction associated with the long-term use (average follow-up: 5 years) of aspirin in apparently healthy male subjects was apparent only in those 50 years of age or older. However, this widely publicized conclusion derives from post-hoc subgroup analysis. Moreover, there were only 51 myocardial infarctions in the 9051 subjects 40 to 49 years of age, i.e., an overall incidence of 0.56%, which would make detection of any aspirin effect in reducing risk an unrealistic exercise.

The recently reported Second Overview of the Antiplatelet Trialists' Collaboration (Second Main Meeting, Oxford, 23-25 March, 1990) failed to detect any statistically significant heterogeneity in the effects of the antiplatelet therapy in reducing the risk of major vascular events (nonfatal stroke, nonfatal myocardial infarction and vascular death) as a function of age. Another popular belief, i.e., of a sex difference in the protective effects of aspirin, is not upheld by the results of this very large overview involving approximately 70,000 patients, of whom individual data were available from 31 randomized clinical trials.

<u>SMOKING</u>: A number of studies have reported increased thromboxane metabolite excretion in apparently healthy chronic cigarette smokers (Fischer et al., 1986; Nowak et al., 1987; Lassila et al., 1988; Barrow et al., 1989).

In the study of Nowak et al. (1987), the difference in excretion of 2,3-dinor-TXB_2 was abolished by the administration of 20 mg aspirin bid for 10 days. After aspirin, the return of the excretion of 2,3-dinor-TXB_2 to pretreatment levels paralleled the recovery of platelet cyclooxygenase activity, consistent with a predominant platelet source of enhanced TXA_2 biosynthesis. In the study of Lassila et al. (1988) involving nine pairs of monozygotic male twins who were discordant for smoking for approximately 20 years, urinary 2,3-dinor-TXB_2 of the smoking twin was significantly higher (on the average 1.8 times higher) in every pair. Moreover, statistically significant correlations were found between thromboxane metabolite excretion and indexes of short-term (cotinine excretion) as well as long-term (pack years) smoking (Lassila et al., 1988). A positive correlation between the average reported cigarette consumption and excretion of thromboxane metabolites was also found by Barrow et al. (1989). In this study, there were comparable increases in the excretion rates of both 2,3-dinor-TXB_2 and 11-dehydro-TXB_2 in the smoking compared to the non-smoking group, consistent with these biochemical changes reflecting increased biosynthesis rather than altered metabolic disposition of TXA_2. In contrast, urinary unmetabolized TXB_2 which is thought to be derived primarily from the kidney was not significantly increased in smokers, nor was it correlated with cigarette consumption. At variance with these data, Uedelhoven et al. (1991) have recently reported that chronic smoking causes an alteration in the metabolism of TXA_2 by shifting the ratio of 11-dehydro-TXB_2 to 2,3-dinor-TXB_2 in urine. A competition between nicotine and TXB_2 for the 11-OH-dehydrogenation reaction has been postulated by the authors. Short-term exposure of normally non-smoking subjects to cigarette smoke did not increase the excretion of thromboxane metabolites, thus suggesting that increased TXA_2 biosynthesis in chronic smokers is unlikely to be a consequence of acute platelet activation (Barrow et al., 1989).

HYPERCHOLESTEROLEMIA: Increased platelet TXA_2 production has been described in Type IIa hypercholesterolemia (see Schrör, 1990 for a review). In order to verify the relevance of these *ex vivo* measurements to the actual rate of TXA_2 biosynthesis *in vivo*, we have assessed the urinary excretion of 11-dehydro-TXB_2 and 2,3-dinor-TXB_2 in 46 patients with type IIa hypercholesterolemia and 20 sex- and age-matched controls. Metabolite excretion was approximately 3-times higher in patients than controls, with 75% of the former having excretory rates in excess of 2 SD from the normal mean (Davì et al., 1991). A statistically significant correlation ($r=0.673$, $p<0.001$, $n=66$) was found between 11-dehydro-TXB_2 excretion and total plasma cholesterol. The HMG-CoA reductase inhibitor simvastatin (20 mg/day for 6 months) reduced significantly both cholesterol levels by 22 to 28% and urinary 11-dehydro-TXB_2 excretion by 32 to 42%, in 10 Type IIa patients. The observed reduction in metabolite excretion was consistent with the expected change that would be predicted by the above correlation, if enhanced TXA_2 biosynthesis was at least in part a consequence of elevated blood cholesterol levels. Selective inhibition of platelet cyclooxygenase activity by low-dose aspirin (50 mg/day for 7 days) was associated with cumulative inhibition of 11-dehydro-TXB_2 excretion by approximately 70%, consistent with a predominant platelet source of enhanced TXA_2 biosynthesis.

DIABETES MELLITUS: At variance with the results of *ex vivo* studies suggesting various abnormalities in platelet biochemistry and function, Alessandrini et al. (1988) have reported that the urinary excretion of 2,3-dinor-TXB_2 did not differ between healthy subjects and patients with Type I diabetes, with or without retinopathy, who lacked clinical evidence of macrovascular disease. In contrast, the excretion rate of 11-dehydro-TXB_2 was approximately 4-times higher in patients with Type II diabetes who had clinical evidence of macrovascular disease than in healthy controls (Davì et al., 1990; GA FitzGerald, personal communication). Enhanced metabolite excretion was present in the vast majority of these patients, irrespective of the type of macrovascular complication. The fractional conversion of exogenously infused TXB_2 to urinary 11-dehydro-TXB_2 was assessed in 4 diabetic patients and found to be comparable to that previously measured in healthy subjects (Ciabattoni et al., 1989). Thus, enhanced metabolite excretion detected in patients with Type II diabetes is likely to reflect increased biosynthesis of TXA_2 rather than a shift in its metabolic disposition. The 80% reduction in 11-dehydro TXB_2 in these patients after they received 50 mg of aspirin daily for one week, as well as the slow rate of recovery of metabolite excretion, was consistent with a role for platelets as a major source of enhanced TXA_2 production (Davì et al., 1990). Both diffuse vascular lesions and metabolic changes associated with the diabetic state might contribute to a persistent alteration in platelet biochemistry and function. As for the former possibility, in half of the patients studied by Davì et al. (1990) the clinical manifestation of macrovascular disease was stable angina pectoris, a condition not associated with enhanced TXA_2 biosynthesis (Fitzgerald et al., 1986). Moreover, elderly nondiabetic patients with peripheral vascular disease and no evidence of ischemic heart disease excreted

11-dehydro-TXB_2 a normal rate (Vejar et al., 1990). As for the second hypothesis, our study has demonstrated that biochemical indexes of platelet activation are cross-sectionally related to the state of metabolic control and that tight metabolic control can prospectively affect the actual rate of TXA_2 biosynthesis *in vivo* (Davì et al., 1990). It is likely that there are two components in the observed changes: one relating to the severity/duration of diabetes; the other, which may well be independent, to the severity/duration of atherosclerosis per se.

BLOOD PRESSURE: In a preliminary study of the rate of TXA_2 biosynthesis in relation to the blood pressure level, Minuz et al. (1990) found no absolute differences between the urinary excretion of 2,3-dinor-TXB_2 in mild hypertensive and control subjects. Moreover, no apparent relation was found between metabolite excretion and blood pressure in patients with mild hypertension (DBP:90 to 118 mmHg). However, the possible occurrence of independent circadian fluctuations in TXA_2 biosynthesis and blood pressure control might have obscured a relation between the two, if indeed it existed.

A special case for a relation between the rate of TXA_2 biosynthesis, the level of blood pressure and vascular occlusive complications is provided by pregnancy-induced hypertension. Fitzgerald et al. (1990) have recently demonstrated that excretion of both 2,3-dinor-TXB_2 and 11-dehydro-TXB_2 was significantly higher in patients with pregnancy-induced hypertension than in normotensive pregnant women. Moreover, thromboxane metabolite excretion correlated positively with mean arterial blood pressure and other indices of the severity of pregnancy-induced hypertension. The demonstration by Benigni et al. (1989) that low-dose aspirin (60 mg/day from the 12th week of gestation until delivery) reduced urinary 2,3-dinor-TXB_2 by approximately 80% in women at risk for pregnancy-induced hypertension is strongly suggestive of a predominant platelet source of enhanced TXA_2 biosynthesis in this setting. The potential beneficial effects of low-dose aspirin, as suggested by earlier small studies, are currently being assessed in at least 3 large multicenter randomized clinical trials.

CONCLUSIONS: The data we have reviewed suggest that enhanced platelet biosynthesis of TXA_2 is closely related to a number of coronary risk factors and is acutely expressed in unstable ischemic syndromes. We would like to propose that this alteration in platelet biochemistry and function represents an important mechanism that amplifies the consequences of acute vascular lesions as well as those of long-standing metabolic or hemodynamic disturbances, and results in increased risk of vascular occlusive events. This hypothesis can be tested under a variety of unexplored clinical conditions (e.g., combined influence of several risk factors) through the biochemical and analytical approach outlined in this review. Moreover the cause-effect relationship of these biochemical changes to vascular occlusive complications can be assessed through the use of inhibitors of TXA_2 synthesis and/or action.

Aknowledgements: The expert editorial assistance of M.L. Bonanomi is gratefully acknowledged.

REFERENCES

Alessandrini P, McRae J, Feman S, and FitzGerald GA (1988) N Engl J Med. 319,208-212.

Barrow SE, Ward PS, Sleightholm MA, Ritter JM, and Dollery CT (1989) Biochim Biophys Acta. 993, 121-127.

Benigni A, Gregorini G, Frusca T, Chiabrando C, Ballerini S, Valcamonico A, Orisio S, Piccinelli A, Pinciroli V, Fanelli R, Gastaldi A, and Remuzzi G (1989) N Engl J Med. 321, 357-362.

Bhagwat SS, Hamann PR, Still WL, Bunting S, and Fitzpatrick FA (1985) Nature. 315, 511-513.

Catella F, and FitzGerald GA (1987) Thromb Res. 47, 647-656.

Ciabattoni G, Pugliese F, Davì G, Pierucci A, Simonetti BM, and Patrono C (1989) Biochim Biophys Acta. 992, 66-70.

Davì G, Catalano I, Averna M, Notarbartolo A, Strano A, Ciabattoni G, and Patrono C (1990) N Engl J Med. 322, 1769-1774.

Davì G, Averna M, Catalano I, Notarbartolo A, Ciabattoni G, and Patrono C (1991) Thromb Haemostas. 65, 1185 (abstract).

Fischer S, Bernutz C, Meier H, and Weber PC (1986) Biochim Biophys Acta. 876, 194-199.

Fitzgerald DJ, Rocki W, Murray R, Mayo G, and FitzGerald GA (1990) Lancet. 335, 751-754.

Hamberg M, Svensson J, and Samuelsson B (1975) Proc Natl Acad Sci USA. 72, 2994-2998.

Hirata M, Hayashi Y, Ushikubi F, Yokota Y, Kageyama R, Nakanishi S, and Narumiya S (1991) Nature. 349, 617-620.

Lassila R, Seyberth HW, Haapanen A, Schweer H, Koskenvuo M, and Laustiola KE (1988) Br Med J. 297, 955-957.

Lawson JA, Patrono C, Ciabattoni G, and FitzGerald GA (1986) Anal Biochem. 155, 198-205.

Minuz P, Barrow SE, Cockcroft JR, and Ritter JM (1990) Hypertension. 15, 469-474.

Nowak J, Murray JJ, Oates JA, and FitzGerald GA (1987) Circulation. 76, 6-14.

Patrignani P, Morton H, Cirino M, Lord A, Charette L, Gillard J, Rokach J, and Patrono C (1989) Biochim Biophys Acta. 992, 71-77.

Patrono C, Ciabattoni G, Pugliese F, Pierucci A, Blair IA, and FitzGerald GA (1986) J Clin Invest. 77, 590-594.

Patrono C, Ciabattoni G, and Patrignani P (1989) In: Platelets and Vascular Occlusion, (Patrono C and FitzGerald GA Eds.), Raven Press, New York, pp 193-212.

Roberts LJ II, Sweetman BJ, and Oates JA (1981) J Biol Chem. 256, 8384-8393.

Schrör K (1990) Eicosanoids. 3, 67-73.

Steering Committee of the Physicians' Health Study Research Group (1989) N Engl J Med. 321, 129-135.

Uedelhoven WM, Rützel A, Meese CO, and Weber PC (1991) Biochim Biophys Acta. 1081, 197-201.

Vejar M, Fragasso G, Hackett D, Lipkin PD, Maseri A, Born GVR, Ciabattoni G, and Patrono C (1990) Thromb Haemostas. 63, 163-168.

AAS 37
Prostaglandins in the
Cardiovascular System

PATHOPHYSIOLOGY OF CRITICAL LEG ISCHAEMIA AND MODE OF ACTION OF PROSTAGLANDINS

Vittorio Bertele'[1], Chiara Cerletti[2], Giovanni de Gaetano[2]

[1]Istituto di Clinica Medica Generale, Ospedale "L. Sacco", Università di Milano and

[2]Istituto di Ricerche Farmacologiche Mario Negri, Consorzio "Mario Negri Sud"
66030 Santa Maria Imbaro, Italy

The purpose of this paper is to review and possibly match some of the alledged pathophysiological aspects of critical limb ischaemia (CLI) and the properties of vasoactive prostaglandins (PGs) (namely PGE_1, and PGI_2) likely counteracting them, thus suggesting a therapeutic role of these PGs in CLI.

PATHOPHYSIOLOGICAL ASPECTS OF CLI

The pathophysiological mechanisms of CLI are still largely undefined. According to the hypothesis proposed by the recent European Consensus Conference on CLI (Second Consensus Document on CLI, 1991), atherosclerosis is still regarded as the underlying pathogenetic process. Possibly complicated by thrombosis, atherosclerosis narrows the lumen of proximal conducting arteries, thus reducing blood flow and perfusion pressure to the distal circulation. Despite compensatory mechanisms, such as arteriolar vasodilation and collateral formation, eventually the blood flow falls down to a level at which nutritive requirements of peripheral tissues cannot be met. This is also due to a maldistribution of peripheral flow, so that flow reduction does not spare even the nutritional vessels, though representing only the 15% of the overall peripheral microcirculation. This sequence of events results in the failure of microcirculation, leading to the typical pathological picture characterized by reduction of the number of perfused capillaries, reduction of blood flow in them, presence of perivascular haemorrhage and of tissue edema.

ANTIATHEROSCLEROTIC EFFECT OF PGs

In respect to the fundamental pathogenetic process of CLI, PGs reportedly exert an antiatherosclerotic effect, mainly due to stimulation of cholesterol metabolism in smooth muscle cells (SMCs) (Hajjar & Weksler, 1983; Orekhov et al., 1986) and macrophages (Willis et al., 1986). PGs exert a hypolipemic activity also by increasing the binding of LDL to apo-B receptors in different animal species (Virgolini et al., 1991). Moreover, the effect of PGI_2 on cholesterol metabolism is potentiated by HDL; this is possibly due to the fact that HDL-associated apolipoprotein A-I reportedly stabilizes PGI_2 in blood (Morishita et al., 1990), an effect apparently reduced in cardiovascular disease (Aoyama et al., 1990).

PGI_2 and its analogues may also act as antiatherosclerotic agents by inhibiting the proliferation of SMCs and fibroblasts either directly or by preventing growth factor release from platelets, endothelial cells and macrophages. The antiproliferative activity of PGs has been questioned by the lack of an effect of iloprost on intimal hyperplasia following endothelial injury in rat carotid arteries (Levitt et al., 1991).

On the other hand - quite interestingly - it was recently reported that another PGI_2 analogue has been shown to selectively inhibit SMC proliferation, while not affecting endothelial proliferation, an effect that could be of advantage in the perspective of the therapeutic use of these agents in the prevention of atherosclerosis progress.

Both antiatherosclerotic activities (stimulation of cholesterol-ester metabolism and inhibition of SMC proliferation) are mediated by cAMP increase. Though short-lasting, this mechanism of action and its biological effects could be reconciled with a delayed and prolonged clinical benefit, because of the particular biochemical and pathogenetic targets involved.

PROFIBRINOLYTIC ACTIVITY

Prostacyclin potential (FitzGerald et al., 1984) and fibrinolytic activity (Dembinska-Kiec et al., 1982; Szczeklik et al., 1983; Musial et al., 1986) are reportedly reduced in atherosclerotic vessels (D'Angelo et al., 1978). This may facilitate thrombus formation at the site of vascular lesions, leading to further reduction of the lumen or even to its acute occlusion. Interestingly enough, defective PGI_2 production and fibrinolytic activity seem to be related. This is suggested by the observation that high dose-aspirin and indobufen limit fibrinolytic response to venous stasis, while both salicylate and low dose-aspirin, which spare the overall and the vascular PGs production respectively, do not (de Gaetano et al., 1986). In healthy volunteers given aspirin we observed a reduced fibrinolytic response to venous stasis measured as euglobuline lysis area. Infusion of iloprost could restore a normal fibrinolytic response similar to that observed in control subjects not given aspirin (Bertele' et al., 1989). Neither aspirin nor iloprost modified tissue plasminogen activator (t-PA) or plasminogen activator inhibitor (PAI-1) antigen levels in our hands, although later on aspirin has been shown to inhibit t-PA antigen release in response to venous stasis (Levin et al., 1989; Iacoviello et al., 1991). We observed a similar fibrinolytic effect of iloprost in patients with peripheral occlusive artery disease with poor fibrinolytic response to venous stasis. The infusion of iloprost restored a normal fibrinolytic response, though without increasing t-PA antigen levels, which were reduced in these patients (Bertele' et al., 1988).

Besides promoting local pathogenetic processes, the distal circulation may be affected by atherosclerosis as peripheral vessels are reached by cells and plasma factors activated by contact with larger atherosclerotic vessels.

Once activated, platelets, leukocytes and endothelial cells release growth factors, which may in turn extend atherosclerotic lesions. Platelets and polymorphonuclear leukocytes (PMNs) may aggregate to each other and form thrombi plugging the microcirculation. Fibrin formation at the surface of activated cells stabilizes the thrombus, whose lysis is hampered by platelet release of PAI-1. Thromboxane, serotonin and leukotriene (C4 and D4) release may cause vasoconstriction. Leukotrienes themselves, free-radicals and lysosomal proteases may mediate ischaemia-induced tissue damage. All these processes are magnified by the loss of endothelial defence mechanisms, which are replaced by the expression of proadhesive, prothrombotic, vasoconstrictory properties. PGs may interfere with these processes at different levels. Their antiplatelet activity, for istance, is known since long. By increasing cyclic AMP, PGs prevent platelet response to different stimuli. The control of overall platelet function by PGs may suggest a far greater advantage of these compounds as compared to other antiplatelet agents, such as aspirin; the latter affects only an amplification pathway of platelet function not necessary to most of the physiologic stimuli to induce full platelet activation. At least theoretically, these properties make inhibitory PGs the most effective antiplatelet agents presently available.

This assumption has been verified since long in "in vivo" models of platelet activation. When prostacyclin had not been discovered yet, PGE_1 as well as some pyrimido-pyrimidine compounds but not aspirin, were shown to prevent the fall in platelet count following ADP infusion in rats (Reyers-Degli Innocenti et al., 1974)

EFFECT ON PMNs AND PMN/PLATELET INTERACTION

Moreover, PGs inhibit platelet activation promoted by stimulated PMNs. Iloprost prevented such an activation (Del Maschio et al., 1990), while several other potential inhibitors of PMN/platelet interaction did not; among the latter compounds, one should include aspirin, dipyridamole, PAF receptor antagonists (unless used in prevention of PMN activation by this specific agonist), superoxide dismutase, catalase and serine protease inhibitors (unless in the absence of cell-interaction, a condition otherwise protecting cathepsin G, released from PMNs on adherent platelets from inactivation by antiproteases (Evangelista et al., 1991).

In a mixed population of PMNs and platelets, iloprost at nanomolar concentrations of inhibited intraplatelet Ca^{2+} rise induced by different stimuli of PMN function. It also inhibited the release of the azurophil granule content, superoxide generation and chemotaxis of PMN stimulated by the chemotactic peptide fMLP (Cerletti et al., 1991).

The inhibitory effects on PMN function, however, were apparent at μmolar concentrations of iloprost, much higher than those required for the inhibition of platelet activation induced by stimulated PMNs. Thus, iloprost interferes with PMN/platelet activation most likely by directly inhibiting platelet function, at least in the range of concentrations achievable "in vivo".

On the other hand, "in vivo" studies using intravital videomicroscopy in rats have shown that both PGE_1 and PGI_2 (as well as its analogues) inhibit leukocyte adhesion to normal (Fricke et al., 1985) and damaged (Müller et al., 1988) vessel wall. The same effect was observed in a model of post-ischaemic vascular damage (Erlansson et al., 1991). Moreover, the reduction of infarct size induced by iloprost in an ischaemia/reperfusion model in dogs has been ascribed to a reduced neutrophil accumulation (Simpson et al., 1987).

PROSTAGLANDINS AS MEDIATORS OF ENDOTHELIUM DEFENCE MECHANISMS

Besides platelets and leukocytes, endothelial cells too play a role in the pathogenesis of CLI. Damage of endothelium brings about a shift from antithrombogenic and vasodilatory properties to prothrombotic and vasoconstrictory mediators and mechanisms. These induce activation of platelets and leukocytes and of their interaction as well. They also promote the expression of procoagulant activity and SMC contraction, proliferation and intimal migration. The exhaustion of PGI_2 "reserve" is of obvious relevance in this shift of properties, because of the loss of its antiplatelet and vasodilatory activity and of its potentiating effect on Endothelium-Derived Relaxing Factor (EDRF).
Actually, PGI_2 and EDRF act in concert in defence of vascular wall: they are released by the same stimuli (De Nucci et al., 1988) and potentiate each other as inhibitors of platelet and leukocyte function and as promoters of thrombolysis but not as relaxants of SMCs (Gryglewski et al., 1989). The cell selectivity of the synergism between adenylate and guanylate cyclases might facilitate the combined use of PGI_2 and EDRF donors in prevention of thrombotic disorders without interference with the overall cardiovascular system function (Gryglewski et al., 1989).
Iloprost has been shown indeed to prevent hypoxia-induced loss of endothelial function mediated by EDRF (Turker et al., 1988), a factor of critical relevance in the microvascular defence system regulation and a pivotal actor in the microvascular flow regulating system .

ANTITHROMBOTIC EFFECT

Do all these physiological and pharmacological activities of PGs result in an actual antithrombotic effect? Apparently, they do. Indeed, not only they limit thrombus formation in different animal models of vascular injury (Witt & Müller, 1987), but are also able to reduce the size of the thrombus once formed (Witt & Baldus, 1988), an effect possibly related to the profibrinolytic activity already mentioned.

EFFECT ON MICROCIRCULATION

Another question is: may inhibitory PGs interfere with processes and mediators possibly counteracting compensatory vasodilation or altering autoregulatory vasomotion?
The evidence that PGI2 and iloprost protect myocardium from reperfusion injury in the absence of haemodynamic effects might question the relevance of a protective role of their vasodilatory activity (Melin & Becker, 1983; Chiariello et al., 1988; Ferrari et al., 1988). However, these observations do not completely dispel a possible beneficial effect of vasodilatory activity of PGs in the peripheral circulation, in contrast with observations at the coronary level. Indeed, PGs can actually protect microvascular flow regulating system: by dilating arterioles and venules, increasing capillary perfusion (Müller et al., 1987), limiting vascular permeability to macromolecules (Erlansson et al., 1991; Müller et al., 1987) and , therefore, tissue edema and even necrosis (Müller & Schmidtke, 1990) following the reduction of blood supply. This latter effect, particularly, could also be ascribed to the so called cytoprotective effect of PGs.

CYTOPROTECTIVE EFFECT

First observed on gastric and intestinal mucosa, this effect is unlikely confined to specific cell or organ targets. Rather, it could involve several tissues, thanks to a general effect on cell membranes, leading to reduction of Ca^{2+} influx into the cell or into mitochondria (thus impairing oxidative peroxidation and energy production) or leading to a reduction of the outflow of dangerous mediators, such as proteolytic enzymes or noradrenaline from perivascular sympathetic nerve fibres (Schrör & Funke, 1985; Ferrari et al., 1988). In several models of tissue damage induced by reperfusion (Tosaki et al., 1990), toxic agents (Sakai et al., 1990) or irradiation (Sinzinger et al., 1991) a protective effect of PGI2 and its analogues has been demonstrated.

FROM PHARMACOLOGICAL ACTIVITIES TO THERAPEUTICAL EFFICACY

PGs may interfere with the pathogenetic events leading to CLI by many different mechanisms. It is difficult to say whether some of them (particularly which ones) are of actual clinical relevance, mostly due to the uncertainties still surrounding the pathophysiology of CLI. There is evidence that biological activities of PGs (antiplatelet, vasodilatory) may result in pharmacological effects (antithrombotic, defence of microvascular system, cytoprotection), all of possible clinical benefit in CLI. Pooling data from homogeneous trials, T. Chalmers has recently shown that iloprost reduces by about a half the amputation rate at 3 to 6 months in patients with CLI (unpublished observation). The combination of two major end-points (amputation and death rate) from the trials, where mortality data were available, strenghtened this suggestion. Indeed, Chalmer's meta-analysis showed that iloprost almost halved the incidence of these combined end-points in patients with CLI.

FUTURE PERSPECTIVES

In conclusion, a better understanding of the pathogenetic events of CLI and the role of prostanoids in this field would improve our means to treat this disease. On the other hand, preliminary findings of a clinical benefit of PGs in CLI may provide a useful basis to further address these questions by a more pragmatic approach. In the Eighties, basic pharmacological investigations on the antiplatelet effect of aspirin were strenghtened by the results of several trials and the meta-analysis of the Anti-Platelet Trialists' collaboration showing the benefit of aspirin in the prevention of cardiovascular events. The evidence of the clinical benefit of aspirin definitively proved the relevance of a mechanism of action (the inhibition of platelet thromboxane production) generally thought too narrow to account for any important therapeutical advantage.

Thus, most likely future randomized clinical trials on the efficacy of PGs on clinically relevant events in CLI will help better understanding of the pathophysiology of this disease and of the pharmacological role of PGs in its treatment.

ACKNOWLEDGEMENTS

We thank Maria Teresa Di Prospero for the preparation of the manuscript.

This work was supported by the C.N.R. (National Research Council, Rome, Italy, Convenzione C.N.R. - Consorzio Mario Negri Sud).

REFERENCES

Aoyama, T., Yui, Y., Morishita, Y., and Kaway, C. (1990) Circulation 81, 1784-1791

Bertele', V., Mussoni, L., Del Rosso, G., Pintucci, G., Carriero, M.R., Merati, M.G., Libretti, A., and de Gaetano, G. (1988) Thromb. Haemost. 60, 141-144.

Bertele', V., Mussoni, L., Pintucci, G., Del Rosso, G. Romano, G., de Gaetano, G., and Libretti, A. (1989) Thromb. Haemost. 61, 286-288

Cerletti, C., Del Maschio, A.,Ursini M., Rajtar G., Evangelista, V., and de Gaetano, G. (1991) Thromb. Res. Suppl. XIII, 49

Chiariello, M., Golino, P., Cappelli-Bagazzi, M., Ambrosio, G., Tritto, I., and Salvatore, M. (1988) Am. Heart J.115, 499-504

D'Angelo, V., Villa S., Mysliwiec, M., and Donati, M.B. (1978) Thromb. Haemost. 39, 535-536

Dembinska-Kiec, A., Kostka-Trabka, E., and Gryglewski, R.J. (1982) Thromb. Haemost. 47, 190

de Gaetano, G., Carriero, M.R., Cerletti, C., and Mussoni, L. (1986) Biochem. Pharmacol. 35, 3147-3150

De Nucci, G., Gryglewski, R.J., Warner, T.D., and Vane, J.R.(1988) Proc. Natl. Acad. Sci. 85, 2334-2338

Del Maschio, A.,Evangelista, A., Rajtar G., Chen, Z.M., Cerletti, C., and de Gaetano, G. (1990) Am. J. Physiol. 258, H870-H879

Erlansson, M., Bergqvist, D., Persson, N.H., and Svensjo, E.(1991) Prostaglandins 41, 157-168

Evangelista, V., Rajtar, G., de Gaetano, G., White, J.G., and Cerletti, C. (1991) Blood 77, 2379-2388

Ferrari, R., Cargnoni, A., Ceconi, C., Curello, S. Belloli, S., Albertini, A., and Visioli O. (1988) J. Mol. Cell Cardiol. 20, 1095-1106

FitzGerald, G.A., Smith, B., Pedersen, A.K., and Brash, A.R. (1984) N. Engl. J. Med. 310, 1065-1068

Fricke, D., Damerau, S., and Vogt, W., (1985) Int. Arch. Allergy Appl. Immunol. 78, 429-437

Gryglewski, R.J., Korbut, R., Trabka-Janik, E., Zembowicz, A. and Trybulec, M. (1989) J. Cardiovasc. Pharmacol. 14 (Suppl.11), S124-S128

Iacoviello L., Amore C., De Curtis A., Cerletti C., and Donati M.B. (1991) Thromb. Haemost. 65, 922

Hajjar, D.P., and Weksler, B.B. (1983) J. Lipid Res. 24, 1176-1185

Levin, R.I., Harpel, P.C., Harpel, J.G., and Recht, P.A. (1989) Blood 4, 1635-1643

Levitt, M.A., Dryjski, M., Tluczek, J., and Bjornsson, T.D. (1991) Prostaglandins 41, 1-6

Melin, J.A., and Becker, L.C. (1983) J. Am. Coll. Cardiol. 2, 279-286

Morishita, H., Yui, Y., Hattori, R., Aoyama, T., and Kawai, C. (1990) J. Clin. Invest. 86, 1885-1891

Müller, B., Schmidtke, M., and Witt, W. (1987) Leukotrienes Med. 29, 187-198

Müller, B., Schmidtke, M., and Witt, W. (1988) Eicosanoids 1, 13-17

Müller, B., and Schmidtke, M. (1990) Prostaglandins Leukotrienes and Essential Fatty Acids 39, 63-64

Musial, J., Wilczynska, M., Sladek, K, Cierniewski, C.S., Nizankowski, R., and Szczeklik, A.(1986) Prostaglandins 31, 61-70

Orekhov, A.N., Tertov, V.V., Mazurov, A.V. Andreeva, E.R.,Repin, V.S., and Smirnov, V.N. (1986) Drug Rev. Res. 9, 189-201

Reyers-Degli Innocenti, I., Poggi, A., and de Gaetano, G. (1974) Scand. J. Haemat. 13, 331-337

Sakai, A., Yajima, M., and Nishio, S. (1990) Life Sciences 47, 711-719

Schrör, K., and Funke, K, (1985) J. Cardiovasc. Pharmacol. 7 (Suppl.5), S50-S54

Second Consensus Document on Critical Limb Ischaemia, (1991) Circulation in press

Simpson, P.J., Michelson, J. Fontane, J.C., Gallagher, K.P., and Lucchesi, B.R. (1987) Circ. Res. 60, 666-673

Sinzinger, H., Zidek, T., Rauscha, F., and Firbas, W. (1991) Prostaglandins 41, 57-65

Szczeklik A., Kopec, M., Sladek, K., Musial, J., Chmielewska, J., Teisseyre, E., Dudek-Wojciechowska, G., and Palester-Chlebowczyk, M. (1983) Thromb. Res. 29, 655-660

Tosaki, A., Koltai, M., and Paubert-Braquet, M. (1990) Eur. J. Pharmacol. 191, 69-81

Turker, R.K., and Demirel, E. (1988) Pharamcology 36, 151-155

Virgolini, I, Li, S.R., Lupattelli, G., Pidlich, J., Angelberger, P., Banyai, M., and Sinzinger, H. (1991) Prostaglandins 42, 81-93

Willis, A.L., Smith, D.L., Vigo, C., and Kluge, A.F. (1986) Lancet 2, 682-683

Witt, W., and Baldus, B. (1988) Fibrinolysis 2, 157

Witt, W., and Müller, B., (1987) In: Advances in Prostaglandin, Thromboxane, and Leukotriene Research (B. Samuelsson, R. Paoletti and P.W. Ramwell Eds), Raven Press, New York, pp 279-284

AAS 37
Prostaglandins in the
Cardiovascular System

INCREASED PRODUCTION OF PLATELET-DERIVED THROMBOXANE IN PATIENTS WITH LUPUS ANTICOAGULANT

J. MACLOUF, F. LELLOUCHE, M. MARTINUZZO[1], P. SAID[2], and L.O. CARRERAS[1,2]

U150 INSERM, Hôpital Lariboisière, 6, rue Guy Patin 75475-Paris Cedex 10 France [1]Haemostasis and Thrombosis Section, Division of Haematology,[2]Department of Clinical Biochemistry, Faculty of Pharmacy and Biochemistry Hospital de Clínicas, University of Buenos Aires, Córdoba 2351, Buenos Aires, Argentina

SUMMARY The in vivo production of thromboxane A_2 and prostacyclin was assessed in 31 samples from 25 patients with lupus anticoagulant and in 32 controls. The urinary excretion of 11-dehydro-thromboxane B_2 (a major thromboxane metabolite of platelet origin) was very significantly increased ($p<0.0003$) in the patients contrasting with a lesser increase of urinary 2,3-dinor-6-keto-prostaglandin $F_{1\alpha}$ reflecting the vascular production of prostacyclin ($p<0.02$). Our study shows that in patients with lupus anticoagulant, platelet activation may occur without a compensatory increment in the vascular biosynthesis of prostacyclin suggesting an increased risk for thrombosis.

Thromboxane (TX)A_2 and prostacyclin (PGI_2) are the major prostanoids respectively formed by platelets and vessel wall. Because of their potent and contrasting effects on platelet activation and vascular tone, an abnormal (i.e. elevated) TXA_2/PGI_2 ratio may predispose affected patients to thrombosis (Moncada and Vane, 1978). Lupus anticoagulant (LA) has been reported to interfere with the production of PGI_2 by vascular tissues *in vitro* (Carreras et al 1981a and b, Carreras and Vermylen, 1982, de Castellarnau et al, 1983, Elias and Eldor, 1984, Schorer et al 1989). This phenomenon could either reflect or play a role in the origin of thrombotic events and obstetric complications in patients with LA (Carreras and Vermylen, 1991). However, controversial results on the effect of the LA on the generation of eicosanoids by cultured endothelial cells and stimulated platelets have been reported (Rustin et al 1987, Petraiulo et al 1988, Hasselaar et al 1988).

Recent studies have shown that urinary metabolites of TX and PGI_2 constitute unique markers of the activation and/or interaction between platelets and vascular cells. The measurement of these metabolites does reflect the *in vivo* production of these mediators and has the advantage of circumventing the artefactual production of eicosanoids occurring during blood or tissue sampling (Granström et al 1984, Catella et al 1986). Thus, such approach could help determine the status of an imbalance of production between TX and PGI_2 in patients with LA.

We have recently developed a technique using thin layer chromatography/enzyme immunoassay for measuring the urinary metabolites of platelet-derived TXA_2 (i.e. 2,3-dinor-TXB_2 and 11-dehydro-TXB_2) and of vascular cell-derived PGI_2 (i.e. 2,3-dinor-6-keto-$PGF_{1\alpha}$) (Lellouche et al 1990). This methodology was used to evaluate the biosynthesis of eicosanoids in patients with LA.

MATERIALS AND METHODS

Patients:

We measured the metabolites of TXA_2 and PGI_2 in the urine of 25 patients (mean age, 33.7 years) with LA and anticardiolipin (aCL) antibodies detected by ELISA as described (Forastiero et al 1990, Loizou et al 1985, Harris 1990). All patients had normal renal function and normal platelet count. Thirty two healthy subjects (mean age 32 years) who had not received any drug for at least 15 days before urine collection served as controls.

Measurement of urinary metabolites of TXA_2 and PGI_2:

Overnight urines were collected in the morning, fractionated in 50 ml aliquots and kept frozen at -70 °C until analysis.

Briefly, urinary PGI_2 and TXA_2 metabolites were extracted from 3-40 ml of urine corresponding to 100 μmoles creatinine using Sep-Pak^R cartridges (Waters, Milford, MA); ^{3}H-TXB_2 (Du-Pont, Paris, France, 3.7-9.25 TBq/mmol) was added for recovery. Metabolites were further purified by thin layer chromatography and quantitation was performed by enzyme immunoassay (Pradelles et al 1985) after correction of the values for losses in recovery. This method has been correlated with the results obtained by GC/MS (r=0.98) (Lellouche et al 1990).

RESULTS

All the patients' sera had aCL antibodies detected by ELISA at high (>100 GPL units or >60 MPL units) or moderate level (20-100 GPL units or 20-60 MPL units) in addition to the LA.

Determination of the urinary excretion of TXA_2 and PGI_2 metabolites showed a significantly increased excretion of 11-dehydro-TXB_2 in 25 patients with LA as compared to 32 healthy individuals (141 ± 25 vs 33.7 ± 2.9 ng/mmol creatinine respectively, $p<0.0003$).

TABLE I
Excretion of the urinary metabolites of TXA_2 and of PGI_2 in patients with lupus anticoagulant (ng/mmol creatinine)

	Controls n=32	Patients n=25
11-dehydro-TXB_2	33.7 ± 2.9	141 ± 25*
dinor-6-keto-$PGF_{1\alpha}$	15.1 ± 1.3	22.3 ± 2.4**

* $p<0.0003$; ** $p<0.02$

We found no significant difference between patients with or without SLE (128±21 vs 107±19 ng/mmol creatinine respectively, p=0.48). In contrast, we found minor modifications of 2,3-dinor-6-keto-$PGF_{1\alpha}$ (22.3 ± 2.4 vs 15.1 ± 1.3 ng/mmol creatinine, $p<0.02$)(Table 1). In 3 patients with LA and aCL antibodies, we measured the urinary eicosanoid metabolites on 3 occasions over a 1 year period. Although there were some intra-individual fluctuations throughout time, the values of 11-dehydro-TXB_2 were consistently elevated whereas 2,3-dinor-6-keto-$PGF_{1\alpha}$ remained within the range of control values.

DISCUSSION

Anticardiolipin antibodies as well as the LA are associated with thromboembolic phenomena, repeated fetal loss and thrombocytopenia (Carreras and Vermylen 1982, Elias and Eldor 1984, Harris et al 1983, Lechner 1987). The term "anticardiolipin antibody syndrome" and more recently "antiphospholipid syndrome" have been proposed to describe this particular group of patients (Hughes et al 1986). In spite of considerable interest in this syndrome over the last few years the mechanisms implicated in the association between antiphospholipid (aPL) antibodies and thrombosis remain unclear (Carreras and Vermylen 1991). Several authors have reported that the LA may interfere with the production of PGI_2 by vascular tissues (Carreras et al 1981a and b, Carreras and Vermylen, 1982, de Castellarnau et al, 1983, Elias and Eldor, 1984, Schorer et al 1989). Such inhibition of PGI_2 production could play a role in the origin of thrombotic events and obstetric complications in these patients (Carreras et al 1981a and b, Carreras and Vermylen, 1982, de Castellarnau et al, 1983, Elias and Eldor 1984). However, controversial results on the effect of the LA on the generation of PGI_2 by endothelial cells in culture have also been reported (Rustin et al 1987, Petraiuolo et al 1988, Hasselaar et al 1988). These data obtained *in vitro* could partially be related to methodological aspects (Carreras and Vermylen 1991). For example, they could be influenced by the source of endothelial cells, the presence or absence of the immunoglobulin containing the LA in the incubation medium during the stimulation experiments, or agents employed to stimulate PGI_2

synthesis.

The present study proves that an abnormal synthesis of eicosanoids occurs *in vivo* in some patients with LA. We found a much higher increase of the urinary excretion of TXA_2 metabolites of platelet origin than that of PGI_2, leading to an imbalance in the TXA_2/PGI_2 ratio. In the present series of patients with SLE, this abnormality may not be attributed to the underlying disease. Patrono et al (1985) have shown earlier that only urinary TXB_2 and 6-keto-$PGF_{1\alpha}$ were affected in patients with SLE but without LA whereas the platelet-derived urinary metabolite 2,3-dinor-TXB_2 was unchanged. Based on earlier studies we can rule out that the marked increase in urinary excretion of these metabolites in our patients as compared with the control group may not be related to differences in sex (Vesterqvist et al 1983, 1984), age distribution (Reilly et al 1986) or platelet count (Ciabattoni et al 1990) (none of the patients was thrombocytopenic at the time of the study). Arfors et al (Arfors et al 1990) have recently reported an increased excretion of 2,3-dinor-TXB_2 in patients with aPL antibodies which, they hypothesized, could be derived from platelets. The present study differs on the fact that all patients were selected because of the presence of LA activity.

In general, a concomitant increase in the biosynthesis of TXA_2 and PGI_2 has been observed in a number of conditions associated with increased platelet turnover (FitzGerald et al 1984, Fitzgerald et al 1986, Reilly et al 1986). Enhanced synthesis of PGI_2 may represent (or reflect) a compensatory response of vascular endothelium to platelet activation (Fitzgerald et al 1986). Moreover, an enhanced *in vivo* biosynthesis of PGI_2 in patients with severe atherosclerosis (FitzGerald et al 1984) occurs despite a reduced capacity of atherosclerotic blood vessels to generate PGI_2 *in vitro* (Sinzinger et al 1979). In this study, the urinary metabolites considered to reflect the vascular production of PGI_2 (FitzGerald et al 1983, Patrono et al 1983) were only slightly increased as compared with normal controls. This may reflect an abnormal compensatory response of the vessel wall to platelet activation. In summary, our study shows that LA would create a rather unique abnormality with concomitant platelet activation and TXA_2 generation associated to a failure of the vessel wall to produce increased amounts of the natural platelet inhibitory compound PGI_2. This phenomenon may be crucial to generate an increased risk for thrombosis in patients with LA (Lellouche et al 1991).

Acknowledgments: Part of this work was supported by a grant from Caisse Nationale d'Assurance Maladie des Travailleurs Salariés/I.N.S.E.R.M (J.M.)and fellowships from INSERM and Ministère de la Recherche et de la Technologie (L.C.) and CONICET (P.S.)

REFERENCES

Arfors L, Vesterqvist O, Johnsson H, Gréen K (1990) Eur. J. Clin. Invest. 20, 607-612

Carreras LO, Defreyn G, Machin SJ, Vermylen J., Deman R., Spitz B., Van Assche A (1981a) Lancet 1, 244-246

Carreras LO, Vermylen J (1982) Thromb Haemostas 48, 38-40

Carreras LO, Vermylen J (1991) In: Phospholipid binding antibodies (Harris EN, Exner T, Hughes GRV, Asherson R, Eds) CRC Press, New York p 231

Carreras LO, Vermylen J, Spitz B, Van Assche A (1981b) Br J Obstet Gynaecol. 88, 890-894

Catella F, Healy D, Lawson JA, FitzGerald GA (1986) Proc Natl Acad Sci USA 83, 5861-5865

Ciabattoni G, Landolfi R, Zappacosta B, Pogliani E, Patrono C (1990) 7th International Conference on Prostaglandins and Related Compounds, Florence, Italy, May 28-June 1, (abstract)

de Castellarnau C, Vila L, Sancho MJ. Borrel M, Fontcuberta J Rutllant ML (1983) Lancet 2, 1137-1138

Elias M, Eldor A (1984) Arch Intern Med 144, 510-515

Fitzgerald DJ, Roy L, Catella F, FitzGerald GA (1986) New Engl J Med 315, 983-989

FitzGerald GA, Pedersen AK, Patrono C (1983) Circulation 67, 1174-1177

FitzGerald GA, Smith B, Pedersen AK, Brash AR (1984) New Engl J Med 310, 1065-1068

Forastiero RR, Falcón CR, Carreras LO (1990) Haemostasis 20, 208-214

Granström E, Westlund P, Kumlin M, Nordenström A (1984) in Drugs affecting leukotrienes and other eicosanoid pathways (Samuelsson B, Berti F, Folco GC, Velo GP eds) Plenum Press, New York pp 5-17
Harris EN (Coordinator) (1990) Am. J. Clin. Pathol. 94, 476
Harris EN, Gharavi AE, Boey ML, Mackworth-Young CG, Loizou S, Hughes GRV (1983) Lancet 2, 1211-1214
Hasselaar P, Derksen RHWM, Blokzijl L, de Groot PG (1988) Thromb. Haemostas 59, 80-85
Hughes GVR, Harris EN, Gharavi AE (1986) J Rheumatol 13, 486-489
Khamashta MA, Harris EN, Gharavi AE, Derve G, Gil A, Vázquez JJ, Hughes GRV (1988) Ann. Rheum. Dis. 47, 849-854
Lechner K (1987) In Verstraete M, Vermylen J, Lijnen HR, Arnout J, (eds): Thrombosis and Haemostasis 1987. Leuven, International Society on Thrombosis and Haemostasis and Leuven University Press, p 525-547
Lellouche F, Fradin A, FitzGerald GA, Maclouf J (1990) Prostaglandins 40,297-310
Lellouche F, Martinuzzo M, Said P, Maclouf J, Carreras LO (1991) Blood in press
Loizou S. Mc Crea JD, Rudge AC, Reynolds R, Boyle CC, Harris EN (1985) Clin Exp Immunol 62, 738-745
Moncada S, Vane JR (1978) Br Med Bull 34, 129-135
Patrono C, Ciabattoni G, Patrignani P, Filabozzi P, Pinca E, Satta MA, Van Dorne D, Cinotti GA, Pugliese F, Pierucci A, Simonetti BM (1983) In Advances in Prostaglandins, Thromboxane and Leukotriene Research (Samuelsson B, Paoletti R, Ramwell P eds). Raven Press, New York, pp 492-498
Patrono C, Ciabattoni G, Remuzzi G, Gotti E, Bombardieri S, Di Munno O, Tartarelli G, Cinotti GA, Simonetti BM, Pierucci A (1985) J. Clin. Invest. 76, 1011-1018
Petraiuolo W, Bovill E, Hoak J (1988) Thromb. Res 50, 847-855
Pradelles P, Grassi J, Maclouf J (1985) Anal Chem 57 ,1170-1173
Reilly IAG, FitzGerald GA (1986) Thromb. Res. 41, 545-554
Reilly IAG, Roy L, FitzGerald GA (1986) Br Med J 292, 1037-1039
Rustin MHA, Bull HA, Machin SJ, Isenberg DA, Snaith MD, Dowd PM (1988) J. Invest. Dermatol. 90, 744-748
Schorer AE, Wickham NWR, Watson KV (1989) Br J Haematol 71, 399-407
Sinzinger H, Feigl W, Silberbauer J (1979) Lancet 2, 469
Vesterqvist O, Gréen K (1984) Prostaglandins 28, 139-154
Vesterqvist O, Gréen K, Lincoln FH, Sebek OK (1983) Thromb. Res. 33, 39-49

AAS 37
Prostaglandins in the
Cardiovascular System

REGULATION OF THE CONCENTRATION OF FREE ARACHIDONIC ACID IN HOMOGENATES OF HUMAN PLATELETS

I. Preuss and H. Patscheke

Institute for Clinical Chemistry, Klinikum Mannheim of the University of Heidelberg, 6800 Mannheim, Germany, and Institute for Medical Diagnostics, Klinikum Karlsruhe, 7500 Karlsruhe, Germany.

SUMMARY: With the intention to study the regulation of the availability of free arachidonic acid through the enzymes of the Lands cycle, we established a model system in homogenates of human platelets. Phospholipase A_2, arachidonoyl-CoA synthetase and lysophosphatidyl acyltransferase proved to be simultaneously active and a steady turnover of arachidonic acid was the consequence. EGTA suppressed the deacylating activity that acted on endogenous membrane phospholipids and prevented eicosanoid formation from previously esterified exogenous arachidonoyl-CoA. The reacylating enzymes took part in the control of eicosanoid biosynthesis by re-esterification of liberated arachidonic acid. Blockade of the reacylation by apyrase made arachidonic acid completely available for further metabolization into 12-HETE and thereby induced an increase in the eicosanoid release.

The biosynthesis of eicosanoids in various cell types including human platelets is controlled by the concentration of free arachidonic acid (Irvine, 1982). Under basal conditions, free arachidonic acid is maintained at low levels (Bills et al., 1977; Broekman et al., 1980). Exogenous arachidonic acid

Abbreviations: AS, arachidonoyl-CoA synthetase; LAT, lysophosphatidyl acyltransferase; 12-HETE, 12(S)-hydroxy-5,8,10,14-eicosatetraenoic acid; GPC, sn-Glycero-3-phosphocholine; GPE, sn-Glycero-3-phosphoethanolamine; EGTA, ethyleneglycol-bis(ß-aminoethyl ether)N,N,N',N'-tetraacetic acid; TLC, thin layer chromatography.

at submicromolar concentrations is efficiently taken up and incorporated into membrane phospholipids without eicosanoid formation (Bills et al., 1977; Neufeld et al., 1983). The entry in the phospholipid pool takes place via reacylation of lysophospholipids (LANDS, 1979) through the sequential actions of AS (Wilson et al., 1982) and LAT (McKean et al., 1982). Upon platelet activation, the eicosanoid precursor is selectively liberated predominantly from GPE and GPC (Bills et al., 1977; Broekman et al., 1980) and metabolized to cyclooxygenase and 12-lipoxygenase products. It is widely believed that the activity of PLA_2 plays the central role in controlling the release of eicosanoids. On the other hand, Lands (1979) described a balanced turnover of arachidonic acid through the deacylation of phospholipids and reacylation of lysophospholipids (Lands cycle). In this model, reacylating activity contributes to arachidonic acid availability. The aim of our study was to investigate, whether the reacylating enzymes could take part in the control of eicosanoid biosynthesis.

MATERIALS AND METHODS

Radiochemicals: [1-^{14}C]arachidonic acid (1.9 GBq/mmol) and [1-^{14}C]arachidonoyl-CoA (1.7 GBq/mmol) were supplied by DuPont (Dreieich, Germany). [^{3}H]$_{8}$12-HETE, 1-acyl-2-[1-^{14}C]arachidonoyl-GPC and 1-acyl-2-[1-^{14}C]arachidonoyl-GPE were purchased from Amersham Buchler (Braunschweig, Germany).

Washed human platelets were prepared from fresh blood according to Patscheke (1981). The platelet-rich plasma was treated with acetylsalicylic acid 5 mmol/l (30 minutes, room temperature). Platelets was sedimented, washed once with acid citrate and resuspended in a suspension solution (NaCl 120 mmol/l, KCl 5 mmol/l, $CaCl_2$ 2 mmol/l, $MgCl_2$ 1 mmol/l, glucose 5 mmol/l, human albumin 2 g/l, apyrase grade V (Sigma Chemie, Deisenhofen, Germany) 50 mg/l, sodium phosphate-NaOH 30 mmol/l, pH 6.5).

Deacylation assay: Washed platelets (2 x 10^9/ml) were incubated (one hour, 37°C) with [^{14}C]arachidonic acid 1.9 μmol/l added in 30 sequential portions. After washing twice with acid citrate, platelets were resuspended in suspension solution. 100 μl of the suspension of prelabeled platelets (1 x 10^{10}/ml) were mixed with 400 μl of the reaction mixture, immediately sonicated on ice with a branson sonifier (3 times for 15 sec, 20 kHz) and incubated at 37°C. The standard reaction mixture was composed of 5 μl of dithiothreitol 100 mmol/l, 50 μl of human albumin, essentially fatty acid free (Sigma Chemie, Deisenhofen, FRG) 10 g/l, 50 μl of $CaCl_2$ 10 mmol/l, 50 μl of $MgCl_2$ 10 mmol/l, 50 μl of CoA 6.7 mmol/l, 50 μl of ATP 67 mmol/l and completed with buffer (Tris-HCl 50 mmol/l, pH 9.0, or TES-NaOH 100 mmol/l, pH 7.4). Homogenates with apyrase grade VII (Sigma Chemie, Deisenhofen, FRG) did not obtain ATP. Incubations in the presence of EGTA (Merck, Darmstadt, FRG) were carried out without addition of $CaCl_2$.

Reacylation assay: The preparation and incubation procedures were virtually the same as described for the deacylation assay. 350 μl of the reaction mixture were mixed with 100 μl of the suspension of unlabeled platelets (1 x 10^{10}/ml) and treated by sonication. [^{14}C]arachidonic acid (50 pmol) or [^{14}C]arachidonoyl-CoA (50 pmol) were added after the first sonication interval in 50 μl of buffer containing human albumin 0.5 g/l.

Analysis: Labeled eicosanoids, phospholipids and triglycerides were extracted from the whole sample according to a modified method of the Bligh & Dyer (1959) procedure (Cohen et al., 1971). The rates of extraction of [^{14}C]arachidonic acid, [^{3}H]12-HETE, [^{14}C]GPE and [^{14}C]GPC was about 95 %; extraction of the hydrophilic [^{14}C]arachidonoyl-CoA yielded approximately 4 %. The organic extracts were dried under nitrogen, redissolved in chloroform/methanol (2:1, by vol) and spotted on Silica gel 60 TLC plates (Merck, Darmstadt, FRG). The plates were developed by chloroform/methanol/acetic acid/water (90:8:1:0.8, by vol). The radioactive spots were evaluated by a Berthold LB 2842 TLC linear analyzer (Berthold, Wildbad, FRG). Peaks were identified and the percentage of radioactivity was calculated for each compound after integration and background subtraction.

RESULTS

Deacylation of [^{14}C]arachidonic acid-labeled phospholipids: Fresh homogenates of platelets prelabeled with [^{14}C]arachidonic acid showed a deacylating activity that acted on the endogenous membrane phospholipids (Table I). While resting platelets did not contain any detectable eicosanoids, [^{14}C]arachidonic acid was continuously released and partly metabolized into [^{14}C]12-HETE within 40 minutes upon cell disruption. The eicosanoid release was significantly reduced in the presence of EGTA. In order to prove whether the deacylation is masked through re-esterification of just liberated arachidonic acid, the reacylation was suppressed by apyrase. Apyrase ensured the breakdown of ATP (Traverso-Cori et al., 1965), one of the cofactors required for AS activity (Wilson et al., 1982). The resulting inhibition led to a significant increase in the released eicosanoids. Arachidonic acid re-esterification was totally blocked by apyrase 2 U/ml. The pure deacylating activity showed virtually no preference in pH 9.0 or pH 7.4.

Table I: Effect of apyrase and EGTA on the eicosanoid release from endogenous membrane phospholipids. Homogenates of platelets prelabeled with [^{14}C]arachidonic acid were incubated at pH 7.4 or pH 9.0 for 40 minutes with all cofactors required for deacylating and reacylating activity (control) or in the presence of apyrase and EGTA, respectively. [^{14}C]Eicosanoids are represented by [^{14}C]arachidonic acid and [^{14}C]12-HETE. Data are given as means ± S.E.M. from n experiments. P-values were calculated by the one-tailed Mann-Whitney test and corrected according to Bonferoni.

Treatment	[^{14}C]Eicosanoids [% of extracted radioactivity]	
	pH 9.0	pH 7.4
Control	4.1 ± 0.2* (n = 10)	5.1 ± 0.2** (n = 6)
Apyrase 2 U/ml	8.0 ± 0.7* (n = 4)	7.6 ± 0.4** (n = 4)
Apyrase 4 U/ml	8.0 ± 0.8* (n = 4)	7.5 ± 0.2** (n = 4)
EGTA 3 mmol/l	0.0 ± 0.0* (n = 4)	2.0 ± 0.4** (n = 4)

* $p \leq 0.012$, ** $p \leq 0.019$

Reacylation with [^{14}C]arachidonic acid: Exogenous [^{14}C]arachidonic acid was employed in homogenates of unlabeled platelets in order to investigate the activities of AS and LAT. Under control conditions most of the substrate was incorporated into phospholipids and some [^{14}C]12-HETE was produced (Fig. 1, left panel). Apyrase 4 U/ml in contrast prevented the synthesis of labeled phospholipids and caused an exclusive [^{14}C]12-HETE formation (Fig. 1, right panel).

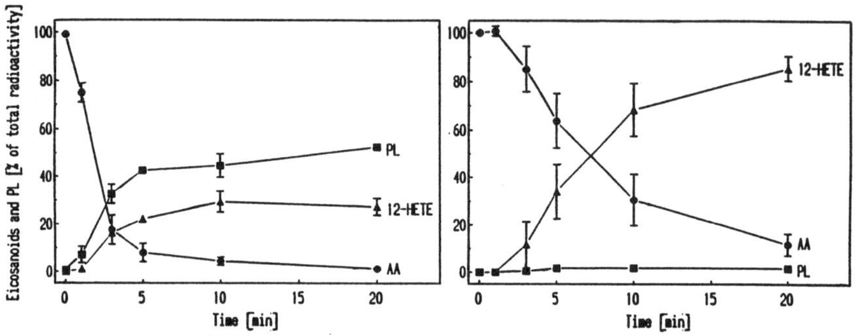

Fig 1: Reaction of [^{14}C]arachidonic acid in platelet homogenates. 500 μl of non-labeled platelets 2 x 10^9/ml were sonicated at 0 minutes and incubated with [^{14}C]arachidonic acid 50 pmol at pH 9.0. Data are given as means ± S.E.M. from three experiments. Radioactivity extracted at 0 minutes was corrected to 100 %. AA, arachidonic acid; PL, phospholipids. Left panel: Control. Right panel: Apyrase 4 U/ml.

Reacylation with [^{14}C]arachidonyl-CoA: Exogenous [^{14}C]arachidonoyl-CoA was partly re-esterified into phospholipids through the action of LAT (Fig. 2, left panel). While the labeled phospholipids soon reached a plateau, [^{14}C]12-HETE steadily increased as result of the deacylating activity. In this process arachidonic acid was liberated from phospholipids that had been previously esterified with [^{14}C]arachidonoyl-CoA. The eicosanoid formation was prevented in the presence of EGTA (Fig. 2, right panel).

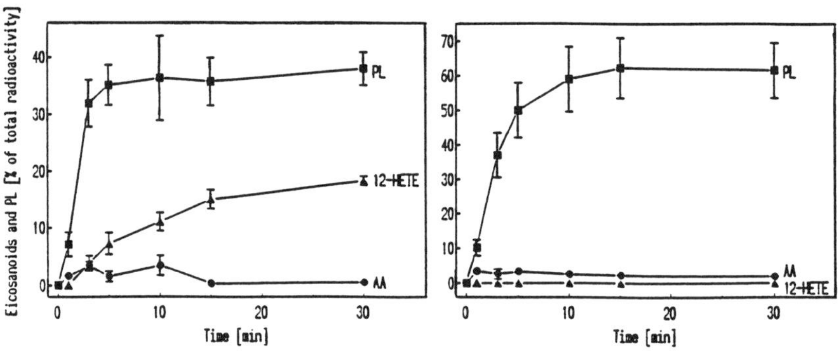

Fig 2: Reaction of [^{14}C]arachidonoyl-CoA in platelet homogenates. 500 μl of non-labeled platelets 2 x 10^9/ml were sonicated at 0 minutes and incubated with [^{14}C]arachidonoyl-CoA 50 pmol at pH 9.0. Data are given as means ± S.E.M. from three experiments. Radioactivity extracted at 0 minutes was corrected to 0 %. AA, arachidonic acid; PL phospholipids. Left panel: Control. Right panel: EGTA 3 mmol/l.

DISCUSSION

Deacylation of arachidonic acid from endogenous membrane phospholipids was demonstrated in homogenates of human platelets prelabeled with [^{14}C]arachidonic acid. On the other hand, exogenous [^{14}C]arachidonic acid as well as arachidonic acid from exogenous [^{14}C]arachidonoyl-CoA were incorporated into unlabeled phospholipids. Moreover, arachidonic acid was liberated from phospholipids that had been previously re-esterified with [^{14}C]arachidonoyl-CoA. These results give clear evidence that the enzymes of the deacylation-reacylation cycle (Lands cycle) are simultaneously active in fresh platelet homogenates. Apyrase blocked the reacylation by depriving the platelet homogenate of ATP. Therefore, in the presence of apyrase the deacylating activity directed to endogenous arachidonic acid could be measured. It was present at pH 7.4 and was not further stimulated by pH 9.0. This is in contrast to Billah et al. (1980), who described an activation of platelet PLA_2 by increasing pH up to 9.5. The discrepancy could be explained by the existence of two forms of PLA_2 (Ballou et al., 1986), one of them with a pH optimum at 7.0 and the other at 9.0.

The net amount of eicosanoids formed depended on the activities of the deacylating and reacylating enzymes PLA_2, AS and LAT which were inversively working. Liberation of arachidonic acid was a Ca^{2+}-dependent process and the release of eicosanoids was strongly inhibited by EGTA. In contrast, the reacylating enzymes counteracted the eicosanoid release. Blockade of the AS activity through apyrase caused a significant increase in the released eicosanoids. These results indicated, that the reacylating enzymes reduced the biosynthesis of eicosanoids by preventing arachidonic acid from further metabolization.

It has been suggested that the reacylating enzymes contribute to the regulation of eicosanoid biosynthesis in intact platelets (Irvine, 1982; Körner et al., 1984; Hornberger & Patscheke, 1989; 1990). Hydrogen peroxide and methyl mercury inhibited the partly purified AS and LAT, respectively, and induced the liberation of arachidonic acid in intact platelets (Hornberger & Patscheke, 1989; 1990). Our observations showing an effective arachidonic acid turnover in platelet homogenates support the concept that the eicosanoid release is not only controlled by an activation of PLA_2 but also by an inhibition of the reacylating enzymes AS and LAT.

Acknowledgement: The expert technical assistance of Ute Thömen is gratefully acknowledged. This work was supported by the Deutsche Forschungsgemeinschaft, PA 263.

REFERENCES

Ballou, L. R., DeWitt, L. M., and Cheung, W. Y. (1986): Substrate-specific forms of human platelet phospholipase A_2. J. Biol. Chem. 261, 3107-3111.

Billah, M. M., Lapetina, E. G., and Cuatrecasas, P. (1980): Phospholipase A_2 and phospholipase C activities of platelets. J. Biol. Chem. 255, 10227-10231.

Bills, T. K., Smith, J. B., and Silver, M. J. (1977): Selective release of arachidonic acid from the phospholipids of human platelets in response to thrombin. J. Clin. Invest. 60, 1-6.

Bligh, E. G. and Dyer, W. J. (1959): A rapid method of total lipid extraction and purification. Can. J. Biochem. Physiol. **37**, 911-919.

Broekman, M. J., Ward, J. W., and Marcus, A. J. (1980): Phospholipid metabolism in stimulated human platelets. J. Clin. Invest. 66, 275-283.

Cohen, P., Broekman, M. J., Verkley, A., Lisman, J. W. W., and Derksen, A. (1971): Quantification of human platelet inositides and the influence of ionic environment on their incorporation of orthophosphate-^{32}P. J. Clin. Invest. 50, 762-772.

Hornberger, W. and Patscheke, H. (1989): Hydrogen peroxide and methyl mercury are primary stimuli of eicosanoid release in human platelets. J. Clin. Chem. Clin. Biochem. 27, 567-575.

Hornberger, W. and Patscheke, H. (1990): Primary stimuli of icosanoid release inhibit arachidonoyl-CoA synthetase and lysophospholipid acyltransferase. Eur. J. Biochem. 187, 175-181.

Irvine, R.F. (1982): How is the level of free arachidonic acid controlled in mammalian cells? Biochem. J. 204, 3-16.

Körner, C. F., Hausmann, G., and Resch, K. (1984): Rate of prostaglandin synthesis is not controlled by phospholipase A activity but by reincorporation of released fatty acids into phospholipids. Agents Actions 15, 28-30.

Lands, W. E. M. (1979). In: Geometrical and positional fatty acid isomers (Emken, E. A. and Dutton, H. J., Eds), American Oil Chemists Society, Champaign IL, pp. 181-212.

McKean, M. L., Smith, J. B., and Silver, M. J. (1982): Phospholipidbiosynthesis in human platelets. J. Biol. Chem. 257, 11278-11283.

Neufeld, E. J., Wilson, D. B., Sprecher, H., and Majerus, P. W. (1983): High affinity esterification of eicosanoid precursor fatty acids by platelets. J. Clin. Invest. 72, 214-220.

Patscheke, H. (1981): Shape and functional properties of human platelets washed with acid citrate. Haemostasis 10, 14-27.

Traverso-Cori, A., Chaimovich, H., and Cori, O. (1965): Kinetic studies and properties of potato apyrase. Arch. Biochim. Biophys. 109, 173-184.

Wilson, D. B., Prescott, S. M., and Majerus, P. W. (1982): Discovery of an arachidonoyl-coenzyme A synthetase in human platelets. J. Biol. Chem. 257, 3510-3515.

AAS 37
Prostaglandins in the
Cardiovascular System

RELEASE OF EICOSANOIDS AND ENDOTHELIN IN AN EXPERIMENTAL MODEL OF ADULT RESPIRATORY DISTRESS SYNDROME

S. Pritze, B.A. Peskar and Th. Simmet

Department of Pharmacology and Toxicology, Ruhr-University, Universitätsstr. 150, D-4630 Bochum 1, F.R.G.

SUMMARY: In an experimental model of adult respiratory distress syndrome (ARDS) we have investigated the release of several vasoactive mediators since the rapid and severe increase in pulmonary arterial pressure is known to be a key feature in this condition. Intravenous injection of oleic acid (OA) into rats resulted in the development of a syndrome similar to ARDS characterized by severe hypoxia. As early as 15 min after OA injection elevated levels of 11-deoxy-15-keto-13,14-dihydro-11,16-cyclo-prostaglandin (PG) E_2 (DKH$_2$-cyclo-PGE$_2$) as an indicator of endogenous PGE$_2$ formation could be observed. Similarly, elevated levels of cysteinyl-leukotrienes (LT), determined as immunoreactive (ir) LTE$_4$, and ir-endothelin (ET) could be detected. These mediators were found to be elevated in plasma samples for at least 3 h. In addition, rather large amounts of ir-ET could be detected in bronchoalveolar lavage (BAL) fluid samples between 1 h and 3 h. Thus, it seems possible that cysteinyl-LT and peptides of the ET family, both known for their vasoactivity, might be involved in the pathophysiological process of ARDS.

INTRODUCTION

In the first description of the adult respiratory distress syndrome (ARDS) Ashbaugh and coworkers (1967) reported that 7 out of 12 patients died. Despite all the progress in intensive care medicine in the past decades, the mortality rate is still in the range of 50 - 75 % and in complicated cases may even reach 90 % (Seidenfeld et al., 1986). One of the obstacles preventing effective treatment might be that the pathophysiological basis for ARDS is still incompletely understood. Since arachidonic acid metabolites may have profound pulmonary microvascular effects (Malik et al., 1985), we have now investigated whether in an experimental model of ARDS, the oleic acid-induced lung injury (Eiermann et al., 1983), there may be increased generation of cysteinyl-LT and prostanoids such as PGE_2. In addition, we have investigated the formation of ET, an endothelium-derived potent pulmonary vasoconstrictor (Horgan et al., 1991).

MATERIALS AND METHODS

Materials: Oleic acid was from Sigma, St. Louis, MO, USA. Chemicals were of analytical grade and the solvents were of HPLC grade.

Experimental procedure: Male Wistar rats (270 - 340 g) were briefly anaesthetized with diethyl ether and were injected intravenously via the penile vein with 300 µl of a vortexed mixture containing bovine serum albumin (BSA) 0.1 % in saline and oleic acid (OA) (5:1, v/v) (Eiermann et al., 1983). At various time points after injection the rats received heparin 600 U/kg i.v., were anaesthetized again and blood additionally anticoagulated in vitro with Na_2EDTA 5.0 mM was collected from the abdominal aorta. Plasma samples were stored frozen at -20°C for radioimmunological analysis.

When BAL fluid was obtained, the lungs of anaesthetized rats were flushed with 5 x 10 ml NaCl 150 mM.

In separate experiments blood gas analysis including pH, $PaCO_2$, PaO_2 was performed before as well as after various time periods after OA/BSA injection. Arterial blood was obtained in awake animals by left ventricular cardiac puncture.

Analytical procedures: The stable bicyclic degradation end product 11-deoxy-15-keto-13,14-dihydro-11,16-cyclo-PGE_2 (DKH_2-cyclo-PGE_2) of the circulating PGE_2 metabolite 15-keto-13,14-dihydro-PGE_2 was determined radioimmunologically (Peskar et al., 1980). Immunoreactive cysteinyl-LT were assayed after enzymatic conversion to LTE_4 (Hoppe et al., 1986) and after C_{18} SEP-PAK extraction. Also after C_{18} SEP-PAK extraction ET was quantitated radioimmunologically as previously described (Simmet et al., 1991).

For reverse phase HPLC of ir-ET the material was loaded onto a C_{18} Nucleosil column eluted with a non-linear gradient from 30 % to 60 % acetonitrile containing trifluoracetic 0.1 % (Simmet et al., 1991).

Statistical analysis: Statistical analysis was performed using Student's t-test for unpaired data corrected by the Bonferroni method.

RESULTS

Intravenous injection of the OA/BSA mixture triggered development of respiratory distress with the most pronounced changes in blood gases at 3 h after injection. At this time-point PaO_2 had dropped from the control value 106.1 ± 2.7 Torr (n=9) to 47.4 ± 10.6 Torr (n=5, $P < 0.001$) and $PaCO_2$ had increased from 28.5 ± 1.1 Torr (n=9) prior to injection to 37.0 ± 2.4 Torr (n=5, $P < 0.005$). By contrast the pH was only slightly lowered (data not shown).

DKH_2-cyclo-PGE_2 as a parameter of PGE_2 biosynthesis was detectable in plasma samples under basal conditions (Fig. 1). At 15 min after OA/BSA injection a large and significant ($P < 0.01$) increase in DKH_2-cyclo-PGE_2 plasma levels could be detected (Fig. 1). Although a decrease in DKH_2-cyclo-PGE_2 levels could be observed during the following 225 min at 240 min the plasma levels were still significantly ($P < 0.001$) elevated (Fig. 1).

As to the plasma levels of ir-LTE_4 significantly ($P < 0.01$) elevated concentrations were already found at 15 min after OA/BSA injection (Fig. 2). A further increase up to 60 min was followed by a slow decrease in ir-LTE_4 (Fig. 2).

Radioimmunological determination of ir-ET in plasma samples revealed a rapid increase in ir-ET reaching peak plasma levels of 114 ± 19 pg/ml (n=8) at 45 min after OA/BSA injection. By contrast, in BAL fluid maximum amounts of ir-ET could be recovered at 120 min after OA/BSA injection (2939 ± 344 pg/50 ml BAL fluid).

Ir-ET from both plasma and BAL-fluid samples coeluted with the retention times of synthetic ET-1 and smaller amounts with that of big ET-1 and ET-2, while only traces comigrated with synthetic ET-3 (data not shown).

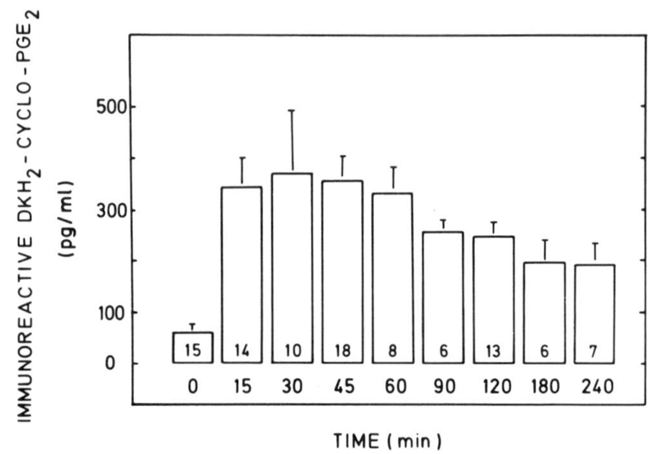

Figure 1: Time-course of immunoreactive 15-keto-13,14-dihydro-11,16-cyclo-PGE_2 in plasma from rats injected i.v. with a OA/BSA mixture at time 0. The number within the columns indicate the number of experiments.

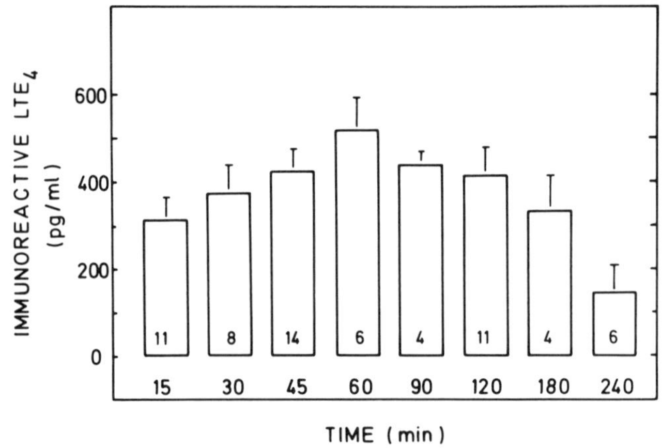

Figure 2: Time-course of immunoreactive LTE_4 in plasma from rats injected i.v. with a OA/BSA mixture at time 0. The numbers within the columns indicate the number of experiments.

DISCUSSION

Our results show that in OA-induced lung injury as an experimental model of ARDS, there is release of ir-DKH$_2$-cyclo-PGE$_2$, which is an indicator of PGE$_2$ biosynthesis. Although widely used in respiration physiology, the biochemical basis of the OA-induced lung edema has not been identified yet. Nevertheless, upon OA injection stimulation of endothelial cells is likely to occur in the pulmonary microcirculation. This point is supported by the increase in DKH$_2$-cyclo-PGE$_2$ plasma levels, since PGE$_2$, but not PGI$_2$, appears to be the major prostanoid synthesized by microvessels (Smith, 1986). PGE$_2$ released in the course of ARDS may counteract the effects of vasoconstrictor mediators, since it can induce pulmonary vasodilation (Voelkel et al., 1989).

Apart from the vasodilator PGE$_2$ we also found elevated circulating levels of ir-LTE$_4$ as an indicator of increased biosynthesis of cysteinyl-LT such as LTC$_4$ and LTD$_4$ which are potent pulmonary vasoconstrictors (Garcia et al., 1987). The edemagenic potential of the compounds seems to be related to an increase in vascular permeability and to their vasoconstrictor properties (Garcia et al., 1987). Increased levels of cysteinyl-LT have previously been detected in BAL fluid from rats injected with OA (Ball et al., 1988) as well as in pulmonary edema fluid from patients with ARDS (Garcia et al., 1987). Pretreatment of rats with the LTD$_4$/E$_4$ antagonist LY 171 1883 attenuated the elevated pulmonary vascular permeability (Ball et al., 1988) stressing the significance of cysteinyl-LT as mediators under these conditions.

In light of the potent vasoconstrictor activity of ET (Yanagisawa and Masaki, 1989) the release of these peptides in an ARDS model is of considerable interest. In in vitro experiments exogenous ET-1 has been shown to be a potent pulmonary vasoconstrictor primarily by increasing pulmonary venous resistance (Horgan et al., 1991). In vitro the edemagenic activity detected was apparently solely due to the increased pulmonary capillary hydrostatic pressure (Horgan et al., 1991). In addition, ET-1 is also able to stimulate 15-HETE production in the rat lung (Nagase et al., 1990) which similarly can induce pulmonary vasoconstriction and edema formation (Burhop et al., 1988). These in vitro findings in combination with our in vivo experiments strongly suggest that ET besides cysteinyl-LT may have a pathophysiological role in ARDS.

Acknowledgements: This work was supported by the Deutsche Forschungsgemeinschaft. We thank Dr. H. Shams, Department of Physiology, Ruhr-University, for the blood gas analysis.

REFERENCES

Ashbaugh, D.G., Bigelow, D.B., Petty, T.L. , and Levine, B.E. (1967) Acute respiratory distress in adults. Lancet II, 319-323.

Ball, H.A., Cook, J.A., Spicer, K.M., Hsu, C.Y., and Halushka, P.V. (1988) Oleic acid-induced pulmonary injury in rats: potential role of sulfidopeptide leukotrienes. Circ. Shock 26, 59-70.

Burhop, K.E., Selig, W.M., and Malik, A.B. (1988) Monohydroxyeicosatetraenoic acids (5-HETE and 15-HETE) induce pulmonary vasoconstriction and edema. Circ. Res. 62, 687-698.

Eiermann, G.J., Dickey, B.F., and Thrall, R.S. (1983) Polymorphonuclear leukocyte participation in acute oleic-acid-induced lung injury. Am. Rev. Respir. Dis. 128, 845-850.

Garcia, J.G.N., Noonan, T.C., Jubiz, W., and Malik, A.B. (1987) Leukotrienes and the pulmonary microcirculation. Am. Rev. Respir. Dis. 136, 161-169.

Hoppe, U., Hoppe, E.M., Peskar, B.M., and Peskar, B.A. (1986) Radioimmunoassay for leukotriene E_4. Use for determination of total sulfidopeptide-leukotriene release from rat gastric mucosa. FEBS Lett. 208, 26-30.

Horgan, M.J., Pinheiro, J.M.B., and Malik, A.B. (1991) Mechanism of endothelin-1-induced pulmonary vasoconstriction. Circ. Res. 69, 157-164.

Malik, A.B., Perlman, M.B., Cooper, J.A., Noonan, T., and Bizios, R. (1985) Pulmonary microvascular effects of arachidonic acid metabolites and their role in lung vascular injury. Fed. Proc. 44, 36-42.

Nagase, T., Fukuchi, Y., Jo, C., Teramoto, S., Uejima, Y., Ishida, K., Shimizu, T., and Orimo, H. (1990) Endothelin-1 stimulates arachidonate 15-lipoxygenase activity and oxygen radical formation in the rat distal lung. Biochem. Biophys. Res. Commun. 168, 485-489.

Peskar, B.M., Günther, B., Steffens, Ch., Kröner, E.E., and Peskar, B.A. (1980) Antibodies against dehydration products of 15-keto-13,14-dihydro-prostaglandin E_2. FEBS Lett. 115, 123-126.

Seidenfeld, J.J., Pohl, D.F., Bell, R.C., Harris, G.D., and Johnson Jr, W.G. (1986) Incidence, site, and outcome of infections in patients with the adult respiratory distress syndrome. Am. Rev. Respir. Dis. 134, 12-16.

Simmet, Th., Pritze, S., Thelen K.I., and Peskar, B.A. (1991) Release of endothelin in the oleic acid-induced respiratory distress syndrome in rats. Eur. J. Pharmacol. in press.

Smith, W.L. (1986) Prostaglandin biosynthesis and its compartmentation in vascular smooth muscle and endothelial cells. Ann. Rev. Physiol. 48, 251-262.

Voelkel, N.F., Stenmark, K.R., Westcott, J.Y., and Chang, S.W. (1989) Lung eicosanoid metabolism. Clin. Chest Med. 10, 95-105.

Yanagisawa, M., and Masaki, T. (1989) Molecular biology and biochemistry of the endothelins. Trends Pharmacol. Sci. 10, 374-378.

AAS 37
Prostaglandins in the
Cardiovascular System

INVOLVEMENT OF ARACHIDONIC ACID AND ITS METABOLITES IN THE INHIBITORY EFFECT OF BETA-ADRENOCEPTOR BLOCKING DRUGS ON BLOOD PLATELETS

Rado Nosáľ, Viera Jančinová and Margita Petríková

Institute of Experimental Pharmacology, Slovak Academy of Sciences, Bratislava, Czecho-Slovakia

SUMMARY: Propranolol (PRO), alprenolol (ALP), metipranolol (MET) and oxprenolol (OXP) inhibited arachidonic acid (AA) liberation from membrane phospholipids, malondialdehyde (MDA) formation and thromboxane B_2 (TXB_2) production in stimulated platelets. The inhibition was dose-dependent and with slight variations followed the rank order of potency: PRO ≥ ALP ≥ MET ≥ OXP. Atenolol (ATE) was without any inhibitory effect. Inhibition of the arachidonic acid pathway in stimulated platelets may significantly contribute to the antiaggregatory effect of beta-adrenoceptor blocking drugs.

INTRODUCTION

Beta-adrenoceptor blocking (BAB) drugs affect stimulated platelet aggregation depending on their liposolubility and the stimulatory pattern involved (Nosáľ et al., 1991). Inhibition of stimulated aggregation was closely related to membrane fluidization in platelets (Nosáľ et al., 1985). Since propranolol inhibited phospholipase A in platelets and other tissues (Vanderhoek & Feinstein, 1979; Pappu et al., 1985) it was of interest to investigate the effect of different BAB drugs on the stimulated arachidonic acid pathway in rat platelets.

METHODS AND MATERIALS

Rat blood platelets were isolated by differential centrifugation as described earlier (Nosál' et al., 1985). The liberation of ^{3}H-AA was studied in isolated platelets pretreated with BAB drugs and stimulated with thrombin (5 NIH units/ml) as published previously (Jančinová & Nosál', 1989). The formation of MDA in isolated platelets (21.8 x $10^5/\mu l$) stimulated with thrombin (20 NIH units/ml) was measured according to McMillan et al. (1977) and Ohkawa et al. (1979) fluorometrically using thiobarbituric acid. Thromboxane B_2 was determined in isolated platelets (5 x $10^4/\mu l$) stimulated with thrombin (2 NIH units/ml) using the TXB_2 kit (Jančinová et al., 1992).

Materials

Atenolol and propranolol: ICI, metipranolol: Spofa, alprenolol: Hässle, oxprenolol: Ciba, arachidonic acid- 5,6,8,9,11,14,15-^{3}H and ^{125}I-thromboxane Ria kit: Izinta, 2-thiobarbituric acid: Serva, human thrombin: Imuna

RESULTS

Figure 1 demonstrates the dose-dependent effect of PRO, ALP, MET, OXP and ATE on thrombin-stimulated liberation of ^{3}H-AA related radioactivity from isolated platelets. PRO and ALP in the concentrations of 0.01, 0.1 and 1 mmol/l significantly decreased ^{3}H-AA liberation from thrombin stimulated platelets by 1.5, 5.4 and 6.7 % , respectively. MET was active in the concentrations of 0.1 and 1 mmol/l (3 and 7.8 %, respectively), OXP was effective only in the concentration of 1 mmol/l (6.8 % decrease). ATE increased stimulated ^{3}H-AA liberation in the concentrations of 0.01 and 0.1 mmol/l by 2.2 and 1.1 %, respectively.

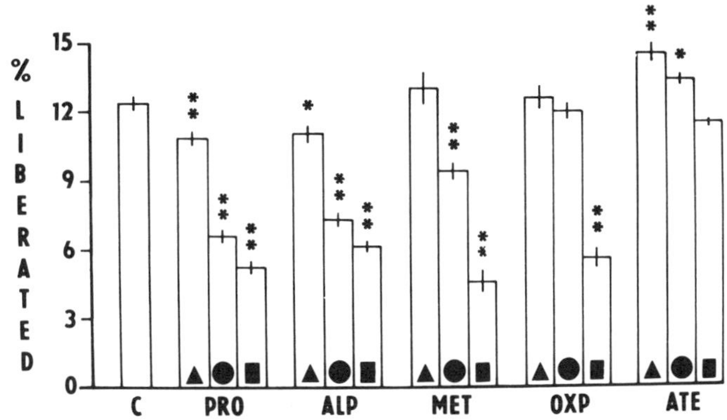

Fig. 1: Effect of BAB drugs in the concentration of 0.01 [▲], 0.1 [●] and 1 mmol/l [■] on thrombin-stimulated liberation of ^{3}H-AA-related radioactivity from blood platelets. Percentage from total arachidonate content (sum of activity in the supernatant and total lipid extract = 100 %) is expressed. n = 6, $\bar{x} \pm$ SEM, $*p \leq 0.05$, $**p \leq 0.01$

The effect of BAB drugs on thrombin-stimulated formation of malondialdehyde is demonstrated in figure 2. In their concentration of 0.1 mmol/l, the respective decrease of MDA formation induced by PRO, ALP and MET was 13, 9 and 7 nmol/10^8 platelets, and in the concentration of 1 mmol/l it amounted to 18, 17 and 20 nmol/10^8 platelets. ATE did not alter the formation of MDA in stimulated platelets.

Figure 3 shows the production of thromboxane B_2 in stimulated platelets. Pretreatment with PRO, ALP, MET and OXP in the concentration of 0.1 mmol/l decreased TXB_2 production by 64, 58, 60 and 45 pg/10^6 platelets, respectively and in the concentration of 1 mmol/l by 66.3, 66.1, 66.7 and 60.8 pg/10^6 platelets, respectively. ATE was without any effect on TXB_2 production in stimulated platelets.

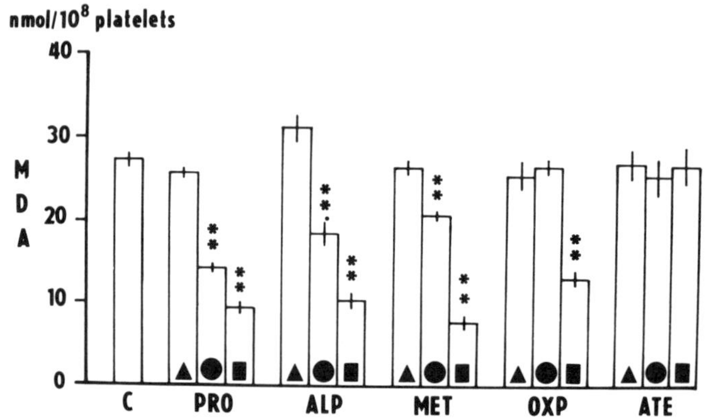

Fig. 2: Effect of BAB drugs in the concentration of 0.01 [▲], 0.1 [●] and 1 mmol/l [■] on thrombin-stimulated production of malondialdehyde in blood platelets.
n = 6, $\bar{x}$ ± SEM, **p ≤ 0.01

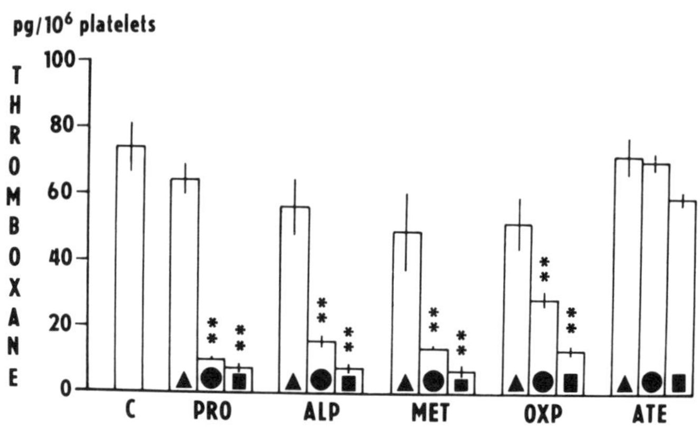

Fig. 3: Effect of BAB drugs in the concentration of 0.01[▲], 0.1[●] and 1 mmol/l[■] on thrombin-stimulated production of thromboxane B_2 in platelets. n = 6, $\bar{x}$ ± SEM, **p ≤ 0.01

DISCUSSION

PRO and ALP decreased in a dose-dependent way the liberation of ^{3}H-AA related radioactivity from thrombin stimulated platelets. MET and OXP were less effective. ^{3}H-AA liberation was predominantly inhibited from platelet membrane phosphatidylcholine (Jančinová & Nosáľ, 1989). Parallel to the interaction with AA liberation, BAB drugs inhibited the formation of MDA in stimulated platelets following the rank order of potency: PRO $\geq$ ALP $\geq$ MET $\geq$ OXP. While MDA is a by-product of cyclooxygenase activation (Vanderhoek & Feinstein, 1979) the inhibitory effect of BAB drugs on thrombin stimulated platelet activation may result from the direct inhibition of prostaglandin synthesis. Similarly to the inhibition of MDA formation, PRO, ALP, MET and OXP inhibited in a dose-dependent way the thrombin stimulated formation of TXB_2 in platelets. Thromboxanes, the end-products of prostaglandin synthesis in platelets, are considered potent autoregulatory platelet stimulators mobilizing intracellular calcium (Gerrard et al., 1981).

The inhibition of arachidonic acid liberation, MDA formation and TXB_2 production induced by the lipophilic BAB drugs PRO, ALP and MET proceeded parallelly with the inhibitory effect of these drugs on stimulated platelet aggregation and intracellular calcium displacement (Nosáľ et al., 1985 and 1991). This inhibitory effect was mediated most probably through the inhibition of activated phospholipase A_2 (Vanderhoek & Feinstein,1979; Pappu et al.,1985). We assume that the degree of the inhibitory effect of BAB drugs depends to a great extent on their liposolubility, which in turn alters the platelet membrane fluidity (Nosáľ et al., 1985 and 1991). The inhibition of intracellular phospholipase activities may be also due to the binding of BAB drugs to membrane acidic phospholipids (Pappu et al., 1985). Hydrophilic ATE, on the other hand, did not affect stimulated platelet aggregation and membrane fluidization (Nosáľ et al., 1985) and did not inhibit stimulated arachidonic acid liberation, MDA formation and TXB_2 production. Our results indicate that the inhibition of stimulated aggregation due to BAB drugs depends, at least partially, on their interaction with the stimulated arachidonic acid pathway in platelets.

REFERENCES

Gerrard, J.M., Peterson, D.A., and White, J.G.(1981): Calcium mobilization. In: Platelets in Biology and Medicine 2 (J.T.Dingle and J.L.Gordon, Eds), Elsevier/North-Holland, New York, pp. 407-436

Jančinová, V., and Nosáľ, R. (1989): Differences among beta-adrenoceptor blocking drugs in modifying platelet aggregation and arachidonic acid liberation under thrombin stimulation. Thromb. Res. 54, 687-698

Jančinová, V., Petríková, M., and Nosáľ, R.(1992): The antihistamine drug cimetidine and arachidonic acid metabolism. Agents Actions - accepted for publication

McMillan, R.M., MacIntyre, D.E., and Gordon, J.L. (1977): Simple sensitive fluorometric assay for malondialdehyde production by blood platelets. Thromb. Res. 11, 425-428

Nosáľ, R., Jančinová, V., Ondriaš, K., Jakubovský, J., and Balgavý, P. (1985): The interaction of beta-adrenoceptor blocking drugs with platelet aggregation, calcium displacement and fluidization of the membrane. Biochim. Biophys. Acta 821, 217-228

Nosáľ, R., Jančinová, V., and Petríková, M. (1991):Antiaggregatory properties of beta-adrenoceptor blocking drugs are related to their physico-chemical properties. Platelets - in press

Ohkawa, H., Ohishi, N., and Yagi, K. (1979): Assay for peroxides in animal tissues by thiobarbituric acid reaction. Analyt. Biochem. 95, 351-358

Pappu, A.S., Yazaki, P.J., and Hostetler, K.Y. (1985): Inhibition of purified lysosomal phospholipase A by beta-adrenoceptor blockers. Biochem. Pharmacol. 34, 521-524

Vanderhoek, J.Y. and Feinstein, M.B. (1979): Local anesthetics, chlorpromazine and propranolol inhibit stimulus-activation of phospholipase A_2 in human platelets. Molec. Pharmacol. 16, 171-180

AAS 37
Prostaglandins in the
Cardiovascular System

Effect of Irradiation on the Prostaglandin System of Human Hypernephroma Cells

Li S.R.*, Irene Virgolini*, E. Wandl**, Qiong Yang*, and H. Sinzinger*

*) Department of Nuclear Medicine, and **) Department of Radiation-Therapy, University of Vienna, Vienna, Austria

SUMMARY: Specific PGE_1-, PGE_2-, PGI_2-binding sites and the eicosanoid production were investigated in cultured human hypernephroma cells. Low numbers of PGE_1-, PGE_2- as well as PGI_2-high-affinity binding sites and high levels of PG-production were found as compared to normal kidney. Treatment with acetylsalicylic acid (ASA) significantly ($p<0.01$) increased PGE_1-, PGE_2- and PGI_2-binding sites and inhibited PG-formation. Following irradiation, PG-receptors and eicosanoid generation were significantly ($p<0.01$) diminished, however, were insignificantly lowered in the ASA-treated group. These findings suggest that ASA may modify the radioresponse of cultured hypernephroma cells by preventing the decrease of PG-receptors induced by irradiation.

INTRODUCTION

Prostaglandins (PGs) are thought to play a pathophysiological role in tumor cell growth and metastasis formation (Honn et al., 1981). Recently, several studies have shown that inhibitors of PG-synthesis may remarkably increase tumor cell radiocurability (Furuta et al., 1988a) which might be dependent on the ability of the tumor to produce PGs (Furuta et al., 1988b). However, the mechanisms by which indomethacin potentiates tumor radioresponse are still unknown. PGs exert their effects through interaction with specific receptors (Virgolini et al., 1988). We have demonstrated in human thyroid cancer (Virgolini et al., 1988) and hepatomas (Virgolini et al., 1989) that the density of PG-receptors significantly correlates with the cellular differentiation of the tumor. In the present study, we have used a similar receptor assay to evaluate the effects of ASA and irradiation on the PG system (PG-receptors, PG-production).

This study was supported by a grant of the Onkologie-Forschungsfond of the University of Vienna

MATERIALS AND METHODS

Hypernephroma tissue was obtained intraoperatively from 12 patients aged 60±12 years (12 males and 2 females) undergoing nephrectomy. From each patient a cell line was cultured, which was routinely maintained in medium consisting of nutrient mixture F12 (Ham) in a humidified atmosphere of 2.5% CO_2, 97.5% O_2 at 37°C. Cells from each cell line were divided into 4 groups: 1. control group, 2. ASA-treated group: cells were cultured in presence of ASA (concentration 0.5 mg/10^6 cells/ml medium for 24 hours), 3. control group irradiated: ^{60}Co irradiation at a dose rate of 1.0 Gy/minute for 10 minutes, and 4. ASA-treated group irradiated: the same irradiation scheme as in group 3. After irradiaton, cellular viability was >97% as assessed by phase-contrast microscopy.

PG-binding studies were done according to the methods described previously (Virgolini et al., 1988; Virgolini et al., 1989). The cells (300 µg protein/ml) were incubated either with different concentrations of ^{3}H-iloprost (a chemically stable PGI_2-analog, Amersham International, Buckinghamshire, UK), ^{3}H-PGE_1 (Amersham) or ^{3}H-PGE_2 (Amersham). The binding reaction was stopped by dilution with 4 ml of 4°C assay buffer and filtered through Whatman GF/B filters. The radioactivity in the samples was counted for 5 minutes in a liquid scintillation counter.

Radiothinlayer chromatography: The tumor cells were incubated with 0.25 µCi ^{14}C-arachidonic acid (AA) for 30 minutes at 37°C. The reaction was stopped with 1 M HCl. After centrifugation the supernatant was extracted with ethylacetate, dried under nitrogen, redissolved in absolute ethanol and stored at -20°C. The samples were then automatically placed onto a silica gel plate together with the standards (PGE_2, $PGF_{2\alpha}$, 12-HETE, TXB_2, PGD_2). The plate was put into a glass chamber with the lower edge in organic phase which consisted of chloroform, acetic acid, H_2O and methanol (90:1:0.7:8) until the organic phase had reached the upper edge. Then the plate was removed and analyzed by an automatic TLC-analyzer coupled with an oscilloscope.

RESULTS

PG-binding study: Scatchard analyses of the binding studies reveal that the binding capacities for PGE_1, PGE_2 and PGI_2 were significantly ($p<0.01$) higher in the ASA-treated group and significantly lower ($P<0.01$) in the irradiation-treated group as compared to the control group. However, insignificant decrease of the binding sites was found in the ASA-treated group irradiated (Table I).

Table I. Effects of ASA and irradiation on PG-binding to human hypernephroma cells.

		PGE_1	iloprost	PGE_2
group 1	B_{max}	715±79	723±128	562±65
	K_d	2.5±1.8	2.8±1.4	1.9±1.0
		**	*	*
group 2	B_{max}	1098±259	1103±412	782±82
	K_d	1.8±1.1	2.5±1.3	1.2±0.8
		**	**	**
group 3	B_{max}	428±62	397±59	318±48
	K_d	2.1±1.5	2.7±1.9	1.7±1.2
		++	+	+
group 4	B_{max}	694±127	708±210	552±82
	K_d	2.0±1.1	2.4±1.7	1.8±0.9

B_{max}: fmol/mg protein, K_d: nM;
*: p<0.05, **: p<0.01, versus the value of group 1;
+: p<0.05, **: p<0.01, versus the value of group 3

Table II. Effects of ASA and irradiation on ^{14}C-AA conversion (in %) by human hypernephroma cells

	TXB_2	PGE_2	PGD_2	$PGF_{2\alpha}$	12-HETE	AA
group 1 (n=7)						
x±S.D.	9.0 ±3.2	13.0 ±5.5	3.8 ±3.6	3.1 ±0.8	3.8 ±1.0	64.8 ±6.7
group 2 (n=7)	***	***	**	***	*	**
x̄±S.D.	1.2 ±0.6	1.6 ±0.5	0.8 ±0.3	0.7 ±0.5	6.5 ±2.6	75.9 ±4.5
group 3 (n=5)	*					
x̄±S.D.	5.2 ±1.1	9.8 ±3.6	3.3 ±0.5	3.3 ±0.3	4.1 ±1.9	67.6 ±7.7
group 4 (n=5)	*** +++	*** +++	*** +++	*** +++		** ++
x̄±S.D.	1.3 ±0.4	1.5 ±0.8	0.9 ±0.5	0.6 ±0.4	4.7 ±0.6	75.3 ±3.1

*:p<0.05, **:p<0.01, ***:p<0.001 versus the value of group 1;
+:p<0.05, ++:p<0.01, +++:p<0.001 versus the value of group 3.

Conversion of ^{14}C-AA to its metabolites: Hypernephroma cells converted exogenous precursor AA to various compounds (HETE, PGD_2, thromboxane B_2, PGE_2, $PGF_{2\alpha}$) (Table II). The main metabolites of AA-conversion of hypernephroma cells were PGE_2 and TXB_2 in the control group as well as in the irradiated group. After ASA-treatment, the main metabolites of AA-conversion, however, were HETE in the ASA-treated group and in the ASA-treated group irradiated.

DISCUSSION

The results of the present study demonstrate that cultured human hypernephroma cells produce various eicosanoids such as PGE_2, $PGF_{2\alpha}$, TXB_2, PGD_2 and 12-HETE. It is shown that PGE_2 is the main product synthezised by human hypernephroma cells. We have identified and described PG-receptors in tumor cells (Virgolini et al., 1988; Viigolini et al., 1989). Human hypernephroma cells have been demonstrated to possess only a small amount of PG-receptors. A significant increase in the density of these PG-receptors was demonstrated after treatment with ASA. This provides evidence for the existence of a down-regulation mechanism of PG-binding sites in human hypernephroma cells.

Recently, Furuta and coworkers have found that indomethacin augments only the radiocurability of tumors which produce PGs (Furuta et al., 1988). However, sofar only little is known about the mechanism. PGs exert their effects through specific cell surface receptors. These experiments show that although the number of PG-receptors is significantly diminished after radiotherapy, the density of PG-receptors on human hypernephroma cells is not altered after preincubation with ASA. The results indicate that the synthesis inhibitor "aspirin" prevents the decrease of PG-receptors induced by irradiation, which may modify the radioresponse of human hypernephroma cells.

CONCLUSION: The results of our study indicate that PGs may modify the radioresponse of human hypernephroma cells by preventing irradiation-induced decrease of PG-receptors. Further studies are necessary to elucidate the role of PGs and possible therapeutic concequences in patients with hypernephromas.

ACKNOWLEGEMENTS. We are grateful to Ingrid Teufel and Regina Haslinger for the expert technical assistance.

REFERENCES

Honn K.V., Bockman R.S., and Marnett L.J. (1981), Prostaglandins 21, 833-864

Furuta Y., Hunter N., Barley T.Jr., Hall E., Milas L.(1988a), Cancer Res 48, 3008-3013

Furuta Y., Hall E., Sanduja S., Barkley T.Jr., Milas L. (1988b), Cancer Res 48:3002-3007

Virgolini I., Herman M., and Sinzinger H. (1988), Br J Cancer 58, 584-588

Virgolini I., Sinzinger H., Müller Ch., Herman M. (1989), Br J Cancer 59, 407-409

AAS 37
Prostaglandins in the
Cardiovascular System

PROSTAGLANDIN (PG) E1 AND 13,14-DIHYDRO(DH)PGE1 ARE DIMINISHING RADIATION-INDUCED ARTERIAL DAMAGE

Irmgard NEUMANN, Waltraud ROGATTI, Irene VIRGOLINI, W.FIRBAS and H.SINZINGER

Departments of Nuclear Medicine and Anatomy, University of Vienna, Wilhelm Auerswald Atherosclerosis Research Group (ASF), Vienna ,Austria

ABSTRACT. Rabbit abdominal aorta was irradiated with single or repeated doses up to 10 Gy. The rabbits were killed at different time intervals after irradiation. 5 µg/kg x 6/hr PGE1 or its biologically active metabolite 13,14-DH-PGE1 were administered either 6 hours before or 6 hours after irradiation. The administration of both PGEs reduced radiation-induced mitotic activity (3H-thymidine incorporation) and extracellular matrix [collagen-(14C-proline) and glycosaminoglycan (35-S-sulphate)]-formation as determined by means of autoradiography. The initial peak increase in vascular PGI2-synthesis was partly abolished, while the long lasting depression was less pronounced.
13,14-DH-PGE1 was only slightly less active as compared to the parent compound. Pre-radiation treatment was more effective than post-irradiation therapy.
These findings suggest that both the PGs exert significant radiation-protective actions on the arterial wall.

INTRODUCTION

It is well known that irradiation causes vasculopathy, which may lead to various clinical symptoms after a delay of many years (3,4).
Proliferation and enhanced extracellular matrix production by vascular smooth muscle cells are accompanied by a variable lipid uptake leading to cellular proliferation as well as to parietal (micro-)thrombus formation which are central mechanisms in radiation-induced vasculopathy (1,2).
We wondered, whether the radiation-induced effects like the enhanced mitotic activity and extracellular matrix formation could be diminished by PGE1-or 13,14-DH-PGE1-treatment demonstrated in a model of experimental irradiation of rabbits.

MATERIALS AND METHODS

Male, one year old New Zealand white rabbits were irradiated with 5 Gy, another group with 10 Gy while a third group of animals was sham-irradiated.

Processing of Vascular Material

The animals were irradiated under general anesthesia (Pentothal; 5-aethyl-5-[1-methylbuthyl]-thiobarbituric acid Na; Abbot Labs, North-Chicago, Hl., USA) to a 10x10 cm area of the abdomen with single doses of 5 or 10 Gy using a gammatron (Siemens, Erlangen, Germany). 1 mCi 3H-thymidine or 100 uCi 14C-proline or 100 uCi 35S-sulphate (Amersham, Int., Buckinghamshire, UK) were administered intravenously one hour prior killing and 100 units of heparin were applicated 30 minutes prior killing to prevent thrombin-induced enhancement of PGI2-liberation in vitro. 1-336 hours after irradiation the animals were killed by a blow onto their neck and both the irradiated abdominal aorta (AA) and the thoracic aorta (AT) were prepared carefully and examined immediately.
Mitotic activity (3 H-thymidine incorporation), collagen-(14C-proline-uptake) and glycosaminoglycan (35S-sulphate incorporation) production from histological samples were #evaluated from all the animals by means of autoradiography.

PGE1-Therapy

One third of the animals received 5 ug PGE1(Prostavasin)/ kg x 6/hr, another third the same dose of 13,14-DH-PGE1 (provided by Schwarz-Pharma, Monheim, Germany), while a third group received the buffer vehicle only. Treatment was applicated to half of the animals starting 6 hours before irradiation each hour and to the other half 6 hours after radiation in the same way.

Autoradiography

For the determination of mitotic activity, collagen-and glycosaminoglycan production aliquots of vascular tissue were fixed in phosphate buffered (pH 7.4) glutaraldehyde and embedded in paraffin. Sections were stained with hematoxylin-eosin and used for autoradiography. After the exposure had lasted 2-3 weeks, positivity was assessed by counting grain positive cells per total cell number (at least 10x1000 cells). Mitotic activity is expressed in o/o (percent) positive cells, collagen-and glycosaminoglycan production in grains per cell.

Statistical Analyses

The values are given as $\bar{x}$±SD; calculations for significance were performed using Student's t-test.

RESULTS

In response to the applied radiation doses (5 and 10 Gy) an enhanced mitotic activity of smooth-muscle cells is observed in all vascular layers (Tables 1 a-c). This pathophysiological mechanism is partly abolished in animals treated either with PGE1 or with 13,14-DH-PGE1, exhibiting that PGE1 is slightly more effective than its metabolite 13,14-DH-PGE1. Prostaglandin-treatment 6 hours before irradiation is generally shown to be more advantageous as compared to treatment 6 hours after radiation (Tables 1 a-c and 2). In parallel, another group of animals which was irradiated with 10 Gy and killed at different time-intertvalls between 1 and 336 hours, a time-dependent enhanced mitotic activity is observed up to a delay od 168 hours. A longer time-intervall of 336 hours does not result in a higher mitotic-rate. Here, too, the mitotic activity is partly depressed by prostaglandin pretreatment (Table 4).
In analogy to the mitotic activity the radiation-induced increased extracellular matrix production is also shown to be decreased by PGE1 and 13,14-DH-PGE1. In this case, too, the most evident effect is gained by applying PGE1 6 hours before radiation (Table 3 a-b).

DISCUSSION

Besides the endothelial damage the cellular proliferation of smooth-muscle cells as well as the enhanced extracellular matrix production are radiation-induced pathophysiological mechanisms, which are responsible for vasculopathy (6,10). This is known to be a rare but severe clinical complication, which might also result in stroke or myocardial infarction (3). PGE1 has been proven to be of clinical benefit in the treatment of peripheral vascular disease, which is also accompanied by an increased mitotic activity and an enhanced extracellular matrix production (7). Our findings demonstrate that PGE1 and 13,14-DH-PGE1 can partly prevent the above mentioned vascular changes. Both prostaglandins have a comparable capacity at decreasing the irradiation-induced enhanced mitotic activity and 14C-prolin and 35S-sulphate precursor incorporation reflecting the collagen and glycosaminoglycan production and so representing the extracellular matrix production. PGE1 is slightly more effective than its metabolite 13,14-DH-PGE1. Concerning the application time we found that prostaglandin-treatment 6 hours before irradiation seems to be advantageous as compared to treatment after radiation. Furthermore radiation-induced mitotic activity showed a time-dependency with an increase until 168 hours after the applied irradiation-dose (10 Gy), which is also abolished by both the prostaglandins PGE1 and 13,14-DH-PGE1. It has to be varified, whether a concomitant PG-treatment could prevent radiation-induced vasculopathy in patients.

Table 1 a Mitotic activity in abdominal aortic intima

Pretreatment with PGE1 and 13,14-DH-PGE1 partly abolishes irradiation-induced increase in mitotic activity

	buffer	PGE1	13,14-DH-PGE1	
sham irrad.	0.56±0.16	0.60±0.17	0.57±0.19	AT
	0.70±0.22	0.63±0.18	0.61±0.21	AA
5 Gy	0.61±0.19	0.62±0.14	0.64±0.18 *)	AT
	1.86±0.54	1.33±0.28	1.37±0.19	AA
10 Gy	0.58±0.22	0.61±0.19	0.64±0.17	AT
	2.07±0.63	1.63±0.36	1.69±0.31	AA

$\bar{x}$±SD; *) p <0.01 (vs. buffer control);
AA...abdominal aorta; AT...thoracic aorta

Table 1 b. Mitotic activity in the media

Pretreatment with both PGE1 and 13,14-DH-PGE1 partly abolishes irradiation-induced increase in mitotic activity

	buffer	PGE1	13,14-DH-PGE1	
sham irrad.	1.25+0.43	1.29+0.27	1.31+0.30	AT
	1.21+0.51	1.24+0.43	1.28+0.36	AA
5 Gy	1.39+0.38	1.38+0.40	1.35+0.27	AT
	3.65+1.14	2.70+0.47	2.81+0.30 *)	AA
10 Gy	1.33+0.49	1.41+0.36	1.39+0.40	AT
	3.88+1,07	3.08+0.74	3.18+0.62	AA

$\bar{x}$±SD; *) p <0.01 (vs. buffer control);
AA...abdominal aorta; AT...thoracic aorta

Table 1 c. Mitotic activity in aortic adventitia

Pretreatment with PGE1 and 13,14-DH-PGE1 partly abolishes irradiation-induced increase in mitotic activity

	buffer	PGE1	13,14-DH-PGE1	
sham irrad.	1.57±0.93	1.60±0.66	1.57±0.29	AT
	1.66±0.82	1.62±0.55	1.64±0.43	AA
5 Gy	1.74±0.71	1.64±0.53	1.58±0,50	AT
	5.76±0.97	5.01±0,49	5.22±0,80	AA
10 Gy	1.66±0.98	1,64±0,46	1.60±0.64	AT
	5.69±0.88	4.50±0,84 *)	4.70±0.93	AA

$\bar{x}$±SD; *) p <0.01 (vs. buffer control);
AA...abdominal aorta; AT...thoracic aorta

Table 2 . Mitotic activity in the rabbit aortic intima

Posttreatment with PGE1 and 13,14-DH-PGE1 partly abolishes irradiation-induced increase in mitotic activity.
The extent is less pronounced as compared to pretreatment.

	buffer	PGE1	13,14-DH-PGE1	
sham irrad.	0.56±0.16	0.61±0.21	0.63±0.20	AT
	0.70±0.22	0.63±0.19	0,65±0.20	AA
5 Gy	0.61±0.19	0.64±0.18	0.62±0.17	AT
	0.86±0.54	0.49±0.23	1.55±0.24	AA
10 Gy	0.58±0.22	0.60±0.22	1.61±0.21	AT
	2.07±0.63	1.82±0.33	1.90±0.40	AA

$\bar{x}$±SD;
AA...abdominal aorta; AT...thoracic aorta

Table 3 a. Radiation-dose dependent induced extracellular matrix formation is diminished by PGE1 and 13,14-DH-PGE1 treatment before irradiation.

	35S		14C		
	PGE1	DH-PGE1	PGE1	DH-PGE1	
sham irrad.	18.6±3.7	18.3±4.6	18.7±4.0	16.9±3.8	+
	25.2±4.1*)	24.6±5.3*)	24.2±5.1*)	23.6±4.2*)	-
5 Gy	29.4±4.8	29.7±5.3	28.0±6.0	27.9±5.1	+
	34.2±7.6	33.7±4.8	32.6±5.8	34.1±5.2*)	-
10 Gy	36.7±2.7	38.6±3.2	35.4±3.8	40.2±6.1	+
	42.6±3.9*)	44.8±6.3	40.8±5.9	43.3±6.6	-

-...not treated group, +...treated group;
$\bar{x}$±SD; *) p <0.01

Table 3 b . Dose dependent induced extracellular matrix formation is diminished by PGE1 and 13,14-DH-PGE1 treatment after irradiation.

	35S		14C		
	PGE1	DH-PGE1	PGE1	DH-PGE1	
sham irrad.	26.3±4.0	24.1±5.3	22.9±3.4	23.7±4.0	+
	25.2±3.6	25.9±4.6	24.8±4.2	24.4±5.1	-
5 Gy	32.4±5.1	31.6±4.7	29.9±4.1	31.6±5.4	+
	35.3±8.1	34.0±5.1	31.4±5.0	33.1±6.0	-
10 Gy	39.8±4.7	40.2±4.0	38.7±3.7	42.2±3.1	+
	42.5±5.5	45.8±5.7	42.7±6.3	43.0±7.1	-

-...not treated group, +...treated group;

1.Table 4. Time-dependent enhanced mitotic activity is partly abolished by PGE1 and 13,14-DH-PGE1 pretreatment.

Intima

hrs		buffer	PGE1	13,14-DH-PGE1
Contr.	AT	0.50±0.19	0.57±0.18	0.55±0.20
	AA	0.47±0.21	0.53±0.20	0.54±0.17
1	AT	0.60±0.23	0.61±0.20	0.60±0.14
	AA	1.56±0.41	1.36±0.42	1.40±0.33
2	AT	0.66±0.24	0.66±0.17	0.62±0.20
	AA	1.44±0.37	1.28±0.15	1.35±0.22
4	AT	0.71±0.31	0.63±0.22	0.70±0.19
	AA	1.68±0.40	1.33±0.24 *)	1.46±0.17
8	AT	0.67±0.33	0.65±0.09	0.62±0.14
	AA	1.57±0.45	1.30±0.36	1.41±0.29
24	AT	0.68±0.33	0.66±0.13	0.65±0.20
	AA	1.94±0.61	1.56±0.60 *)	1.73±0.71
48	AT	0.84±0.35	0,71±0.20	0.70±0.24
	AA	2.06±0.69	1.82±0.54	1.99±0.62
168	AT	0.78±0.34	0.75±0.19	0.72±0.20
	AA	2.41±0.79	1.96±0.60 *)	2.17±0.60
336	AT	0.88±0.35	0.76±0.22	0.71±0.17
	AA	2.24±0.86	1.83±0.74	2.06±0.74

AA...irradiated (10 Gy) abdominal aorta; AT...thoracic aorta
$\bar{x}$±SD; *) p <0.01 (versus control at same time interval)

1 Baluda, V.P., Sushekewich, G.N., Parkshkow, E.M., and Lukoyanava, T.I. (1982) Influence of p-rays 60 Co and fast neutrons on intravascular platelet aggregation and prostacyclin-like activing of the vascular wall. Zbl. Med. 62, 243-247

2 Darmody, W.R., Thomas, L.M., and Gurdjian, E.S. (1967) Postirradiation vascular insufficiency syndrome. Neurology 17, 1190-1192

3 Fajardo, L.F., and Steward, J.R. (1972) Coronary artery disease after radiation. New Engl. J. Med. 286, 1265-1267.

4 Fajardo, L.F., and Brown, M.J. (1973) Cardiac mural thrombi caused by radiation. Radiation Res. 55, 387-389

5 Sheehan, J.F. (1944) Foam cell plaques in the intima of irradiated small arteries (one hundered to five hundered microns in external diameter). Arch. Path. 37, 297-303

6 Silberbauer K., Sinzinger H., Feigl W., and Leithner ,Ch. (1977) Arterielle Strahlenschädigungen. VASA 6, 183-187

7 Sinzinger, H., Zidek T., Rauscha F., and Firbas W. (1991) Enhanced mitotic activity induced by irradiation is abolished by PGI2 pretreatment. Prostaglandins 41, 57.

8 Sinzinger, H., Firbas W., and Cromwell M. (1982) Radiation induced alterations in rabbit aortic prostacyclin formation. Prostaglandins 24, 323-329.

9 Sinzinger, H., Cromwell M., and Firbas W. (1984) Long-lasting depression of rabbit aortic prostacyclin formation by single-dose irradiation. Rad. Res. 97, 533.

10 Sinzinger, H., Firbas W., and Cromwell M. (1983) Strahlenvasculopathie - bedingt durch Änderung der gefäßeigenen Prostaglandinsynthese ? Wr. klin. Wschr. 21, 761.

AAS 37
Prostaglandins in the
Cardiovascular System

PHARMACOKINETICS OF INTRAGRAFT ILOPROST INFUSION DURING FEMORO-CRURAL RECONSTRUCTION.

FCT Smith, M Hildebrand, HR Watson, CP Shearman.

Department of Vascular Surgery, Queen Elizabeth Hospital, Birmingham B15 2TH, UK. and Research Laboratories Schering AG, Muellerstrasse 170-178, D-1000 Berlin 65.

SUMMARY: Pharmacokinetics of a single intra-graft infusion of 3000ng iloprost during femoro-crural bypass surgery have been investigated. Plasma iloprost concentrations, biphasic half-lives, and total drug clearances were found to occur within ranges demonstrated for IV infusion dose regimens.

INTRODUCTION

Iloprost is a stable PGI_2-mimetic used to augment blood flow in femoro-crural arterial bypass grafts, which are prone to early thrombosis. Early results have shown that an optimal dose of 3000ng of iloprost, infused into the graft at completion of surgery, produces long-lasting haemodynamic effects (Shearman et al, 1990; Hickey et al, 1991). However the pharmacokinetics of this intra-arterially administered dose of iloprost have not previously been determined. The aim of the present preliminary study was to establish pharmacokinetic parameters of a single bolus infusion of 3000ng iloprost into the graft, at the completion of femoro-crural bypass surgery.

MATERIALS AND METHODS

This was an open non-comparative study involving sequential sampling of plasma from four patients, after administration of iloprost during femoro-crural bypass.

Ethical committee permission and informed consent of patients were obtained. All patients underwent vascular reconstruction for critical limb ischaemia, using in-situ long saphenous vein as a bypass conduit, with distal anastomosis to a single calf vessel. Normal renal and hepatic function were established pre-operatively.

On completion of the distal anastomosis patients received 3000ng of iloprost, in 15ml of saline, infused into the graft via an unligated side-branch, at a constant rate, over 2 minutes. Graft blood flow, peripheral resistance and systemic blood pressure were measured pre- and post-infusion. Blood samples for iloprost assay were taken from an antecubital vein before drug injection and at 1,3,5,10,15,30,60,120,240 and 480 minutes after infusion. Blood samples were placed in heparinised tubes and centrifuged at 2200g for 15mins. 2ml of plasma from each sample was stored at -20°C until assay.

Bioanalyses of Iloprost: Iloprost was measured by a sensitive and specific scintillation proximity assay (SPA) (Hildebrand et al, 1990). An antiserum raised against "iloprost-9-pentynyl"-BSA in rabbits was employed. Iloprost-[^{3}H]-methylester with a specific activity of 66.9 Ci/mmol was used as a tracer. SPA-analyses were carried out with 0.2ml plasma adjusted to pH2 with 1 *N* HCl and extracted with 2.5ml diethyl-ether. The organic layer was separated after ethanol/dry ice solidification. The residue was redissolved in 0.21 ml of BSA buffer, and tracer (4000 cpm; 1:15000 dilution), as well as anti-rabbit-protein SPA reagent suspended in BSA, were added. The samples were shaken overnight and measured in a Pharmacia Beta-Plate counter. Calibration samples were obtained with drug-free human plasma containing 0-1000 pg/ml. Control samples containing 0, 12.5, 25, 100 and 200 pg/ml were also estimated as above.

Evaluation of pharmacokinetic data was carried out by TOPFIT (Schering, Gödecke, Thomae) using an open two compartment model.

RESULTS

Patient details and pharmacokinetic parameters of iloprost after single intragraft infusion of 3000ng are summarised in Table 1. No adverse effects following infusion of iloprost were recorded.

Patient	1.	2.	3.	4.
Age (yrs)	62	62	70	77
Weight/kg	75	76	64.5	62.5
Sex	F	M	M	F
$C_{1\,min}$ (pg/ml)	320	381	588	771
AUC_{0-t} (pg·h/ml)	2710	2520	1930	2750
$AUC_{0-\infty}$ (pg·h/ml)	3730	4170	2390	3130
$T\frac{1}{2}$ α (min)	1.7	2.0	1.0	0.7
$T\frac{1}{2}$ β (min)	17	30	5.7	3.5
Clearance ml/min/kg	10.7	9.5	19.5	15.3

Table 1 Pharmacokinetic parameters of intra-graft infusion of 3000ng of iloprost during femoro-crural reconstruction.

Maximal plasma concentrations of iloprost were measured one minute following infusion (mean $C_{1\,min}$ 515 pg/ml, range 320-771). Iloprost concentrations declined biphasically with half lives 0.7-2 mins (α phase) and 4-30 mins (β phase). Mean area under the measured plasma level curves, AUC_{0-t}, was 2478 ± 379 pg·h/ml. and mean extrapolated $AUC_{0-\infty}$ amounted to 3355 ± 772 pg·h/ml. Mean total drug clearance was 13.8 ± 4.6 ml/min/kg.

Following iloprost infusion, mean graft blood increased by 34% from 134-180 ml/min and mean peripheral resistance decreased by 46% from 1.02-0.55 mmHg/ml/min. Haemodynamic changes persisted to skin closure at 20 minutes.

DISCUSSION

The present preliminary study was undertaken to determine the pharmacokinetic parameters of a single dose of 3000ng iloprost in a specific clinical situation, in which the drug is used to augment arterial bypass graft blood flow in the early post-operative period.

An apparent difference existed between samples from patients 1,2 and 3,4. This may have been due to some difference in plasma storage conditions prior to assay. Nonetheless, mean total drug clearance was similar to that seen in previous patient and volunteer groups (Krause and Krais 1986, 1987). Analysis of half-life data revealed a short term (α) half-life phase of $T\frac{1}{2}$= 1-2 mins. The second (β) phase exhibited patient dependency and was characterised by by $T\frac{1}{2}$ 4-6 mins (patients 1,2) and 17-30 mins (patients 3,4). However half-life data were in the range seen for an IV infusion dose regimen.

Although plasma concentrations of iloprost decrease rapidly, haemodynamic effects, decreased peripheral resistance and increased graft blood flow, persist for prolonged periods (Shearman et al 1990, Hickey et al 1991). This suggests that beneficial local effects initiated by iloprost are subsequently sustained through other mechanisms.

REFERENCES

Hickey NC, Shearman CP, Crowson MC, Simms MH, Watson HR. (1991) Iloprost improves femoro-distal graft flow after a single bolus injection. Eur J Vasc Surg 5, 19-22.

Hildebrand M, Nieuweboer B, Biere H, Klar U, Seemann G, Krause W, Jakobs U. (1990). Development, validation and practical use of a sensitive and specific radioimmunoassay for the determination of iloprost. Eicosanoids 3, 165-169.

Krause W, Krais Th. (1986) Pharmacokinetics and pharmacodynamics of the prostacyclin analogue Iloprost in man. Eur J Clin Pharmacol. 30, 61-68.

Krause W, Krais Th. (1987) Pharmacokinetics and pharmacodynamics of radiolabelled Iloprost in elderly volunteers. Eur J Clin Pharmacol. 32, 597-605.

Shearman CP, Hickey NC, Simms MH. (1990) Femoro-distal graft flow augmentation with the prostacyclin analogue Iloprost. Eur J Vasc Surg 4, 455-457.

AAS 37
Prostaglandins in the
Cardiovascular System

SYNERGISTIC PLATELET INHIBITORY EFFECT OF THE PHOSPHODIESTERASE INHIBITOR PIROXIMONE AND ILOPROST

M. Buerke, H.A. Dieterich, J. Meyer, H. Darius

II. Medizinische Klinik, Direktor: Prof. Dr. J. Meyer,
J. Gutenberg-Universität, Langenbeckstr., Mainz, FRG.

Platelet activity is regulated through synthesis and degradation of the intracellular second messengers cAMP or cGMP. The antiplatelet effect of the phosphodiesterase (PDE) III inhibitor Piroximone (PIR) was studied in vitro in platelet rich plasma. ADP induced aggregation was inhibited by PIR with an IC_{50} of 67±43μM. The inhibitory effect was time and dose dependent.
The antiaggregatory effects in vivo were studied in anaesthetised rats. Reduction of platelet count following injection of 100μg/kg bw collagen was measured after bolus injection of PIR and vehicle. Piroximone bolus 2mg/kg bw resulted in a 50% inhibition of platelet aggregation in rats.
Cyclic AMP levels in washed platelets rose time and dose dependently after PIR. Coincubation of PDE III inhibitor PIR and adenylate cyclase activator Iloprost (ILO) resulted in a significant synergistic enhancement of the antiaggregatory effect.
The PDE III inhibitor PIR exerted an effective inhibition of platelet aggregation in vivo and in vitro. The inhibitory effects in vitro were synergistically augmented by the prostacyclin analog Iloprost. These platelet inhibitory effects might be of clinical importance.

Introduction

The platelet function cascade from platelet shape change, to secretion, to adhesion or aggregation is inhibited, when the intracellular concentration of the second messenger cAMP is

increased (1,2,3,4,6). The intracellular concentration of cAMP is regulated by balance of adenylate cyclase activity and phosphodiesterase activity (3,4). Prostacyclin and its synthetic derivates increase platelet cyclic AMP by adenylate cyclase activation. Inhibiton of platelet phosphodiesterase results in cyclic AMP accumulation (5). Prostacyclin or its stable analogs and phosphodiesterase inhibitors act synergistically to increase cyclic AMP in platelets and to inhibit platelet aggregation.
The purpose of the present study was to determine the antiaggregatory effect of the new phosphodiesterase III inhibitor Piroximone (Merrel Dow, Rüsselsheim, FRG) in vitro and in vivo and a synergistic enhancement with the adenylate cyclase activator and stable prostacyclin analog Iloprost. The experiments were performed as ADP induced aggregation in platelet rich plasma and collagen induced reduction of platelet count in anaesthetized rats.

Methods

Platelet Aggregation in vitro. Platelet aggregation was measured as described by Born (7). Changes in light transmission characterised the degree of platelet aggregation. Blood samples were withdrawn from human volunteers. Platelet rich plasma was prepared by centrifugation (1200 rpm, 10 min). Aggregation was measured in a aggregometer (APACT, Hamburg, FRG) by addition of ADP (Boehringer Mannheim, FRG) (0.1-10μM).

Platelet Aggregation in vivo. Male Wistar rats (270-320 g) were anaesthetized by chloroform. A tracheal canula was introduced, and the animals were allowed to breathe spontaneously. A polyethylene catheter was inserted into the left carotoid artery to monitor heart rate, blood pressure and platelet count. A catheter was inserted into the right jugular vein for administration of pentobarbital (15mg/kg/h), collagen, the test compounds or its vehicles. The degree of platelet aggregation was measured as a decrease in peripheral platelet count induced by intravenous injection of 100µg/kg bw collagen (8). Platelet count was measured before and after collagen bolus. Injections of collagen were made before, 30 and 60 min following bolus injection of test compounds. Intravenous bolus of 2mg/kg bw Piroximone vs saline was tested.

cAMP-Assay. Human platelets were isolated from platelet rich plasma and washed two times in phosphate buffered saline solution. Platelet count was adjusted to 300000 platelets/µl. The samples were incubated for defined time period at 37°C with Piroximone. The reaction was stopped by addition of trichloroacetic acid (TCA) (15%, 2:1=v:v). TCA was eliminated by ether extraction. Samples were lyophilised and cyclic AMP levels determined by the use of a commercially available cyclic AMP-RIA (Amersham).

Statistical Analysis of Data. All results are given as mean ± STD of n observations. Comparison between groups were made by Student's t-test for paired data and $p<0.05$ was accepted as statistical significance.

Results

ADP induced aggregation in vitro

The phosphodiesterase inhibitor Piroximone significantly inhibited platelet aggregation in response to ADP. The inhibitory effect of PIR was concentration dependent with an IC_{50} of 67±43 µM (Fig.1).

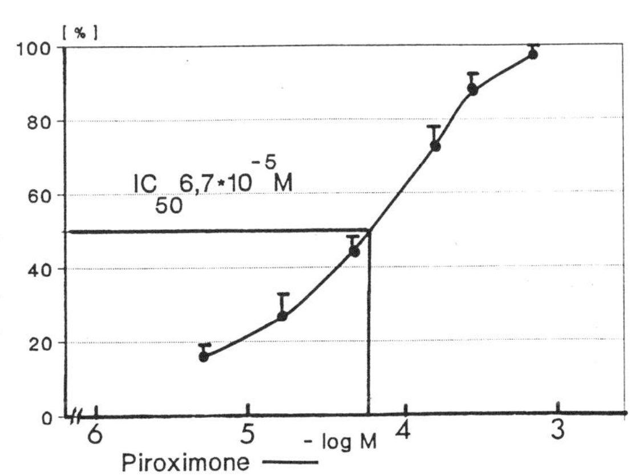

Figure 1: Piroximone induced inhibition of platelet aggregation
PRP was incubated with PIR for 1 min. Aggre-gation was induced by ADP. Results were calculated as percent inhibition of control ag-gregations incubated with vehicle. (mean±STD, n=8)

Incubation of platelet rich plasma between 1 and 120 min by Piroximone resulted in a time dependent inhibition of platelet aggregation. 50μM Piroximone exerted platelet inhibitory effects from 38±15 % for 1 min incubation to 97±3 % for 120 min incubation period.

Following coincubation of PRP with the phosphodiesterase inhibitor Piroximone and the adenylate cyclase activator Iloprost resulted in a statisticaly significant synergistic inhibition of platelet aggregation in vitro. 15μM PIR and 0.3 nM Iloprost inhibited platelet aggregation each by about 18±8 % following 1 min incubation. The combination of both drugs resulted in an inhibition by 52±14 %. (Fig.2)

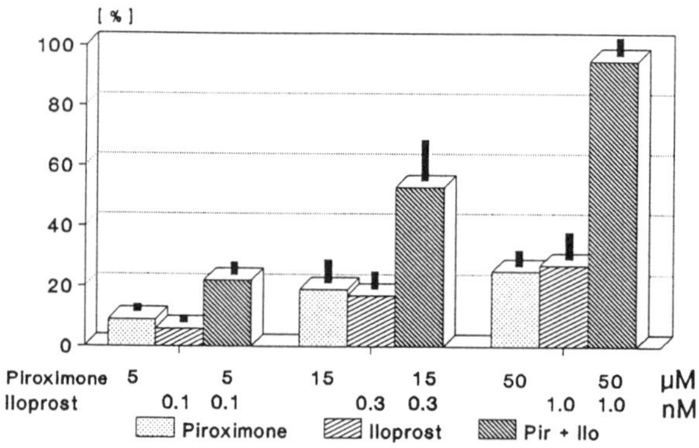

Figure 2: Synergistic effect of Piroximone and Iloprost. Piroximone and Iloprost were added simultaneously 1 min before aggregation was induced by ADP. Coincubation of PIR and ILO resulted in more than additive inhibition of aggregation. The figure depicts the PIR and ILO effects vs combination of both drug. (mean±STD, n=8)

<u>Collagen induced aggregation in vivo</u>

The initial decrease in platelet count following the first collagen injection for all rats were 47±5 %, and there was no significant difference between the means of the two groups receiving Piroximone or vehicle. In the vehicle treated group there was no change in collagen induced platelet count reduction following 30 and 60 min after the vehicle bolus (Fig. 3). The collagen induced decrease in platelet count was markedly attenuated when the rats were treated with the 2mg/kg Piroximone bolus before the second challenge. The inhibition was about 50% 30 and 60 min following PIR bolus. the difference was statisticaly significant from vehicle treated rats (Fig. 3).

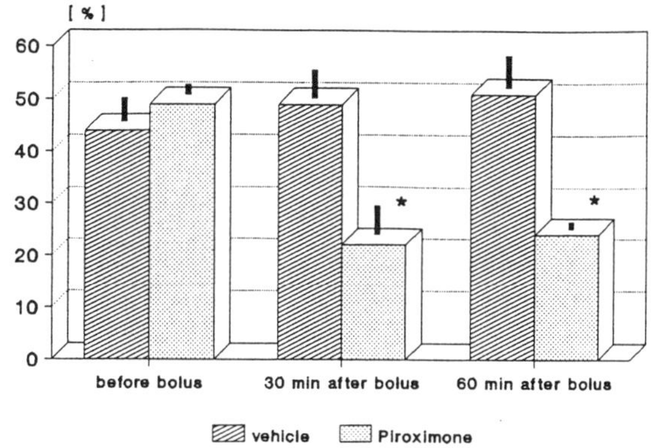

Figure 3: Anti-aggregatory effect of Piroximone in vivo. The platelet effect in vivo was studied in anaesthetised rats. Aggregation was induced by collagen. Reduction in platelet count represented the degree of aggregation. Collagen was injected before, 30 and 60 min after bolus of the test compounds. (mean±STD, n=8,)

Cyclic AMP levels in washed platelets

Cyclic AMP levels in washed platelets were increased time dependently between 1 and 30 min. Cyclic AMP-levels rose from 6±3 pmol cyclic AMP/10^8 platelets after 1 min incubation up to 12±2 pmol cyclic AMP/10^8 platelets following 30 min incubation (Fig. 4)

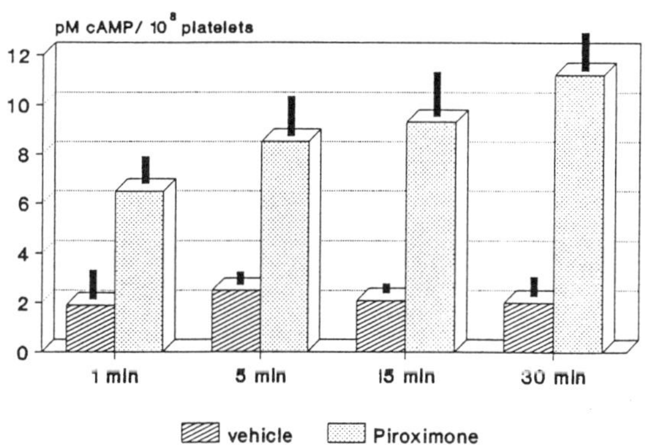

Figure 4: Effect of Piroximone on cyclic AMP levels in washed platelets. Washed platelets were incubated with 250μM Piroximone or vehicle. Piroximone resulted in a significant increase in cAMP levels. Results are expressed as pmol cyclic AMP/10^8 platelets and represent means ± STD of 6 experiments.

Incubation of washed platelets with saline, 150, 250 and 500 μM Piroximone for 5 min resulted in a concentration dependent increase in cyclic AMP levels from an initial level of 3±1 to 6±2, 9±2, and 12±3 pmol cyclic AMP/10^8 platelets.

Discussion

The results of this study demonstrate the potent antiaggregatory effect of the phosphodiesterase inhibitor

Piroximone in vivo and in vitro. In washed platelets Piroximone induced a time and concentration dependent increase in cyclic AMP levels. The antiaggregatory effect in PRP was also time and concentration dependent. The inhibitory effect was significantly enhanced by coincubation of the phosphodiesterase inhibitor PIR and the stable prostacyclin analog Iloprost.

The new phosphodiesterase type III inhibitor Piroximone possesses positive inotropic and vasodilatory effects in patients with congestive heart disease by selective inhibition of PDE III and elevation of intracellular cyclic AMP in the heart and smooth muscle of blood vessels. Platelet function is also regulated by the second messenger cyclic AMP.

The antiaggregatory effect of Piroximone demonstrated in vitro and in vivo might be of clinical importance in patients with congestive heart disease by reducing the thromboembolic risk.

By combining stable PGI_2 analogs and phosphodiesterase inhibitors it is possible to potentiate the platelet inhibitory effect. This might be of importance in patients with congestive heart failure due to coronary heart disease, which exert a marked increase in platelet activity. The results with Piroximone are specifially interesting because in contrast to other experimental studies using IBMX or HL 725 (3) as phosphodiesterase inhibitors, Piroximone is a drug under clinical study for the treatment of patients with congestive heart failure.

References

1. **Moncada, S. and Korbut, S.** (1978) Dipyridamole and other phosphodiesterase inhibitors act as antithrombotic agent by potentiating endogenous prostacyclin. Lancet 1, 1286-9.
2. **Darius, H. Lefer, A.M., Lepran, I., and Smith, B.** (1985) In vivo interaction of prostacyclin with an inhibitor of cyclic nucleotide phosphodiesterase, HL 725. Br. J. Pharmac. 84, 735-41.
3. **Smith, J.B.** (1982) Effect of thromboxane synthetase inhibitors on platelet function: enhancement by inhibition of phosphodiesterase. Thromb. Res. 28, 477-85.
5. **Data, J.L., Molony, B.A., Meinzinger, M.M. and Gormann, R.R.** (1981) Intravenous infusion of prostacyclin sodium in

man: clinical effects and influence on platelet adenosine diphosphate sensitivity and adenosine 3'-5'-cyclic monophosphate levels. Circulation 64, 4-12.
6. **Gormann, R.R., Bunting, S. and Miller, O.V.** (1977) Modulation of human platelet adenylate cyclase by prostacyclin (PGX). Prostaglandins 13, 377-388.
7. **Mills, D.C.B. and Smith, J.B.** (1971) The influence on platelet aggregation of drugs that affect the accumulation of 3':5'-cyclic monophosphate in platelets. Biochem. J. 121, 185-196.
8. **Born, G.V.R.** (1962) Aggregation of blood platelets by adenosine diphosphate and its reversal. Nature 194, 927-929.
9. **Darius, H., Lefer, A.M.** (1985) Antiaggregatory effects of thromboxane receptor antagonists in vivo. Thromb. Res. 40, 663-675.

AAS 37
Prostaglandins in the
Cardiovascular System

IDENTIFICATION OF OXIDATIVELY MODIFIED LIPIDS IN ATHEROSCLEROTIC LESIONS OF HUMAN AORTAS

J. Belkner, R. Wiesner and H. Kühn

Institute of Biochemistry, Medical School (Charité), Humboldt Universitity Berlin, Germany

SUMMARY: The oxygenated lipids of human aortas with atherosclerotic lesions were analysed by RP-, SP- and Chiral Phase-HPLC and compared with those obtained after treatment of human LDL with pure 15-lipoxygenase (LOX) of rabbit reticulocytes. The data suggest an indirect role of 15-LOX in the atherogenesis in aortas.

INTRODUCTION

Atherosclerosis is a complex multifactoral disease which leads to excessive deposition of lipids in the vascular wall (Ross, 1986; Steinberg et al., 1990). Even though the sequence of events leading to the formation of atherosclerotic plaques is still unclear, lipid peroxidation is known to be involved in the pathogenesis of atherosclerosis (Takano & Mineo, 1990). Recent research has established that oxidative modification of LDL is a key process in atherogenesis (Steinberg et al., 1989). Several studies suggested a role of 15-lipoxygenase in this process (Simon et al., 1989; Parthasarathy et al., 1989). This enzyme may exert its action by two different ways:

- direct oxygenation of extracellular LDL after release of the enzyme upon damage to cells
- indirect action via intracellular production of hydroperoxy compounds which are released and trigger free-radical induced non-enzymatic lipid peroxidation and oxidative modification of LDL.

While the first way preferably leads to stereospecific lipid oxygenation products, with the second way exclusively racemic mixtures may be anticipated.

For this reason, we analyzed the oxygenated polyenoic fatty acids in human atherosclerotic lesions of different stages and compared the product pattern with that of human LDL treated with a mammalian 15-lipoxygenase in vitro.

MATERIALS AND METHODS

Tissue samples: The abdominal aortas of 14 male patients (age 50 - 82 years) with chronic ischaemic heart disease, who died in the hospital, were removed during post-mortem exams within 24 h after death. From each aorta regions representing different stages of atherosclerosis were prepared:
I - "healthy looking" regions
II - fatty streaks (stage a according to WHO-classification)
III - advanced atherosclerotic plaques (stage b and c).
Control studies: aorta specimens of male and female, 22 and 32 years resp., who died from suicide. All tissue samples were frozen in liquid nitrogen and stored at -20°C.

Work-up of samples: Tissue samples (1 g) were thawed, shopped into small pieces in 2 ml of 0.1 M phosphate buffer, pH 7.4 and homogenized in a suspension of 2.5 ml chloroform and 5 ml methanol with an Ultraturrax homogenizer three times for 15 sec. 15S-hydroxy-11Z,13E-eicosadienoic acid was added as internal standard. The lipids were extracted according to (Bligh & Dyer, 1959) and aliquots were subjected to alkaline hydrolysis for 30 min at 60°C under argon.

Preparation and oxygenation of LDL: LDL (ζ = 1.019 - 1.063 g/ml) was obtained from EDTA-plasma of human healthy donors by sequential floatating ultracentrifugation (Havel et al., 1955) and dialyzed against 0.15 M NaCl - 1 mM EDTA. The oxygenation (6 - 10 mg LDL-protein/ml) was carried out with 15-lipoxygenase from rabbit reticulocytes. After reduction of the hydroperoxy lipids with sodium borohydride the lipids were extracted as described.

Analytics: HPLC-analyses was performed on a Shimadzu instrument coupled with a Hewlett-Packard diode array detector 1040 A. Estimation of free and esterified cholesterol species, determination and structure elucidation of oxygenated fatty acids were carried out according to (Kühn et al., 1990).

RESULTS

Analyses of the free and esterified cholesterol in human atherosclerotic lesions revealed a sizable portion of oxygenated cholesteryl esters (Fig. 1). With progredience of atherosclerosis there was a significant increase in the contents of free and esterified cholesterol as well as in the percentage of oxygenated cholesteryl esters ($p<0.01$).

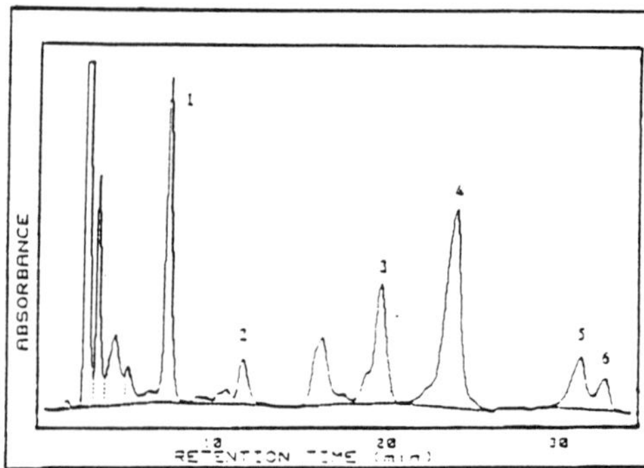

Stage of atherosclerosis	free cholesterol (mg/g protein) (peak 1)	ox.chol.esters / cholesteryl linoleate % (peak 2/4)
I	20.4	5.3
II	59.4	7.0
III	83.4	15.9

Fig. 1: SP-HPLC of nonhydrolyzed lipid extracts of human aortas with atherosclerotic lesions. The table showes the contents of cholesterol and oxygenated cholesteryl esters of different stages.
(1)free cholesterol 2)oxygenated cholesteryl esters
3)cholesteryl arachidonate
4)cholesteryl linoleate
5)cholesteryl oleate
6) cholesteryl palmitate)

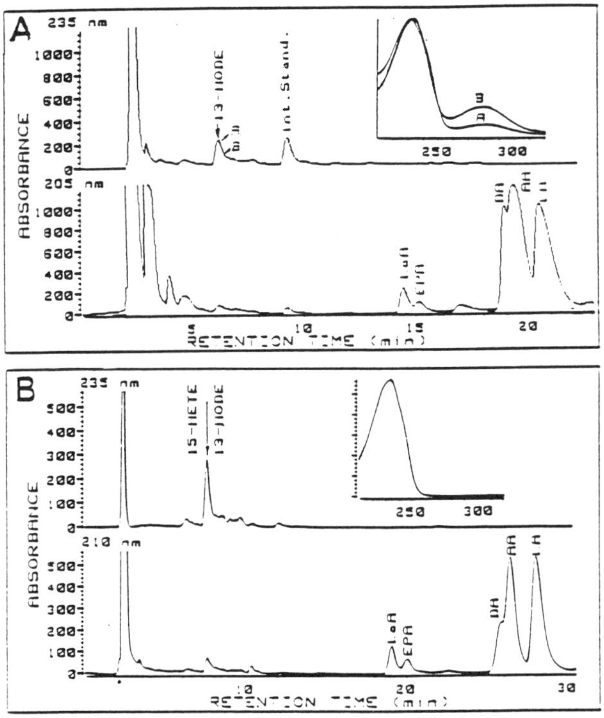

Fig. 2: RP-HPLC of hydrolyzed lipid extracts of human atherosclerotic lesions and LOX-treated LDL
A) Atherosclerotic aorta (stage III)
B) lipoxygenase trated LDL (Insert: uv-spectrum taken at the times indicated)
(LeA: linolenoic acid, EPA: eicosapentaenoic acid, DA: docosahexaenoic acid, AA: Arachidonic acid, LA: linoleic acid)

After alkaline hydrolysis of the lipids a large portion of oxygenated fatty acids co-eluted with 13-HODE in RP-HPLC (Fig. 2A). The ratio of hydroxy fatty acids (absorbance at 235 nm) and non-oxygenated fatty acids (absorbance at 210 nm) as a measure of oxidative modification of lipids significantly increased with the degree of atherosclerosis from 1.5 to 5.9 in the stage I to III (paired t-test: $p<0.001$ for I - II and <0.01 for II - III). Analyses of the lipids before and after alkaline hydrolysis revealed that more than 90 % of the oxygenated fatty acids were esterified. Non-involved aorta from healthy persons beings contained only traces of hydroxy fatty acids.

The uv-spectrum of the HPLC peak co-eluting with oxygenated polyenoic fatty acids proved to be inhomogeneous and showed conjugated keto diene chromophore (absorbance maximum at 270 nm) in addition to the conjugated diene chromophore (absorbance at 234 nm) indicating KODE-isomers.

In further experiments human LDL was treated with the pure 15-LOX from rabbit reticulocytes and analyzed for oxygenated lipids. Sizable amounts of hydroxy polyenoic fatty acids were

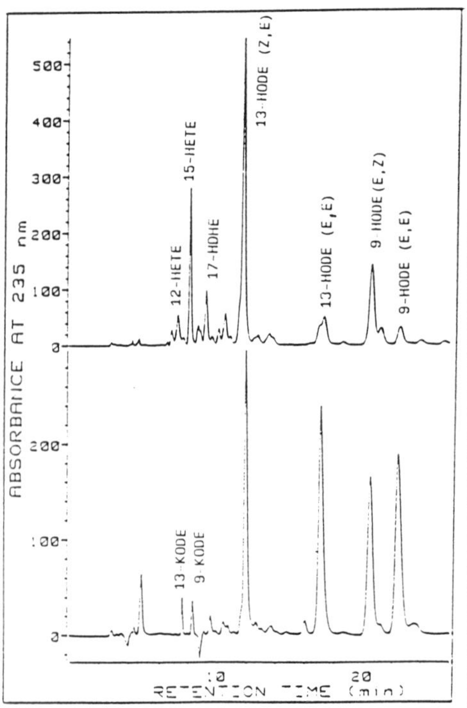

Fig 3.: SP-HPLC of oxygenated fatty acids of the hydrolyzed lipid extracts of LOX-treated LDL and human atherosclerotic lesions (upper trace: LDL; lower trace: atherosclerotic lesion - stage III)

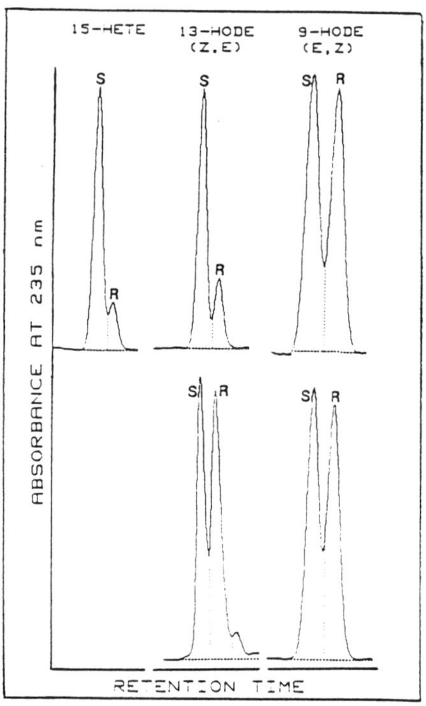

Fig 4.: Enantiomer composition of HETE and HODEs of LOX-treated LDL and atherosclerotic aortas (upper trace: LDL; lower trace: atherosclerotic aorta

formed in an esterified state as judged from the fact that they were only detectable after alkaline hydrolysis of the lipids; keto-polyenoic fatty acids could not be observed in LOX-treated LDL (Fig. 2B).

Fig. 3 shows the patterns of hydroxy fatty acids of human LDL oxygenated in vitro in comparison with those of atherosclerotic aortas. In contrast to the in vitro system, in Atherosclerotic aortas a large portion of unspecific lipid peroxidation products ocurred. In addition, only in aortas 13- and 9-KODE were identified probably originating from a secondary decomposition of hydroperoxy lipids. Chiral phase-HPLC of HETE and HODEs confirmed the difference in the specificity of lipid oxygenation (Fig. 4). 15-HETE and 13-HODE of LOX-treated LDL were found to be predominantly the S-enantiomers, whereas the HODE-isomers from aortas turned out to be racemic mixtures.

CONCLUSIONS

1) The degree of the oxygenation of cholesterol-attached polyenoic fatty acids significantly increases during the development of atherosclerotic lesions.
2) The patterns of the oxygenated fatty acids from atherosclerotic lesions and of that of LOX-treated LDL differ from each other with respect to the regio- and enantiomer specificity.
3) The proposed role of 15-LOX in the formation of atherosclerotic lesions in human aortas appears to be restricted to triggering of non-enzymatic lipid peroxidation.

REFERENCES

Bligh, E.G., and Dyer, W.J. (1959) A rapid method for total lipid extraction and purification. Can J. Biochem. Physiol. 37, 911-917.

Havel, R., Eder, H.A., and Bragdon, H.J. (1955) J. Clin. Invest. 34, 1345-1353.

Kühn, H., Belkner, J., Wiesner, R., and Brash, A.R. (1990) Oxygenation of biologgical membranes by the pure reticulocyte lipoxygenase. J. Biol. Chem. 265, 18351-18361.

Parthasarathy, S., Wieland, E., and Steinberg, D. (1989) A role for endothelial lipoxygenase in the oxidative modification of low density lipoprotein. Proc. Natl. Acad. Sci. USA 86, 1046-1050.

Ross, R. (1986) The pathogenesis of Atherosclerosis - an update. N. Engl. J. Med. 314, 488-500.

Simon, T.C., Makheja, A.N., and Bailey, J.M. (1989) Formation of 15-hydroxyeicosatetraenoic acid (15-HETE) as the predominant eicosanoid in aorta from Watanabe heritable hyperlipidemic and cholesterol-fed rabbits. Atherosclerosis 75, 31-38.

Steinberg, D., Parthasarathy, S., Carew, T.E., Khoo, J.C., and Witztum, J.L. (1989) Beyond cholesterol. Modification of density lipoprotein that increase its atherogenicity. N. Engl. J. Med. 320, 915-924.

Steinberg, D., Witztum, J.L. (1990) Lipoproteins and atherogenesis. Current concepts. JAMA 246, 3047-3052.

Takano, T., and Mineo, C. (1990). Atherosclerosis and molecular pathology: Mechanism of cholesteryl ester accumulation in foam cells and in extracellular space of atherosclerotic lesions. J. Pharmacobio-Dyn. 13, 385-413.

World health organization. Technical reports series, No 143 (1958) Classification of atherosclerotic lesions. Geneva 3 pp.

AAS 37
Prostaglandins in the
Cardiovascular System

EFFECT OF PROSTAGLANDINS AND CAPSAICIN ON GASTRIC VASCULAR FLOW AND MUCOSAL INJURY IN ENDOTHELIN-1-TREATED RATS

B. M. Peskar, P. Nowak and N. Lambrecht

Department of Experimental Clinical Medicine, Ruhr-University of Bochum, D-4630 Bochum 1, Germany

SUMMARY: Infusion of endothelin-1 reduced vascular flow in the isolated perfused rat stomach. Concurrent infusion of iloprost and capsaicin, respectively, did not counteract the flow-reduction caused by endothelin-1. Infusion of prostaglandin (PG)$F_{2\alpha}$ caused vasoconstriction and significantly augmented the endothelin-1-induced flow reduction. In vivo, i.v. infusion of endothelin-1 (50 pmol/kg//min for 10 min) did not cause gastric mucosal damage, but enhanced injury produced by intragastric instillation of 20% ethanol. Intragastric administration of iloprost or $PGF_{2\alpha}$ prevented the pro-ulcerogenic effect of endothelin-1. Similarly, stimulation of afferent sensory neurons by intragastric capsaicin (0.5 mg/kg) protected against damage caused by endothelin-1 and 20% ethanol. Functional ablation of afferent sensory neurons by s.c. administration of 125 mg/kg capsaicin markedly enhanced gastric mucosal damage by intraluminal 20% ethanol. This damage was, however, not further increased by infusion of endothelin-1. These findings show that protection against the pro-ulcerogenic effect of endothelin-1 can occur without antagonism of vasoconstriction. The findings also show that parameters involved in protection such as afferent sensory neurons do not contribute to the pro-ulcerogenic effects of endothelin-1 suggesting that protection against and potentiation of damage rely on different mechanisms.

INTRODUCTION

Adequate mucosal blood flow plays a crucial role in the ability of the gastric mucosa to maintain integrity despite the presence of potentially noxious agents in the gastric lumen. Blood flow ensures the delivery of oxygen and nutrients and facilitates the removal of toxic agents such as influxing hydrogen ions or oxygen radicals generated during mucosal tissue injury. Compounds with vasoconstricting properties have been found to potentiate damage to the gastric mucosa caused by various ulcerogens, while agents which increase gastric mucosal blood flow such as intragastric capsaicin (Holzer, et al., 1990 a) protect against injury. Endothelin-1 is a 21 amino acid residue peptide with two sets of intra-chain disulfide linkages initially isolated from porcine endothelial cells (Yanagisawa et al., 1988 a). Endothelin-1 has potent constrictor actions on vascular smooth muscle in vitro (Yanagisawa et al., 1988 a,b) and in vivo (Yanagisawa et al., 1988 a; Whittle et el., 1989). Local intra-arterial infusion of endothelin-1 causes hemorrhagic and necrotic damage in the rat gastric mucosa (Whittle and

Esplugues, 1988). High specific binding for endothelins was found in the rat gastrointestinal tract suggesting a possible physiological role in the control of gastrointestinal function (Takahashi et al., 1990). We have investigated the ulcerogenic effect of i.v. infusion of endothelin-1 in the absence and presence, respectively, of a weak noxious agent in the gastric lumen. In addition, we have studied whether compounds which protect against gastric mucosal injury caused by endothelin-1 antagonize its vasoconstrictor action.

METHODS AND MATERIALS

The vasoconstriction by endothelin-1 and its modification by iloprost, $PGF_{2\alpha}$ and capsaicin was studied in the isolated in situ perfused rat stomach. This preparation was described in detail previously (Dembinska-Kiec et al., 1989). Briefly, male Wistar rats, fasted overnight, were anesthetized with urethane. The abdomen was opened by a midline incision. All vessels to the abdominal organs except to the stomach were ligated. A cannula was inserted into the abdominal aorta and the proximal part of the body was completely removed. Then the portal vein was cannulated. A polyethylene catheter was also inserted into the gastric lumen via the pylorus. The gastric vascular bed was perfused under constant pressure (80 cm H_2O) with prewarmed oxygenated Krebs-Henseleit buffer containing dextran (30 g/l) via the aortic cannula. The effluent was collected from the portal vein in 2 min fractions. After a 20 min equilibration period endothelin-1 was infused into the arterial supply for 4 min. Infusions of protective agents were started 10 min prior to infusion of endothelin-1 and were continued throughout the experiment (24 min).

In the ulcer studies rats were pretreated with indomethacin (5 mg/kg, s.c., 60 min) to suppress endogenous prostaglandin formation. Endothelin-1 was infused i.v. for 10 min. Simultaneously, 1.5 ml of ethanol (20%) or water was introduced intragastrically and mucosal damage was assessed 10 min after the end of the infusion by calculation of a lesion index. In additional experiments, iloprost, $PGF_{2\alpha}$ or capsaicin were administered p.o. 30 min prior to infusion of endothelin-1. In a separate set of experiments, functional ablation of afferent sensory neurons was achieved by s.c. injection of a total dose of 125 mg/kg capsaicin 14 days before the experiments.

Endothelin-1 was purchased from Bachem-GmbH, Heidelberg, Germany. Capsaicin and $PGF_{2\alpha}$ were from Sigma Chemicals Co., St. Louis, MO, USA. Iloprost was a generous gift from Prof. Loosert, Schering Co., Berlin, Germany. Endothelin-1 was dissolved in saline containing 0.25% bovine serum albumin. Comparison between the groups was made by Student's t test for unpaired data, where $P<0.05$ was taken as significant.

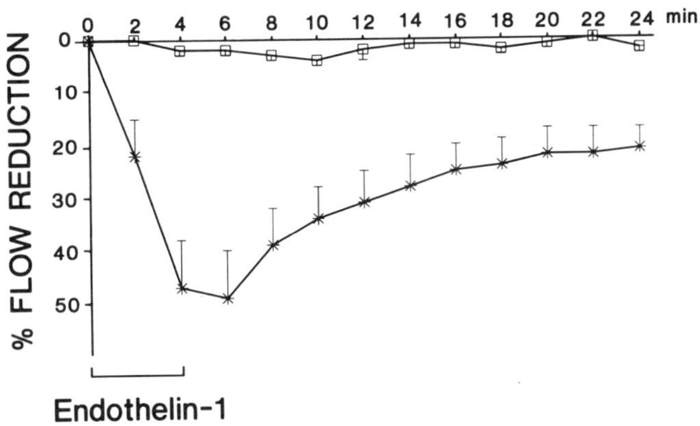

Figure 1: Reduction of vascular flow by endothelin-1 in the isolated in situ perfused rat stomach. After a 20 min equilibration period endothelin-1 (1 pmol/min) was infused into the arterial supply for 4 min (—✱—). Controls were infused with the corresponding volume of vehicle (—□—). Basal flow was 3.9±2 ml/min. Values represent the percent flow reduction compared to basal flow and are expressed as mean ± SEM of 4-6 experiments.

RESULTS

Effect of endothelin-1 on rat gastric vascular flow: Infusion of endothelin-1 (3 nmol/min) for 4 min into the arterial supply of the isolated perfused rat stomach rapidly reduced vascular flow (Fig. 1). The endothelin-1-induced reduction of flow and its recovery was not affected by concurrent infusion of iloprost (0.3 nmol/min) or capsaicin (30 nmol/min). Concurrent infusion of $PGF_{2\alpha}$ (3 nmol/min) even significantly augmented the flow reduction caused by endothelin-1 (Table I).

Effect of endothelin-1 on gastric mucosal integrity in the rat in vivo: Infusion of endothelin-1 (50 pmol/kg/min for 10 min) did not cause gastric mucosal damage in the absence of intraluminal ethanol. Likewise, intragastric instillation of 20% ethanol did not damage the gastric mucosa. However, when endothelin-1 was infused in the presence of intraluminal 20% ethanol marked damage of the gastric mucosa was observed (Fig. 2). Iloprost (20 μg/kg), $PGF_{2\alpha}$ (500 μg/kg) and capsaicin (500 μg/kg) protected against gastric mucosal damage caused by combined treatment with endothelin-1 and 20% ethanol (Fig. 2).

Table I Effect of iloprost, $PGF_{2\alpha}$ and capsaicin on endothelin-1-induced flow reduction in the isolated perfused rat stomach

Compound	Flow reduction (%)	
	Maximum (6 min)	End of experiment (24 min)
Endothelin-1	49±7	21±1
Endothelin-1 + capsaicin	46±4	23±7
Endothelin-1 + iloprost	54±6	18±5
Endothelin-1 + $PGF_{2\alpha}$	73±7*	36±6*

Capsaicin (30 nmol/min), iloprost (0.3 nmol/min) or $PGF_{2\alpha}$ (3 nmol/min) were infused throughout the experiment. Ten min after starting infusion of protective agents endothelin-1 (1 pmol/min) was co-infused for 4 min. Basal flow was 3.3±1 ml/min (mean ± SEM, n=24). Values are given as percent flow reduction compared to basal flow at the maximum flow reduction (6 min after starting the endothelin-1 infusion) and at the end of the experiment (24 min after starting the endothelin-1 infusion), respectively, and represent the mean ± SEM of 6 experiments for each infusion regimen. * $P<0.05$, compared to infusion of endothelin-1 alone.

Effect of ablation of afferent sensory neurons: S.c. injection of 125 mg/kg of capsaicin resulted in functional ablation of afferent sensory neurons as demonstrated by the loss of the wiping reflex after intraocular instillation of 0.1% capsaicin. As shown in Fig. 3, intragastric instillation of 20% ethanol caused substantial mucosal damage in capsaicin-denervated rats. In contrast to control rats, in denervated rats infusion of endothelin-1 (50 pmol/kg/min for 10 min) did not further increase the damage produced by topical 20% ethanol.

DISCUSSION

Endothelin-1 is a potent vasoconstrictor in the gastric vascular bed confirming previous reports (Wallace et al., 1989). Concurrent infusion of iloprost or capsaicin did not counteract the flow reduction caused by endothelin-1 in the in vitro pefused rat stomach. We have previously shown that the dose of capsaicin used in our experiments elicits release of immunoreactive calcitonin gene-related peptide into the venous effluent of the isolated perfused rat stomach indicating stimulation of afferent sensory neurons (Holzer et al., 1990 b). Infusion of $PGF_{2\alpha}$ induced vascular constriction and significantly augmented the endothelin-1-induced flow reduction. Thus, none of the compounds studied antagonized the vasoconstrictor action of endothelin-1 in the in vitro perfused rat stomach.

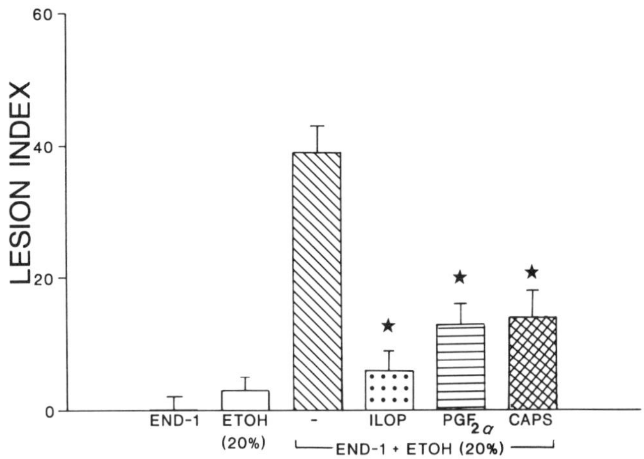

Figure 2: Effect of endothelin-1 on gastric mucosal integrity in vivo. Rats were treated with i.v. infusion of endothelin-1 (50 pmol/kg/min for 10 min) in the absence or presence of intragastric ethanol (20%) and were sacrificed 10 min after the end of the infusion. In additional experiments, iloprost (20 μg/kg), $PGF_{2\alpha}$ (500 μg/kg) or capsaicin (500 μg/kg) were administered orally 30 min prior to infusion of endothelin-1 and intragastric instillation of ethanol (20%). Mucosal damage was assessed by calculating a lesion index and is expressed as mean ± SEM of 6 experiments each group. * $P<0.05$ vs. rats treated with endothelin-1 and intragastric ethanol in the absence of protective compounds.

In vivo, infusion of endothelin-1 in the dose used did not cause gastric mucosal damage. Likewise, intragastric instillation of 20% ethanol in the absence of endothelin-1 infusion produced negligible gastric mucosal injury only. However, during simultaneous infusion of endothelin-1 intragastric instillation of 20% ethanol caused substantial gastric mucosal injury. Local intra-arterial infusion of endothelin has been reported to damage the rat gastric mucosa even in the absence of intraluminal ethanol (Whittle and Esplugues, 1988). Our results, however, show a clear dissociation between the production of gastric mucosal damage in the absence of 20% ethanol and the potentiation of damage caused by this weak ulcerogen by endothelin-1. These findings indicate that the gastric mucosa is by far more sensitive against the pro-ulcerogenic effect of a vasoconstrictor when exposed to a weak noxious agent. Ulceration of the gastric mucosa in the absence of local irritation obviously requires more pronounced vasoconstriction.

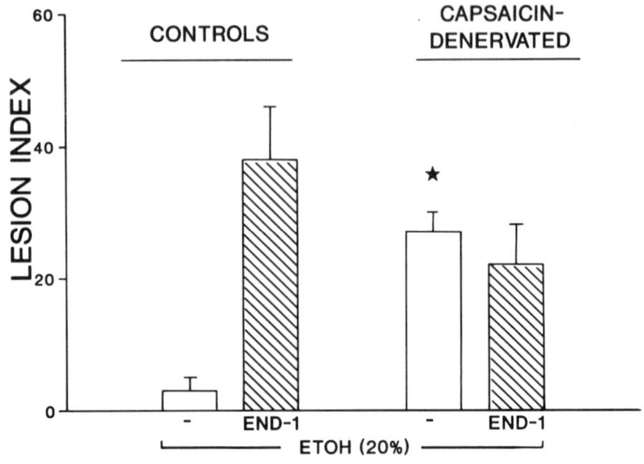

Figure 3: Effect of ablation of afferent sensory neurons on the pro-ulcerogenic action of endothelin-1. Rats were treated with 125 mg/kg capsaicin to denervate afferent sensory neurons. Two weeks later denervated or vehicle-treated control rats received i.g. 1.5 ml of ethanol (20%). Additional groups of rats were treated with i.v. infusions of endothelin-1 (50 pmol/kg/min) or saline for 10 min and were sacrificed 10 min after the end of infusions. Gastric mucosal damage was assessed by calculating a lesion index. In capsaicin-denervated rats intragastric 20% ethanol caused substantial mucosal damage which was not further increased by infusion of endothelin-1. Values are given as mean ± SEM of 6-8 rats per group. * $P<0.05$ vs. rats receiving 20% ethanol without endothelin-1 infusion in non-denervated rats.

Although iloprost, $PGF_{2\alpha}$ and capsaicin did not antagonize the vasoconstrictor action of endothelin-1 in the in vitro perfused rat stomach, all three compounds protected against the pro-ulcerogenic effect of endothelin-1 infusion in vivo. Our results do not exclude the possibility that iloprost, $PGF_{2\alpha}$ and capsaicin counteract effects of endothelin-1 on the gastric mucosal microcirculation in vivo. However, $PGF_{2\alpha}$ has been reported to cause vasoconstriction in the rat gastric mucosal microcirculation in vivo when applied topically to the exposed submucosa (Whittle et al., 1985) and to increase gastric vascular resistance in the blood-perfused chambered segment of the canine stomach following local intra-arterial administration in vivo (Kauffman and Whittle, 1982). Antagonism of vasoconstrictor actions of endothelin-1 in the gastric macrocirculation may thus not be the major mechanism of protection against the pro-ulcerogenic effect of this vasoconstrictor.

Stimulation of afferent sensory neurons by intragastric administration of a low dose of capsaicin was reported to protect against damage caused by ethanol or aspirin (for review see Holzer, 1988). Our findings show that capsaicin also antagonizes the pro-ulcerogenic action of endothelin-1 suggesting that stimulation of afferent sensory neurons can inhibit the deleterious effect of a vasoconstrictor. While 20% ethanol caused only negligible damage in control rats, damage in capsaicin-denervated rats was substantial and resembled the injury elicited by topical absolute ethanol. It has been suggested that the afferent sensory neuronal system represents an endogenous defense mechanism limiting injury to the gastric mucosa (Holzer et al., 1991). Interestingly, infusion of endothelin-1 did not further increase damage caused by 20% ethanol in capsaicin-denervated rats. Functional ablation of afferent sensory neurons has been found to prevent the increase in gastric mucosal blood flow elicited by exposure of the gastric mucosa to 15% ethanol plus HCl resulting in severe mucosal damage (Holzer et al., 1991). Our results show that the vasoconstrictor action of endothelin-1 and the suppression of the compensatory increase in gastric mucosal blood flow achieved by capsaicin-induced denervation are not additive. The findings also indicate that afferent sensory neurons which mediate the capsaicin-induced protection against damage caused by endothelin-1 are not involved in the pro-ulcerogenic effect of the vasoconstrictor suggesting that protection against and potentiation of damage rely on different mechanisms.

REFERENCES

Dembinska-Kiec, A., Peskar, B.A., Müller, M.K., and Peskar, B.M. (1989) Prostaglandins 37, 69-91.

Holzer, P. (1988) Neuroscience 24, 739-768.

Holzer, P., Livingston, E.H., and Guth, P.H. (1991) Gastroenterology 101, 416-423.

Holzer, P., Pabst, M.A., Lippe, I.Th., Peskar, B.M., Peskar, B.A., Livingston, E.H., and Guth, P.H. (1990a) Gastroenterology 98, 838-848.

Holzer, P., Peskar, B.M., Peskar, B.A., and Amann, R. (1990b) Neurosci. Lett. 108, 195-200.

Kauffman, G.L., and Whittle, B.J.R. (1982) Am. J. Physiol. 242, G582-G587.

Takahashi, K., Jones, P.M., Kanse,S.M., Lam, H.-C., Spokes, R.A., Ghatei, M.A., and Bloom, S.R. (1990) Gastroenterology 99, 1660- 1667.

Wallace, J.L., Cirino, G., De Nucci, G., McKnight, W., Wallace, K., and McNaughton, W.K. (1989) Am. J. Physiol. 256, G661-G666.

Whittle, B.J.R., and Esplugues, J.V. (1988) Br. J. Pharmacol. 95, 1011-1013.

Whittle, B.J.R., Oren-Wolman, N., and Guth, P.H. (1985) Am. J. Physiol. 248, G580-G586.

Whittle, B.J.R., Payne, A.N., and Esplugues, J.V. (1989) J. Cardiovasc. Pharmacol. 13, S103-S107.

Yanagisawa, M., Kurihara, H., Kimura, S., Tomobe, Y., Kobayashi, M., Mitsue, Y., Yazaki, Y., Goto, K., and Masaki, T. (1988a) Nature 332, 411-415.

Yanagisawa, M., Inoue, A., Ishikawa, T., Kasuya, Y., Kimura, S., Kumagaye, S., Nakajima, K., Watanabe, T.X., Sakakibara, S., Goto, K., and Masaki, T. (1988b) Proc. Natl. Acad. Sci., U.S.A. 85, 6964-6967.

AAS 37
Prostaglandins in the
Cardiovascular System

PURIFICATION TO HOMOGENITY OF AN NAD DEPENDENT 11-HYDROXYTHROMBOXANE B_2 DEHYDROGENASE FROM PORCINE KIDNEY

Pår Westlund

Department of Reproductive Endocrinology, Karolinska Hospital
Box 60500, S-104 01 Stockholm, Sweden

SUMMARY: A protein with NAD dependent 11-hydroxythromboxane B_2 dehydrogenase activity was purified to homogeniety from porcine kidney using a simple purification procedure, involving precipitation, anion exchange chromatography (DE-52), affinity chromatography (5'-AMP-Sepharose) and gel filtration chromatography (Protein Pak 300SW). The dehydrogenase was found to have a molecular mass of 50 kDa and 42 kDa as determined by comparison with standards on SDS/PAGE and gel filtration chromatography respectively. The apparent K_m and V_{max} values for thromboxane B_2 were 220-250 μM and 15-30 nmol min^{-1} mg^{-1} respectively. The enzyme was clearly separated from the proteins with 15-hydroxyprostaglandin dehydrogenase activity also present in the kidney. Furthermore it was found that 11-hydroxythromboxane B_2 dehydrogenase did not utilize prostaglandin D_2 prostaglandin E_2 or prostaglandin $F_{2\alpha}$ as substrate, and that the enzyme did not catalyze the reverse reaction, conversion of 11-dehydrothromboxane B_2 to thromboxane B_2.

INTRODUCTION

One of the initial metabolic steps in the degradation of the prostaglandins is dehydrogenation of the 15-hydroxyl group, a reaction which in general also leads to an inactivation of the molecule (Änggård, 1966; Granström & Kumlin, 1987). The enzymatic activity has been found to be widely distributed and several dehydrogenases catalyzing this reaction has been purified from different sources (Ängård et al., 1971; Hansen, 1976).

The major metabolic route of a thromboxane A_2 (TXA_2) is though to be non-enzymatic degradation to thromboxane B_2 (TXB_2), and subsequently degradation of TXB_2 via β-oxidation to dinor and tetranor compounds, and/or via oxidation of C-11 and/or C-15 (Roberts el al., 1981). Recently, the focus was turned to 11-dehydro-TXB_2, when it was found to be a prominent circulating metabolite of TXB_2 in the rabbit and human (Westlund et al. 1986a and b; Catella et al., 1986). A recent report measuring both 11-dehydro-TXB_2 and dinor-TXB_2 in human urine showed, in contrast to earlier studies, that 11-dehydro-TXB_2 was the major metabolite also in this body fluid (Catella & FitzGerald, 1987). It is thus of importance to characterize the enzymes involved in TXB_2 metabolism since their activity and localization might influence the rate of formation and proportion of the excreted metabolites. Part of this study has been presented in a preliminary form (Westlund 1988).

MATERIALS AND METHODS

Arachidonic acid was from NuChek Prep, Elysian, MN., USA. [1-^{14}C]-Arachidonic acid (57 Ci/mmol) was from Amersham and [$^3H_8$]-thromboxane B_2 (140 Ci/mmol) and [$^3H_7$]-prostaglandin D_2 (185 Ci/mmol) were from New England Nuclear. Sodium EDTA, NAD, NADH, NADP and NADPH were obtained from Sigma and Coomassie Brilliant Blue G-250 and TLC plates (20 x 20 cm, silica gel 60) were from Merck. DE-52 (diethylaminoethyl cellulose) was from Whatman, Kent, England, 5'-AMP-Sepharose was from Pharmacia, Sweden and Protein Pak 300SW (gelfiltration HPLC) was from Waters. A ConstaMetric 3000 (Milton Roy) HPLC-pump equiped with a Reodyne injector and a Lambda-Max Model 481 Spectrophotometer (Waters) were used for the HPLC. TXB_2, 11-dehydro-TXB_2, 15-keto-13,14-dihydro-TXB_2, prostaglandins E_2 and $F_{2\alpha}$ and their 15-keto-13,14-dihydro metabolites were generous gifts from the Upjohn Company, Kalamazo, MI, USA. [$^3H_7$]- and [1-^{14}C]-11-dehydro-TXB_2 were prepared by methods described in earlier studies (Westlund et al., 1986a and b). [1-^{14}C]-TXB_2 (specific activity, 50 Ci/mmol) was prepared by incubation of labeled arachidonic acid with human washed platelets. [1-^{14}C]-$PGF_{2\alpha}$ and [1-^{14}C]-PGE_2 (final specific activity 0.5 mCi/mmol) were prepared by incubations of arachidonic acid with the microsomal fraction from sheep vesicular glands. The final purity of the compounds were better than 99% as judged by TLC and HPLC.

ENZYME ASSAY: Enzymatic activity was measured at 37 °C by incubating protein fractions (0.1 ml) with radiolabeled substrate and different cofactors for 5-30 min. The incubations were terminated with 2 vols of methanol, diluted with water and extracted with ethyl acetate. The ethyl acetate extract was evaporated to dryness, dissolved in HPLC-grade methanol and subjected to TLC analysis. The metabolic pattern was analyzed by scanning of the TLC plates with a Berthold LB, TLC-scanner II. The enzymatic activity was calculated by peak area measurement (TLC-scan) and by scraping out the zones with radiolabeled material and determination of the radioactivity with scintillation counting. One unit of enzyme activity was defined as oxidation of 1nmol substrate per minute.

Estimations of protein concentration were made by the method described by Bradford (Bradford, 1976).

GEL ELECTROPHORESIS: Sodium dodecyl sulphate polyacrylamide gel electrophoresis (SDS/PAGE) was performed using an 8% acrylamide gel and 3% stacking gel, according to the method of Laemmli (Laemmli, 1970), using a Protein Slab Gel Apparatus (Bio-Rad). All buffers contained 0.1 % SDS and the samples were reduced with mercaptoethanol prior to gel electrophoresis. Bovine serum albumin (BSA, molecular mass≈67,000), ovalbumin (OA, molecular mass≈42,000) and soybean trypsin inhibitor (STI, molecular mass≈22,000) were used as standards. The gel was stained with 0.25 % Coomassie Brilliant Blue w/v, in water/methanol/acetic acid (83:10:7 by vol) (1-2 h). The gel was destained (6-12 h), in methanol/water/glycerol (55:43:2, by vol).

ENZYME PURIFICATION: Normal fresh porcine kidneys obtained 15-20 min after slaughter were kept on dry ice for about one hour. Thereafter they were cut in pieces and kept deep frozen (-70 °C) in 100 g portions which were used as starting material for each preparation. All purification steps were carried out at 0-4 °C, except for the HPLC, Protein Pak 300SW, which was performed at 15-20 °C.

The starting material was thawed and homogenized in 250 ml 25 mM Tris-HCl buffer, pH 8.0, containing 1 mM EDTA (buffer A). After centrifugation at 10.000 x g for 30 min, streptomycin sulphate (final conc. 0.7%) was added to the supernatant and the mixture was stirred for 30 min. Thereafter the mixture was centrifuged at 100.000 x g for 60 min. The proteins in the 100.000 x g supernatant were precipitated with ammonium sulphate (60% saturation). The precipitate was dissolved in buffer A (50 ml) and dialyzed 12 hours against 2 x 2 liter of buffer A (buffer exchange after 5 h). The dialyzed solution was applied to a 3.5 x 20 cm DE-52-column (diethylaminoethyl cellulose), equilibrated with buffer A. Two large fractions were collected from the DE-52 chromatography: proteins not retained by the resin (pass through fraction), and proteins eluted with 0.2 M KCl (0.2 M KCl fraction). The pass through fraction was concentrated (final vol 10-15 ml) by ultrafiltration on Diaflo PM-10 and applied to a 5'-AMP-Sepharose column (5g dry material) equilibrated with buffer A. The sample was left on the column for 30 min. Then the column was eluted with; 40 ml of buffer A (pass through fraction), 40 ml 1 mM NAD in 5 mM Tris-HCl (NAD fraction), pH 8.0, and with 0.5 M KCl in 25 mM Tris-HCl, pH 8.0, (0.5 M KCl fraction). The fractions were concentrated by ultrafiltration on Diaflo PM-10.

Aliquots of the NAD-fraction obtained from the 5'-AMP-Sepharose was applied to a Protein Pak 300SW column equilibrated with 125 mM Tris-HCl buffer pH 8.0 with addition of EDTA (final conc. 1 mM). Samples and standars were injected in a volume of 1-300 µl.

KINETIC EXPERIMENTS AND ANALYSIS OF ENZYMATIC ACTIVITY IN DIFFERENT PROTEIN FRACTIONS: Several of the protein fractions were incubated (final vol 0.1 ml) with TXB_2 (either $^3H_8$ or 1-^{14}C labeled, final conc. 100-1000 µM), 11-dehydro-TXB_2 ($^3H_7$ or 1-^{14}C, final conc. 120 µM), PGD_2 ($^3H_7$, tracer amounts) PGE_2 (1-^{14}C, final conc 60 µM) and $PGF_{2\alpha}$ (1-^{14}C, final conc. 60 µM) as substrates and with different cofactors, NAD (1-10 mM), NADH (2 mM), NADP (2 mM) and NADPH (2 mM).

Table I. Purification of 11-Hydroxythromboanoate B_2 dehydrogenase from porcine kidney. Aliquots of the protein fractions from each purification step were incubated with 200 µM TXB_2 (specific activity 0.25 mCi/mmol) and 1 mM NAD. Analysis and quantification of formed 11-dehydro-TXB_2 was performed with TLC and scintillation counting of scrape material. 1 unit of enzyme activity is equivalent to oxidation of 1nmol TXB_2 per min.

Fraction	Total protein mg	Total activity units	Specific activity units/mg	Yield %	Purification fold
Supernatant (100,000xg)	3063	153	0.05	100	
DE-52, pass through fraction	272	103	0.38	67	7
5'AMP-Sepharose, 1 mM NAD	17	122	7.2	80	140
Protein Pak 300SW	9	92	10.2	60	204

RESULTS AND DISCUSSION

ENZYME PURIFICATION: The protein fractions before the DE-52 column, i.e. 100,000 x g supernatant and dialyzed ammonium sulphate precipitate, converted [1-^{14}C]-TXB_2 to several products. After the DE-52 chromatography, the enzyme activity responsible for the formation of the major peak of radioactivity in the earlier protein fractions eluted in the pass through fraction, whereas material from the 0.2 M KCl fraction converted labeled TXB_2 to less polar material.

The major peak was characterized as 11-dehydro-TXB_2. This identification was based on its cochromatography with material of known structure.

The pass through fraction from DE-52 was concentrated and applied to a 5'-AMP-Sepharose column. Three fractions, viz. pass through, 1 mM NAD and 0.5 M KCl were collected. The NAD fraction contained the major part of the enzyme activity.

After concentration, aliquots (1-300 µl) of the NAD-fraction was applied to a Protein Pak 300SW column. Two major UV-absorbing (280 nm) peaks were detected, I and II, with a few minor contaminants. Material from peak I showed 11-hydroxythromboxane B_2 dehydrogenase activity. Peak II corresponded to the elution of NAD and did not contain any protein. Material from peak I was collected from several injections and was concentrated on Diaflo PM 10 to a final volume of 0.5-1 ml. This material was used for the kinetic experiments.

The purification of 11-hydroxythromboxane B_2 dehydrogenase was 200 fold with an overall yield of 60% (Table I), starting with 100,000 x g supernatant set as 100%.

The molecular mass was determined by comparison with standards, and was found to be 42-44 kDa on gel filtration chromatography and 50-55 kDa SDS/Page (Fig. 1). The purity was controlled on SDS/Page (Fig. 1).

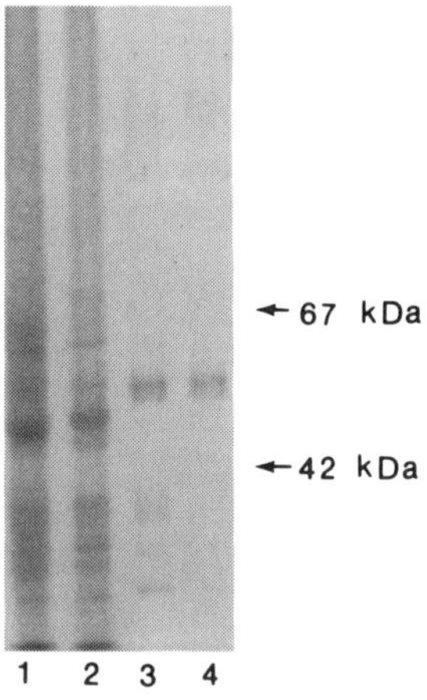

Figure 1. SDS/page of different protein fractions. Lane 1) 100.000 x g supernatante, 2) DE-52, pass through fraction, 3) 1 mM NAD fraction from 5'-AMP-Sepharose and 4) Peak I from Protein Pak 300SW. Standards BSA and OV.

ENZYME CHARACTERISTICS OF 11-HYDROXYTHROMBOXANE B_2 DEHYDROGENASE: The kinetic experiments were performed in duplicate. The apparent K_m and V_{max} values were calculated from a Lineweaver-Burk plot and were found to be 220-250 mM and 15-30 nmol min^{-1} mg^{-1} for TXB_2. The values were comparable to other prostaglandin metabolizing enzymes, except for the 15-hydroxyprostaglandin dehydrogenase from placenta which shows a considerably higher V_{max} value (Hansen, 1976). However, preliminary data indicates that the K_m and V_{max} values were dependent of the ionic strengt of the buffer. The pH optimum was found to be rather broad with a maximum around pH 8.0.

Furthermore it was found that the 11-hydroxythromboxane B_2 dehydrogenase only could use NAD and not NADP as cofactor (Table II). The enzyme was also unable to catalyze the reversed reaction, 11-hydroxy-TXB_2 to TXB_2 or any other metabolite with NADH or NADPH as cofactor (Table II).

ANALYSIS OF ENZYME ACTIVITY AND SPECIFICITY IN DIFFERENT PROTEIN FRACTIONS: The pass through fraction (DE-52) and the NAD-fraction (5′-AMP-Sepharose) only converted TXB_2 (Table II). On the other hand, the 0.2 M KCl fraction from the DE-52 chromatography contained enzyme activity that converted both TXB_2, PGD_2, PGE_2 and $PGF_{2\alpha}$ to less polar compounds. The product formed from PGE_2 corresponded to 15-keto-13,14-dihydro-PGE_2 indicating the presence of both the 15-hydroxyprostaglandin dehydrogenase and the prostaglandin Δ^{13}-reductase. The three poorly resolved TXB_2 metabolites formed by this protein fraction have not yet been identified. However, they showed R_f-values comparable to 15-dehydro-13,14-dihydro-TXB_2.

The 11-hydroxythromboxane B_2 dehydrogenase was thus clearly distinguished from other prostaglandin metabolizing enzymes since the enzyme only

Table II. Conversion of radiolabeled substances by different protein fractions.The enzymatic activity was analysed by TLC-scanning and area calculations of radioactive peaks. Conversion, i.e., more than 10 %. Not detectable, i.e. less than 1 %.

Substrate	Cofactor	Protein fractions	
		0.2 M KCl (DE-52)	NAD (5′-AMP-Sepharose)
TXB_2	NAD	conversin	conversion
TXB_2	NADP	not analysed	not detectable
11-dehydro-TXB_2	NADH	not analysed	not detectable
11-dehydro-TXB_2	NADPH	not analysed	not detectable
PGD_2	NAD	conversion	not detectable
PGE_2	NAD	conversion	not detectable
$PGF_{2\alpha}$	NAD	conversion	not detectable

metabolized TXB_2. The 11-hydroxythromboxane B_2 dehydrogenase also seemed to be position specific since it only attacked the 11-hydroxyl group of TXB_2.

A paper by Wu et al. also describes the purification of a NAD dependent dehydrogenase, from porcine liver, that catalyzes the oxidation of TXB_2 at C-11 (Wu et al., 1990). However, Wu et al. have not conclusively shown that 11-dehydro-TXB_2 was the formed product and furthermore they have not shown that the liver enzyme was destinguished from a 15-hydroxyprostaglandin dehydrogenase.

The enzyme described by Wu et al. differ from the enzyme described in this paper concerning the K_m and V_{max} values, molecular mass of the native enzyme, 110 kDa dimer Wu et al. versus 42 kDa monomer in the present work. Furthermore the enzyme purified from liver was able to catalyze the reversed reaction, e.g. conversion of 11-dehydro-TXB_2 to TXB_2, a reaction which could not be shown for the enzyme purified from kidney using radiolabeled 11-dehdro-TXB_2.

Whether this is to different enzymes with different catalytic specificity have to be shown by future investigations.

Acknowledgments: This study was supported by grants from Petrus and Augusta Hedlund's Foundation, The Swedish Medical Research Council (proj. No. B92-03x-09910-01A), the Swedish Society of Medicine, the Funds of L. Hierta, OE and E Johansson, and Karolinska Institutet. The author is greatly indebted to Mrs. Eva Ohlson for excellent technical assistance.

REFERENCES

Änggård, E. (1966) Acta Physiol. Scand. 66, 509-510.
Änggård, E., Larsson, C. and Samuelsson, B. (1971) Acta Physiol. Scand. 81, 396-404
Bradford, M.M. (1976) Anal. Biochem. 72, 248-254.
Catella, F., Healy, D., Lawson, J.A. and FitzGerald, G.A. (1986) Proc. Natl. Acad. Sci. USA 83, 5861-5865.
Catella, F. and FitzGerald, G.A. (1987) Thromb. Res. 47, 647-656.
Granström, E. and Kumlin, M. (1987) In: Prostaglandins and Related Substances: A Practical Approach. (Benedetto, C., McDonald-Gibson, R.G., Nigham, S. and Slater, T.F., eds) pp. 5-27, IRL Press, Oxford.
Hansen, H.S. (1976) Prostaglandins 12, 647-679.
Laemmli, U.K. (1970) Nature (London) 227, 680-685.
Roberts, II, L.J., Sweetman, B.J. and Oates, J.A. (1981) J. Biol. Chem. 256, 8384-8393.
Westlund, P., Kumlin, M., Nordenström, A. and Granström, E. (1986a) Prostaglandins 31, 413-443.
Westlund, P., Granström, E., Kumlin, M. and Nordenström, A. (1986b) Prostaglandins 31,929-960.
Westlund, P. (1988) Studies on the biosynthesis and metabolism of platelet derived eicosanoids. Thesis ISBN 91-7900-525-X.
Wu, P., Fritzo, M. and Tai, H.-H. (1990) Biochim. Biophys.Acta 1036, 55-63.

AAS 37
Prostaglandins in the
Cardiovascular System

BIOSYNTHESIS OF TXB_2 AND 6-OXO-PGF_{1alpha} IN THE HEART AND OTHER TISSUES UNDER PATHOPHYSIOLOGICAL CONDITIONS

P. Mentz and Ch. Giessler

Department of Pharmacology and Toxicology, Martin-Luther-University Halle, Leninallee 4, 0-4020 Halle/S.

SUMMARY: Many organs have the capacity to form prostanoids. Under pathophysiological conditions the biosynthesis of TXB_2 and 6-oxo-PGF_{1alpha} is markedly increased in the myocardium and the gastric mucosa. Tumor growth is linked with an enhanced prostanoid formation. Furthermore a rise of the PG content could be found in the liquor, aqueous humor and urine under diseases of the related organs. These results could be of some significance for diagnosis and therapy control.

INTRODUCTION

Recent investigations demonstrated the close connection between the prostanoid biosynthesis and several pathophysiological conditions in many organs. Especially in the myocardium the formation of these substances is markedly influenced by ischemia (Karmazyn, 1989), acute pressure overlood (Mentz et al., 1988) and heart failure (Newman et al., 1983). Obviously the begin of a pathophysiological process is paralleled by an increased formation of prostanoids. Under this aspect we proved the liberation of TXB_2 and 6-oxo-PGF_{1alpha} from the myocardium, the gastric mucosa and tissue of different tumors and the concentration of these prostanoids in liquor, aqueous humor and urine under pathophysiological states of the related organs.

MATERIAL AND METHODS

Investigations in the myocardium were carried out in isolated perfused guinea pig hearts. The cardiac function was registered by strain gauge transducers and the coronary flow by electrical drop counting. Furthermore small tissue probes, 50-100 mg in weight, served as material for the experiments. They were incubated for 3 min in O_2-gassed Tyrode solution at 37°C using adequate amounts (10-100 µl) of the incubation medium for analysis.Body fluids derived from the organism were directly applied for PG estimation in small amounts of 10-50 µl. The analysis of the prostanoids was performed by a sensitive and specific enzyme immunoassay (Giessler et al., 1988). All investigations were carried out in close cooperation with several clinics of the universities in Halle and Leipzig.

RESULTS

Tissue probes of different organs of guinea pigs showed marked differences of the prostanoid liberation into the incubation medium. Great amounts (76-302 pg TXB_2/mg wet weight and 75-265 pg 6-oxo-PGF_{1alpha}/mg wet weight) could be found with lung, stomach and renal medulla, but heart, liver and skin formed considerably smaller quantities (11-22 pg TXB_2/mg wet weight and 17-19 pg 6-oxo-PGF_{1alpha}/mg wet weight) of the PG mediators. In isolated organs of animals sensibilized with ovalbumine the application of the antigen is followed by a 2-6 fold increase ($p<0.01$) of the prostanoid release. In the same manner the platelet activating factor (PAF-acether) induced a marked increase of the TXB_2-biosynthesis in the heart (13 to 127 pg/mg wet weight), the lung (615 to 5439 pg/mg wet weight) and the aorta (234 to 676 pg/mg wet weight) ($p<0.01$), while the formation of 6-oxo-PGF_{1alpha} remained unchanged or even reduced. After an ischemia of 20 min and following reperfusion isolated perfused hearts showed an enhanced release of TXB_2 and 6-oxo-PGF_{1alpha}, that could be inhibited by indomethacin (Fig. 1).

Changes of gastric mucosa in cases of portal hypertension and chronic gastritis were linked with an increased formation of 6-oxo-PGF_{1alpha} from 113 $\pm$ 19 to 221 $\pm$ 32 and 344 $\pm$ 49 pg/mg wet weight, respectively ($p<0.01$). The TXB_2-biosynthesis increased to a smaller extent (49 $\pm$ 8 to 61 $\pm$ 16 and 82 $\pm$ 25 pg/mg wet weight, respectively).

Malignant tumors of the skin showed a marked increase of the prostanoid biosynthesis of the tissue. Especially tissue from basalioma could produce significantly more prostanoids in comparison with controls (Fig. 2).

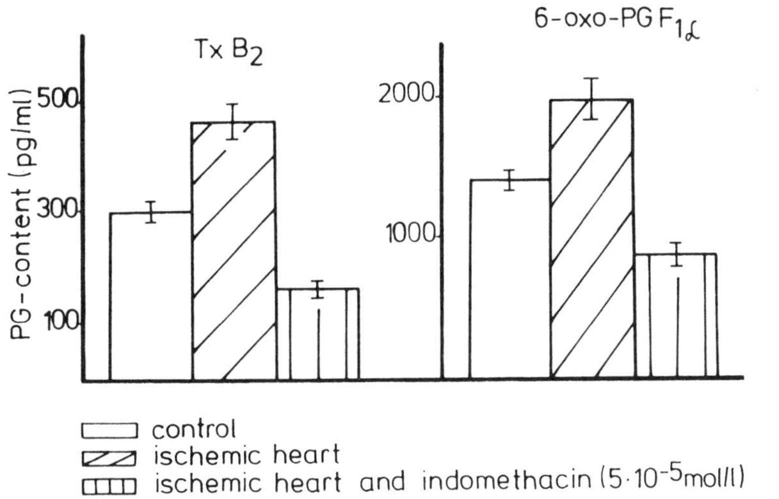

Fig. 1: Changes of the prostanoid content in perfusates of isolated guinea pig hearts after ischemia and reperfusion

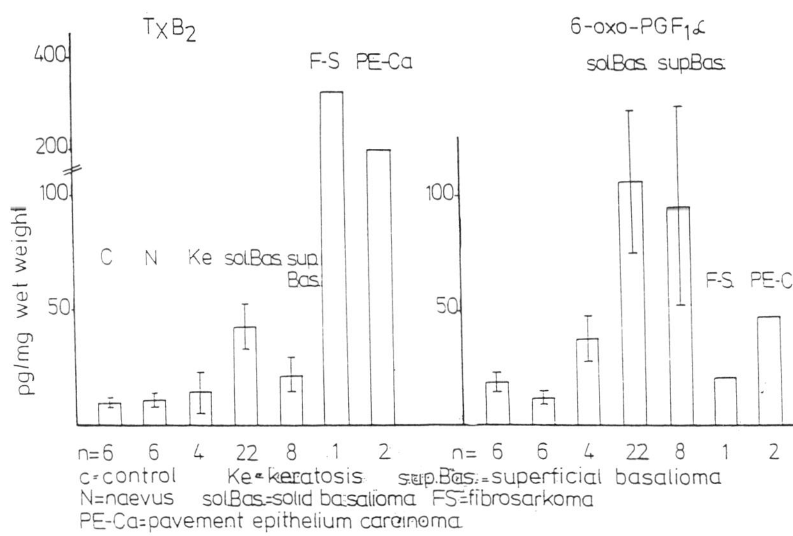

Fig. 2: Prostanoid biosynthesis in the tissue of the skin tumors

In the liquor cerebrospinalis of the children as a rule the prostanoid content remained under the detection level of the method (3-10 pg). On the other side a significant increase could be observed in cases of meningitis, encephalitis and hydrocephalus. The liquor concentration of 6-oxo-PGF_{1alpha} arose up to 511-1340 pg/ml (Fig.3).

An extracapsular cataract extraction in eyes induced a marked rise of the TXB_2- and 6-oxo-PGF_{1alpha} concentration in the aqueous humor, that is inhibited by indomethacin (Tab. I).

Tab. I: Effect of indomethacin on TXB_2- and 6-oxo-PGF_{1alpha} concentration in aqueous humor during cataract extraction

Groups of treatment	Patients (n)	Number of probes under detection limit	Number of probes over detection limit	Range of concentrations (pg/ml)
		TXB_2		
Control	20	6	14	330 - 4830
Indomethacin (1%)	8	6	2	190 - 390
		6 - oxo - PGF_{1alpha}		
Control	20	0	20	520 - 16140
Indomethacin (1%)	8	2	6	1800 - 2860

After a renal transplantation the content of both prostanoids in the daily urine continuously rose up to the 18. day (289 to 1859 ng TXB_2 and 303 to 2073 ng 6-oxo-PGF_{1alpha}) followed by decrease till day 31. (Fig. 4). Under these conditions low prostanoid concentrations in the urine (not shown) seem to indicate a rejection of the transplanted organ.

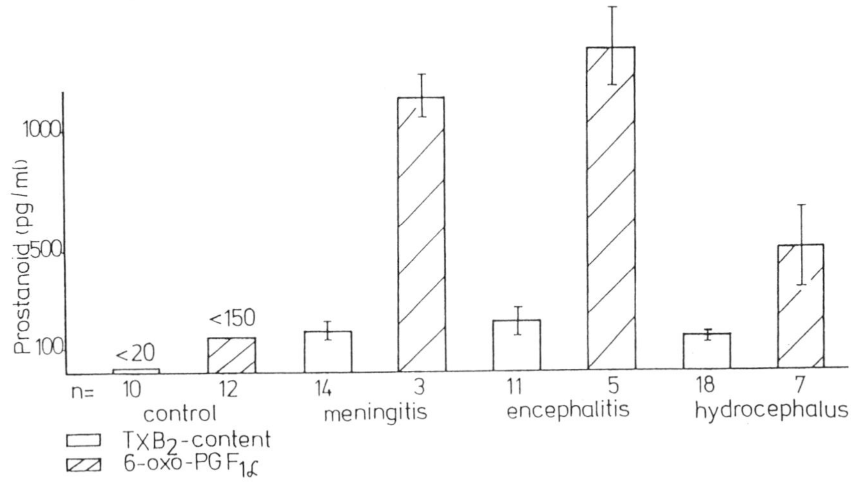

Fig. 3: Prostanoid content (TXB_2 and 6-oxo-PGF_{1alpha}) of the liquor of children in cases of brain diseases (meningitis, encephalitis, hydrocephalus)

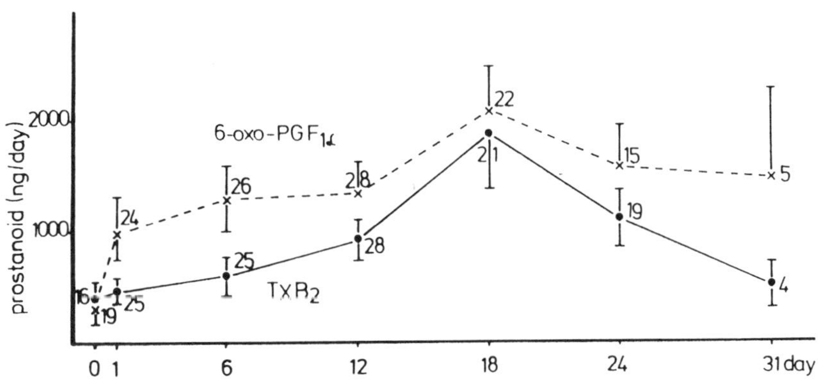

Fig. 4: Daily excretion of TXB_2 and 6-oxo-PGF_{1alpha} into the urine after renal transplantation (n=number of probes)

DISCUSSION

The results suggest, that pathophysiological conditions or a pathological damage of organs were connected with an increased formation of prostanoids. This view is supported by findings of other authors. Ischemia (Engels et al., 1990) or application of the platelet activating factor (Lefort et al., 1984) induced an enhanced formation of eicosanoids in the isolated hearts.
Damage of the gastric mucosa increased the intrinsic prostanoids (Tsuji et al., 1989). Tumor growth is connected with a marked rise of the prostanoid formation (Castelli et al., 1989; Porteder et al., 1986). Furthermore pathological conditions, especially meningitis, enhanced the prostanoid content in the cerebrospinal fluid (Mustafa et al., 1990). Cyclooxygenase and 5-lipoxygenase products have been detected in the anterior chamber during the course of experimentally induced ocular inflammation and in human with uveitis, but whether their presence is incidental or causal is not to be established (Bhattacherjee, 1989; Srinivasan and Kulkarni, 1989). In untreated dogs renal allograft tissue production of TXB_2 and 6-oxo-PGF_{1alpha} was significantly elevated (Mangino et al., 1989).
The cause for the altered PG formation is obviously due to changes or injuries of the cellular membrane and its content of phospholipids. Under this view the significance of the related enzyme activities or an enhanced availability of arachidonic acid as a substrate for the prostanoid biosynthesis should be taken into account. On the other side a decline of the tissue is consecutively characterized by a reduced prostanoid formation.

CONCLUSION: As the prostanoid biosynthesis of the tissue depends on the pathophysiological conditions of the related organs the analysis of these mediators should be of some interest for the diagnosis and opens new possibilities to control therapeutic effects.

REFERENCES

Bhattacherjee, P. (1989) The role of arachidonate metabolites in ocular inflammation, Clin. Biol. Res. 312, 211-227.

Castelli, M.G., Chiabrando, C., Fanelli, R., Martelli, L., Butti, G., Gaetani, P., and Paoletti, P. (1989) Prostaglandin and thromboxane synthesis by human intracranial tumors, Cancer. Res. 49, 1505-1508.

Engels, W., Van Bilsen, M., De Groot, M.J., Lemmens, P.J., Willemsen, P.H., Reneman, R.S., and Van-der Vusse, G.J. (1990) Ischemia and reperfusion induced formation of eicosanoids in isolated rat hearts, Am. J. Physiol. 258, H 1865-1871.

Giessler, Ch., Panse, M., Mentz, P., and Hellthaler, G., (1988) An enzyme-linked immunoassay for thromboxane B_2 and 6-oxo-PGF_{1alpha} using peroxidase as label, Biomed. Biochim. Acta 47, 137-139.

Karmazyn, M. (1989) Synthesis and relevance of cardiac eicosanoids with particular emphasis on ischemia and reperfusion, Can. J. Physiol. Pharmacol. 67, 912-921.

Lefort, J., Rotilio, D., and Vargaftig, B.B. (1984) The platelet-independent release of thromboxane A_2 by PAF-acether from guinea pig lungs involves mechanisms distinct from those for leukocytes, Br. J. Pharmacol. 82, 565-575.

Mangino, M.J., Brunt, E.M., Von Dörsten, P., and Anderson, C.B. (1989) Effects of the thromboxane synthesis inhibitor CGS-12970 on experimental acute renal allograft rejection, J. Pharmacol. Exp. Ther. 248, 23-28.

Mentz, P.,Pawelski, K.E., Giessler, Ch., Mest, H.-J., Mannes, F., and Rotzoll, S. (1988) Myocardial biosynthesis of prostacyclin and the influence of cardiac loading and drugs, Biomed. Biochim. Acta 47, 244-247.

Mustafa, M.M., Ramilo, D., Saez-Lloress, X., Olsen, K.D., Magness, R.R., and Mc Crackn, G.W. (1990) Cerebrospinal fluid prostaglandins, interleukin 1β, and tumor necrosis factor in bacterial meningitis, AJDC 144, 883-887.

Newman, W.H., Fronkis, M.B., and Halushka, P.V. (1983) Increased myocardial release of prostaglandin in dogs with heart failure, J. Cardiovasc. Pharmacol. 5, 194-201.

Porteder, H., Matejka, M., Ulrich, W., Kment, G., and Sinzinger, H. (1986) Immunhistochemischer Nachweis von Prostaglandinen im Stroma oraler Plattenepithelkarzinome Z. Stomatol. 83, 333-345.

Srinivasan, B.B., and Kulkarni, P.S. (1989) Inhibitors of the arachidonic acid cascade in the management of ocular inflammation, Prog. Clin. Biol. Res. 312, 229-249.

Tsuji, S., Kawano, S., Matsunaga, T., Tsujii, M., Hayashi, N., Sakura, H., Tanimura, H., Ogihara, T., Sato, N., and Kamada, T. (1989) Roles of intrinsic prostaglandins and leukotrienes in gastric mucosal damage, Nippon-Shokakibyo-Gakkai Zasski 86, 694-699.

The investigations were performed in cooperation with

- Department of Dermatology, University Leipzig (H.A. Gitt, Th. Walther)
- Department of Internal Medicine, Martin-Luther-University Halle (B. Zipprich, H. Wache)
- Department of Urology, Martin-Luther-University Halle (J. Schabel)
- Department of Ophthalmology, Martin-Luther-University (H.G. Struck, S. Giessler)
- Department of Pädiatrics, Martin-Luther-University Halle (M. John)

AAS 37
Prostaglandins in the
Cardiovascular System

EFFECTS OF DALTROBAN, A THROMBOXANE (TX) A_2 RECEPTOR ANTAGONIST, ON LIPID METABOLISM AND ATHEROSCLEROSIS+

Pill, J., J. Metz*, K. Stegmeier and F. Hartig

Preclinical Research Department, Boehringer Mannheim GmbH, D-6800 Mannheim and *Department of Anatomy and Cell Biology, University of Heidelberg, D-6900 Heidelberg, FRG

SUMMARY: In rat hepatocyte cultures daltroban reduced ^{14}C-acetate incorporation stronger into cholesterol (CH) esters than into free CH. Further data suggest that the reduction of cellular sterols by daltroban is independent from its TXA_2 receptor antagonistic activity and caused by reduced capacity of ACAT depending CH esterification.

In rabbits fed CH-enriched diet treatment with daltroban led to an inhibition of platelet aggregation and to a significant reduction of progression of atherosclerosis. Both reduced CH esterification and TXA_2 receptor antagonism may contribute to the diminution of progression of atherosclerosis by daltroban.

INTRODUCTION:

Among several pathogenic factors, CH-ester accumulation in plaques as well as TX-mediated processes are suggested to contribute to the progression of atherosclerosis. Compounds inhibiting not only one event may offer a superior therapeutic approach to prevent atherosclerosis in man.

+ Supported by the SFB 320

Daltroban, characterized as TXA_2 receptor antagonist, inhibits platelet aggregation in vitro and in vivo (Stegmeier et al., 1986). In a screening experiment the substance was also found to reduce ^{14}C-acetate incorporation into CH ester in rat hepatocyte cultures. In this study we compared the effect of daltroban with that of dazmegrel, an inhibitor of the TX synthase (Fischer et al., 1983;) and with that of U 46619, a TXA_2 mimetic (Coleman et al., 1981) in order to get information whether the effect of daltroban is mediated by the TXA_2/endoperoxide receptor antagonistic activity. Furthermore, we investigated the effect of daltroban on CH oleate formation and on neutral and acid CH ester hydrolases.

Considering that the accumulation of CH ester as well as deposition and aggregation of platelets occur in atherosclerosis daltroban might have an inhibiting activity. We therefore conducted a study in CH-diet induced hypercholestolemic rabbits.

MATERIALS AND METHODS:

Chemicals: Daltroban (4-(2-(4-chlorobenzenesulfonamide)ethyl-benzene acetic acid) was synthesized from Boehringer Mannheim, FRG. Dazmegrel was a generous gift from Pfizer, Munich, FRG.

Primary rat liver cell cultures: Liver cells from male Lewis rats were obtained using the collagenase perfusion technique (Berry & Friend, 1969) and cultivated as described previously (Aufenanger et al., 1986). Investigating de novo synthesis of free and esterified CH cultures were incubated after addition of 2-^{14}C-acetate (37 kBq/ml) in 100 μM acetate for 48 h. To measure incorporation of ^{14}C-oleate into CH ^{14}C-oleate and triglycerides cultures were used after a preincubation period of 24 h with and without daltroban. Cultures were terminated 4 h after addition of ^{14}C-oleate. Neutral and acid CH ester hydrolayse activity was determined according Hoeg et al.(1982).

Acyl-CoA: cholesterol acyl transferase (ACAT) catalyzed CH esterification in microsomes: CH ^{14}C-oleate formation was investigated in a microsome fraction from rat liver using blood serum from diet-induced hypercholesterolemic rabbits as source of CH for esterification (Billheimer et al., 1981).

Separation and determination of radio-labelled lipids: After incubation the monolayer was removed and sonicated in 1 ml water and 2 ml ethanol. Microsomal fractions were terminated by addition of 2 ml ethanol. The neutral lipophilic substances were separated using columns packed with large pore kieselgur (Pill et al., 1985). The solvent was evaporated under nitrogen at 40°C. The residue was dissolved in 2 ml n-heptane and applied to aminopropyl bonded face columns (Bond Elut^{R}, Baker). CH esters, acylglycerols and CH were separated with solvent mixtures with increasing polarity (Kaluzny et al., 1985).

Diet-induced atherosclerosis in male white New Zealand (WNZ) rabbits: Animals were fed a diet (Altromin C2000, Altromin GmbH, Lage, FRG) supplemented with 0.5% CH for 42 (n=6) and 96 (n=15) days. From the letter group 8 animals were treated with daltroban as an admixture to the drinking water from day 42 onwards. U 46619-induced platelet aggregation was investigated in platelet-rich plasma from rabbits at day 50 on CH-enriched diet (Born, 1962). For morphometric analysis of atherosclerosis 10 segments from aorta were fixed in 4% buffered formalin for 4 hours and embedded in Historesin (LKB). The degree of atherosclerosis was evaluated by a computer assisted image analysis of cross sections of the aorta (Metz et al., 1991).

RESULTS:

In vitro: The ^{14}-acetate incorporation (Table I) into CH and its esters in rat hepatocyte monolayer cultures was reduced by daltroban. The effect was stronger on CH esters than free CH.

Table I: Incorporation of ^{14}C-acetate into cholesteryl ester (CH-E) and cholesterol (CH) in rat hepatocyte cultures

	Conc. [M]	Inhibition [%] CH-E			CH		
Daltroban	6 x 10^{-5}	69	±	1.6	49	±	3.7
Dazmegrel	10^{-5}	10	±	1.2	2	±	1.0
Daz + Dal	10^{-5}+6x10^{-5}	69	±	2.5	49	±	3.8
U 46619	10^{-5}	16	±	0.6	0	±	2.7
U 46 + Dal	10^{-5}+6x10^{-5}	69	±	1.9	46	±	4.5

Inhibition in % of solvent-treated controls, Dal: Daltroban, Daz:Dazmengrel, U 46: U 46619, $\bar{\bar{x}}$ ± SEM, n=6 from 3 preparations

The TXA_2-synthase inhibitor dazmegrel as well as the TXA_2-mimetic U 46619 did not show any effect on ^{14}C-acetate incorporation into esterified or free CH. The concommitant incubation of both compounds with daltroban did not affect the daltroban-induced inhibiton of ^{14}C-acetate incorporation.

Daltroban in a concentration range of 10^{-5}-10^{-4}M had no effect on ACAT catalysed CH oleate formation in a microsomal fraction from at liver; diazepam, an ACAT inhibitor (Bell, 1984), reduced the esterification about 55% (2.5x10^{-4}). In rat hepatocyte monolayer cultures (Tab. II) the incorporation of ^{14}C-oleate into CH oleate was clearly reduced when cultures were preincubated with daltroban (A) but not when daltroban and label were added simultaneously (B). The ^{14}C-incorporation into triglycerides was unaffected under both conditions. The activity of neutral and acid CH ester hydrolase was not changed by daltroban under conditions of reduced CH oleate formation.

Table II: Incorporation of ^{14}C-oleate in rat hepatocyte culture

Daltroban [$6x10^{-5}$M]	Cholesteryl ^{14}C-oleate [% inhibition]	^{14}C-Triglycerides [% inhibition]
A	48 ± 1.0	5 ± 2.2
B	18 ± 4.8	6 ± 7.7

Inhibition in % of solvent-treated controls
A: Preincubtion with daltroban for 24 h followed by 4 h incubation with ^{14}C-oleate additionally
B: Preincubation for 24 h followed by 4 h incubation with daltroban and ^{14}C-oleate
$\bar{x}$ ± SEM, 7 culture dishes from 3 preparations

<u>In vivo</u>: The CH-enriched diet increased serum CH in rabbits up to levels of about 2000 mg/100 ml. Daltroban did not show any effect on serum CH concentration. In platetet rich plasma an increased sensitivity of U 46619-induced aggregation was found when rabbits were fed CH-D compared to animals fed standard chow (ED_{50}: $2.4x10^{-7}$M and $6x10^{-7}$M respectively). An about 10 fold higher U 46619 concentration [ED_{50}: $3x10^{-6}$M] was required when rabbits were treated with daltroban.

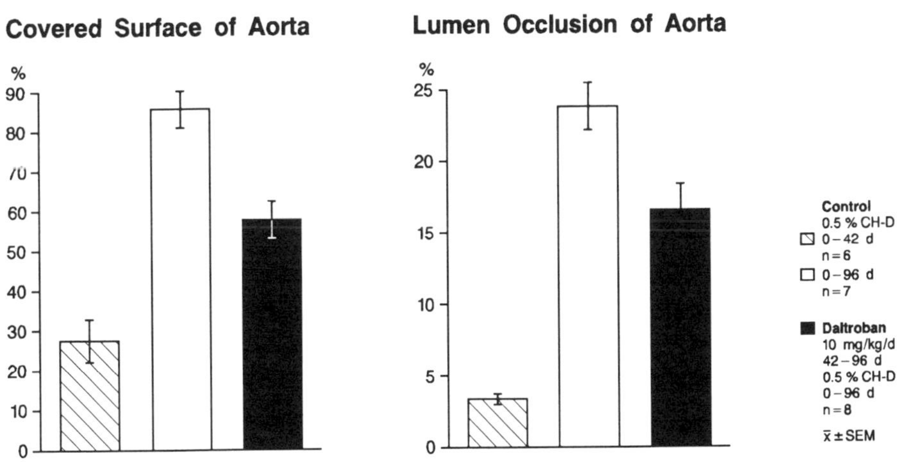

Fig.1: Covered surface and lumen occlusion by plaques in aorta of male WNZ rabbits fed 0.5% CH-enriched diet (CH-D).

Covered surface as well as lumen occlusion of aorta by plaques was significantly lower after daltroban treatment (Fig. 1).

DISCUSSION

The results from rabbits with CH diet-induced atherosclerosis demonstrate clearly that daltroban slows down the progression of atherosclerosis at a dosage intended for use in man. The experimental design, namely the effect on the progression of an already preexisting atherosclerosis, was chosen because it approaches most closely the situation in man with respect to therapeutic application. Under these test conditions suppression of atherosclerotic changes has rarely been found with calcium antagonists (Jackson et al., 1989).

An influence of daltroban on cellular CH ester pool is indicated by the stronger inhibition of ^{14}C-acetate incorporation into CH esters compared to free CH. The loss of effect of TXA_2 synthase inhibitor dazmegrel (Fischer et al., 1983) and of the TXA_2-mimetic U 46619 (Coleman et al., 1981) on synthesis of CH esters and free CH suggests, that the effect of daltroban on cellular sterols is independent from its TXA_2 receptor antagonistic activity. The necessity of preincubation with daltroban to reduce CH ^{14}C-oleate formation in hepatocytes and the lack of effect on esterases as well as on ACAT in microsomes indicates, that daltroban reduces the capacity of the ACAT-depending CH esterification system on cellular level. The unaffected incorporation of radio-label into triglycerides indicates no alterations of other reactions e.g. uptake or CoA thioesterification of ^{14}C-oleate and is an hint of specificity of daltroban-induced reduction of CH esters.

REFERENCES

Aufenanger, J., Pill, J., Schmidt, F.H., and Stegmeier, K. (1986) The effects of BM 15.766, an inhibitor of 7-dehydrocholesterol 7-reductase, on cholesterol biosynthesis in primary rat hepatocytes.
Biochem. Pharmacol. 35, 911-916.

Bell, F.P. (1984) Diazepam inhibits cholesterol esterification by arterial ACAT and plasma LCAT, in vitro.
Atherosclerosis 50, 345-352.

Berry, M.N., and Friend, D.S. (1969) High-yield preparation of isolated rat liver parenchymal cells.
J. Cell Biol. 43, 506-520.

Billheimer, J.T., Tavani, D., and Nes, W.R. (1981) Effect of dispersion of cholesterol in triton WR-1339 on acryl CoA: cholesterol acyltransferase in rat liver microsomes.
Anal. Biochem. 111, 331-335.

Born, G.V.R. (1962) Aggregation of blood platelets by adenosine diphosphate and its reversal.
Nature 194, 927-929.

Coleman, R., Humphrey, P., Kennedy, I., Levy, G., and Lumley, P. (1981) Comparison of the actions of U 46619, a prostaglandin H_2 analogue, with those of prostaglandin H_2 and thromboxane A_2 on some isolated smooth muscle preparations.
Br. J. Pharmacol. 73, 773-778.

Fischer, S., Struppler, M., Böhlig, B., Bernutz, C., Wober, W., and Weber, P.C. (1983) The influence of selective thromboxane synthetase inhibition with a novel imidazole derivate, UK-38,485, on prostanoid formation in man.
Circulation 68, 821-826.

Hoeg, J.M., Demosky, S.J., and Brewer, H.B. (1982) Characterization of neutral and acid ester hydrolase in Wolman's disease.
Biochim. Biophys. Acta 711, 59-65.

Jackson, C.L., Bush, R.C., and Bowyer, D.E. (1989) Mechanism of antiatherogenic action of calcium antagonists.
Atherosclerosis 80, 17-26.

Kaluzny, M.A., Duncan, L.A., Merritt, M.V., and Epps, D.E. (1985) Rapid separation of lipid classes in high yield and purity using bonded phase columns.
J. Lipid Res. 26, 135-140.

Metz, J., Schmelz, A., and Pavlov, P., (1991) Morphologische Untersuchungen zur Quantifizierung der Arteriosklerose.
Zschr. Gerontologie (in press)

Pill, J., Johne, G., Stegmeier, K., Frey, A., Frey, B., and Schmidt, F.H. (1985) New, rapid method for the separation of labelled sterols synthesized by cell cultures by means of Extrelut.
Fresenius Z. Anal. Chem. 322, 512-513.

Stegmeier, K., Pill, J., and Patscheke, H., (1986) BM 13.505, a selective and potent TXA_2 receptor antagonist.
Naunyn-Schmiedeberg's Arch. Pharmacol. 332 (Suppl), R 36.

AAS 37
Prostaglandins in the
Cardiovascular System

EFFECT OF 3-MORPHOLINOSYDNONIMINE (SIN-1), N^G-NITRO-L-ARGININE (NNA) AND N^G-MONOMETHYL-L-ARGININE (NMMA) ON ISOLATED ANAPHYLACTIC GUINEA-PIG HEARTS

D. Pallapies, K. Thelen, A. Dembińska-Kieć*, Th. Simmet and B.A. Peskar

Department of Pharmacology and Toxicology, Ruhr-University of Bochum, Universitätsstr. 150, D-4630 Bochum 1, Germany

*present address: Department of Pharmacology, N. Copernicus Academy of Medicine, Grzegórzecka 16, PL-31531 Cracow, Poland

Summary: In isolated perfused ovalbumin-sensitized guinea-pig hearts modulating effects of nitric oxide (NO) on cardiac function and eicosanoid release were investigated. While the NO-donor SIN-1 exhibited a protective effect during cardiac anaphylaxis, inhibition of NO biosynthesis by NNA or NMMA aggravated anaphylactic changes of cardiac functions. Exogenous and endogenous NO seems to functionally antagonize the effects of vasoconstrictor mediators released during the anaphylactic reaction. In addition, inhibition of cysteinyl-leukotriene (cys-LT) release could contribute to the protective effect of SIN-1 observed.

INTRODUCTION

NO formed endogenously from L-arginine (Palmer et al., 1988a) has been suggested to regulate vascular tone and reactivity in the coronary circulation (Amezcua et al., 1989). It could functionally antagonize the vasoconstrictor effects of eicosanoids and other mediators, which are released during cardiac anaphylaxis. In fact, the cardiac anaphylactic reaction has been shown to be associated with release of nitrite, an oxidation product of NO, into the coronary effluent (Lamparter et al., 1990).

Biosynthesis of NO can be inhibited by the L-arginine analogues NNA (Ishii et al., 1990; Moore et al., 1990; Mülsch and Busse, 1990) and NMMA (Palmer et al., 1988b). We have investigated the effects of the NO-donor SIN-1 and of NNA and NMMA on cardiac functions as well as on eicosanoid release in isolated perfused anaphylactic guinea-pig hearts.

METHODS

Isolated hearts from ovalbumin-sensitized male guinea-pigs (500-700g) were perfused with prewarmed (37°C) oxygenated Tyrode solution at a constant pressure of 45 cm H_2O. After an equilibration period of 25 to 30 min infusions of SIN-1 (final concentration 1.0 mM), NNA, NMMA (final concentration 0.1 mM each) or the appropriate solvents were started. 4 min after start of SIN-1 and 20 min after start of NNA or NMMA infusions hearts were challenged by injection of 1 mg ovalbumin into the aortic inflow cannula.

Coronary flow and heart rate were continuously measured up to 15 min after antigen challenge. Release of cys-LT and 6-keto-prostaglandin (PG) $F_{1\alpha}$ into the coronary effluents was determined radioimmunologically as described previously (Aehringhaus et al., 1983).

MATERIALS

SIN-1 was kindly provided by Cassella-Riedel, Frankfurt, Germany. NNA, NMMA and ovalbumin grade V were from Sigma Chemicals Co., St. Louis, MO, USA. SIN-1 was dissolved in distilled water acidified to pH 5.2 with 1N HCl; all other chemicals were dissolved in 0.9% NaCl.

RESULTS

Cardiac functions before antigen challenge: Infusion of SIN-1 (final concentration 1.0 mM) caused a significant increase in coronary flow (Fig. 1), while NNA or NMMA (final concentration 0.1 mM each) infusions resulted in a significant reduction (Fig. 2, 3). Neither SIN-1 nor NNA nor NMMA had any effect on spontaneous heart rate.

Cardiac functions after antigen challenge: Injection of ovalbumin into the sensitized hearts was followed by an initial more severe and a later less pronounced coronary flow reduction (Fig. 1). An initial tachycardia was followed by arrhythmias. The time-dependent profile of the anaphylactic coronary reaction was basically unchanged during infusion of the NO-donor SIN-1 or the inhibitors of NO biosynthesis NNA and NMMA. However, this profile occurred at a markedly elevated level of coronary flow with SIN-1

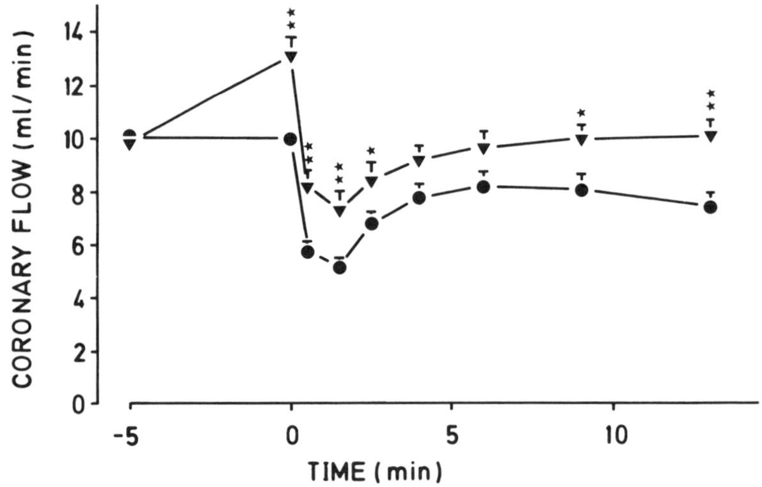

Figure 1: Coronary flow before and after antigen challenge of sensitized guinea-pig hearts infused with solvent (●, n=14) or with SIN-1 (▼, final perfusate concentration 1.0 mM, n=7). Antigen was injected at time 0. ** $P < 0.01$, * $P < 0.05$ as compared to solvent-infused hearts.

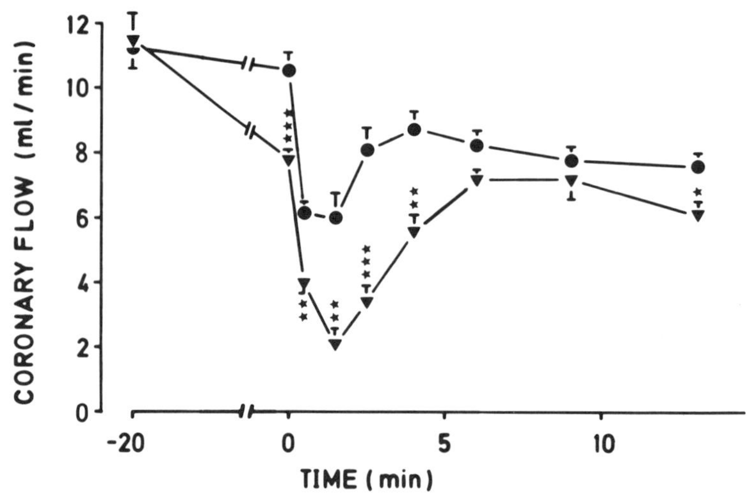

Figure 2: Coronary flow before and after antigen challenge of sensitized guinea-pig hearts infused with solvent (●, n=6) or with NNA (▼, final perfusate concentration 0.1 mM, n=6). Antigen was injected at time 0. *** $P < 0.001$, ** $P < 0.01$, * $P < 0.05$ as compared to solvent-infused hearts.

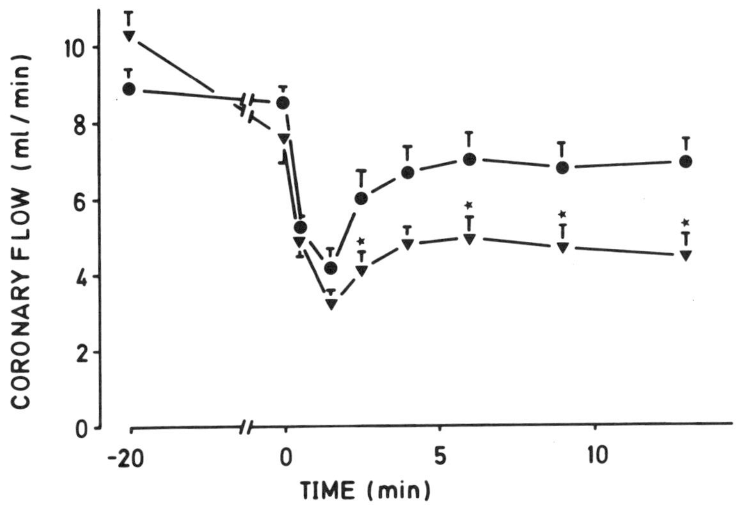

Figure 3: Coronary flow before and after antigen challenge of sensitized guinea-pig hearts infused with solvent (●, n=6) or with NMMA (▼, final perfusate concentration 0.1 mM, n=6). Antigen was injected at time 0. * $P < 0.05$ as compared to solvent-infused hearts.

infusions (Fig. 1) and at a decreased level with NNA and NMMA infusions (Fig. 2, 3). After antigen challenge the typical changes in heart rate were not significantly altered by infusions of SIN-1, NNA or NMMA. The average duration of arrhythmias (509 $\pm$ 76 s in controls, n=14) was significantly reduced by SIN-1 (1.0 mM) to 286 $\pm$ 73 s (n=7, $P < 0.05$), while NNA and NMMA (0.1 mM each) tended to prolong the arrhythmic phase, but the effects were not significant ($P > 0.05$).

Eicosanoid release: Under basal conditions levels of cys-LT and 6-keto-$PGF_{1\alpha}$ in the coronary effluents were close to or below the detection limits of the radioimmunoassays (cys-LT 52 pg/ml; 6-keto-$PGF_{1\alpha}$ 15 pg/ml) and not measurably changed by infusions of SIN-1, NNA or NMMA. However, release of cys-LT into the coronary effluent after antigen challenge was inhibited by infusion of SIN-1. In the presence of SIN-1 (1.0 M) the total release of cys-LT during the 15 min observation period after antigen challenge was decreased to 31.1 $\pm$ 16.8% (n=7, $P < 0.05$) of the control release. By contrast, NNA and NMMA (0.1 mM each) did not significantly affect the release of cys-LT after antigen challenge. However, total release tended to be higher in the presence of NNA (81.5 ± 24.3 ng/15 min) but not of NMMA (45.3 ± 10.7 ng/15 min) as compared to the corresponding control groups (61.9 ± 12.9 ng/15 min and 47.2 ± 15.9 ng/15 min, respectively).

SIN-1 (1.0 mM) caused a significant decrease by 69 ± 6% (n=7, $P < 0.05$) of the total release of 6-keto-PGF$_{1\alpha}$ during the 15 min period after antigen challenge. Conversely, in the presence of NNA or NMMA the total release of 6-keto-PGF$_{1\alpha}$ tended to be increased as compared to the corresponding control groups, but the increases by 52 ± 30% (NNA 0.1 mM) and 27 ± 22% (NMMA 0.1 mM), respectively, were not significant ($P > 0.05$).

DISCUSSION

Coronary flow under basal conditions and after antigen challenge was increased by the exogenous NO-donor SIN-1, but decreased by the inhibitors of endogenous NO biosynthesis NNA and NMMA. These findings suggest a role for NO in the regulation of coronary vascular tone resulting in a protective effect during cardiac anaphylaxis. This hypothesis is supported by the shortened duration of arrhythmias during SIN-1 infusion. The anaphylactic reaction of isolated sensitized guinea-pig hearts is accompanied by the release of mediators such as histamine, platelet-activating factor and eicosanoids (Levi et al., 1984; Simmet and Peskar, 1986; Piper et al., 1989). In our study, release of cys-LT, which are potent coronary vasoconstrictors (Letts and Piper, 1982), after antigen challenge was significantly decreased by SIN-1 and slightly increased by NNA. The reduced release of 6-keto-PGF$_{1\alpha}$ in the presence of SIN-1 could be a consequence of the reduction in cys-LT release (Aehringhaus et al., 1983).

Our results suggest that exogenous and endogenous NO functionally antagonizes the effects of vasoconstrictor mediators released during cardiac anaphylaxis. While, in addition, inhibition of eicosanoid release could contribute to the effects of a high concentration of SIN-1, the possible interaction of endogenous NO with eicosanoid biosynthesis, release and metabolism remains to be further investigated.

REFERENCES

Aehringhaus, U., Peskar, B.A., Wittenberg, H.R. and Wölbling, R.H. (1983) Effect of inhibition of synthesis and receptor antagonism of SRS-A in cardiac anaphylaxis. Br. J. Pharmacol. 80, 73-80.

Amezcua, J.L., Palmer, R.M.J., de Souza, B.M., Moncada, S. (1989) Nitric oxide synthesized from L-arginine regulates vascular tone in the coronary circulation of the rabbit. Br. J. Pharmacol. 97, 1119-1124.

Ishii, K., Chang, B., Kerwin, J.F., Huang, Z.-J. and Murad, F. (1990) N^G-nitro-L-arginine: a potent inhibitor of endothelium-derived relaxing factor formation. Eur. J. Pharmacol. 176, 219-233.

Lamparter, B., Gross, S.S., Griffith, O.W. and Levi, R. (1990) Endothelium-derived nitric oxide plays a role in cardiac anaphylaxis. Arch. Int. Pharmacodyn. Ther. 305, 261.

Letts, L.G. and Piper, P.J. (1982) The actions of leukotrienes C_4 and D_4 on guinea-pig isolated hearts. Br. J. Pharmacol. 76, 169-176.

Levi, R. (1972) Effect of exogenous and immunologically released histamine on the isolated heart: a quantitative comparison. J. Pharmacol. Exp. Ther. 182, 227-238.

Moore, P.K., al-Swayeh, O.A., Chong, N.W.S., Evans, R.A. and Gibson, A. (1990) L-N^G-nitro-arginine (L-NOARG), a novel, L-arginine reversible inhibitor of endothelium-dependent vasodilatation in vitro. Br. J. Pharmacol. 99, 408-412.

Mülsch, A. and Busse, R. (1990) N^G-nitro-L-arginine (N^5-[imino(nitroamino) methyl]-L-ornithine) impairs endothelium-dependent dilations by inhibiting cytosolic nitric oxide synthesis from L-arginine, Naunyn-Schmiedeberg's Arch. Pharmacol. 341, 143-147.

Palmer, R.M.J., Ashton, D.S. and Moncada, S. (1988a) Vascular endothelial cells synthesize nitric oxide from L-arginine. Nature 333, 664-666.

Palmer, R.M.J., Rees, D.D., Ashton, D.S. and Moncada, S. (1988b) L-arginine is the physiological precursor for the formation of nitric oxide in endothelium-dependent relaxation. Biochem. Biophys. Res. Commun. 153, 1251-1256.

Piper, P.J., Yaacob, H.B. and McLeod, J.D. (1989) Interactions of leukotrienes, platelet-activating factor and thromboxane A_2 in cardiac anaphylaxis. New Trend Lipid Mediator Res. 3, 252-256.

Simmet, Th. and Peskar, B.A. (1986) Eicosanoids and the coronary circulation. Rev. Physiol. Biochem. Pharmacol. 104, 1-64.

AAS 37
Prostaglandins in the
Cardiovascular System

THE USE OF GAMMA-LINOLENIC ACID IN DIABETIC NEUROPATHY

D F Horrobin, Efamol Research Institute, P O Box 818, Kentville, Nova Scotia, B4N 4H8, Canada.

SUMMARY

EF4 is an entirely new approach to the management of diabetic neuropathy. EF4 (providing gamma-linolenic acid or gamolenic acid, GLA) has been shown to reverse existing diabetic neuropathy in trials in seven centres. Diabetic animals and humans have a reduced ability to convert dietary linoleic acid to GLA. GLA and its metabolites are required for normal neuronal structure and function and a normal microcirculation. The lack of GLA and its metabolites may play a major role in the development of the neuropathy. EF4 helps to correct the biochemical defects, restores levels of GLA metabolites towards normal and produces highly significant clinical and neurophysiological improvements in diabetic neuropathy.

INTRODUCTION

Diabetic neuropathy is probably the most common complication of diabetes. It eventually causes clinical symptoms in about 50% of all diabetics [1]. But nerve conduction studies indicate that over 95% of diabetics have evidence of nerve damage [2,3].

In diabetic neuropathy, many peripheral nerve fibres degenerate for reasons which are by no means certain although there are many hypotheses. The main types of neuropathy which are characteristic of diabetes are distal somatic polyneuropathy particularly affecting sensory nerves and also neuropathy affecting autonomic nerves.

The main symptoms of somatic polyneuropathy are loss of sensation, weakness, paraesthesia and pain [2]. Autonomic neuropathy which is almost always found to some degree in patients with somatic neuropathy can cause a very wide range of symptoms and signs including instability of control of cardiac rhythm and blood pressure, loss of normal control of the gastro-intestinal tract, loss of normal control of the bladder, and impotence[2]. Sudden death in diabetics appears to be strongly associated with the presence of autonomic neuropathy [4].

It is generally believed that good diabetic control will reduce the risk of development of progressive neuropathy [5]. However, this proposition has been difficult to prove and there are as yet no wholly convincing studies. Every diabetologist has patients who develop severe neuropathy in spite of the best efforts of patient and doctor to ensure good diabetic control.

Every diabetologist also has patients who remain free of symptoms of neuropathy even though they are careless about control of diabetes. There is some evidence that patients who have neuropathy at diagnosis and whose HbA_{1c} levels come down indicating improved control also show improvements in neuropathy [6]. On the other hand, the phenomenon of a rapid worsening of symptoms when tight diabetic control is instituted is also well described [2].

Most diabetologists recommend that diabetics at risk of progressive neuropathy should control their diabetes as tightly as possible. But the idea that this will be effective has more hope than promise since there can be no certainty that good diabetic control will work.

AETIOLOGY

The aetiology of diabetic neuropathy is unknown but there is no shortage of competing hypotheses, most of which interlock at one or more levels. Most of the hypotheses can be grouped into two broad categories, those which emphasize hyperglycaemia, and those which emphasize microvascular problems leading to defective supplies of oxygen and nutrients to the nerve.

The hyperglycaemia hypothesis suggests that all the complications ultimately relate to exposure of tissues to elevated levels of glucose. Under this umbrella are two main sub-hypotheses. The first suggests that the neuropathy is related to covalent glycosylation of proteins which may damage nerves directly and also cause microvascular damage, especially to basement membranes [2]. The second suggests that the main problem is the accumulation of sorbitol, formed from glucose as a result of the action of the enzyme aldose reductase [2]. It has been proposed that this will lead to a range of problems including changes in micro-osmostic balances in the vicinity of neurons, alterations in inositol metabolism and in ATPases and abnormalities in axonal transport.

To date the protein glycosylation concept has not generated any clinical therapies for diabetic neuropathy other than to indicate that better control of glucose may be beneficial. In contrast the aldose reductase concept has led to an explosion of both academic and pharmaceutical research, with many companies aiming to develop aldose reductase inhibitors (ARls). ARls proved encouraging in some animal experiments [7,8] but have largely failed in humans either because of the toxicity of some of the compounds or because of weak or absent efficacy [9-11]. As a result drug company interest in this field is declining rapidly.

The microvascular hypothesis has many possible components, but these components all propose that nerve damage results from inadequate supply of nutrients and especially of oxygen to the nerve [12]. These microvascular problems might result from the loss of normal capillary permeability with accumulation of fluid and protein in the extracellular space, from thickening of capillary basement membranes, from increased blood viscosity due to stiffened red cells or plasma fractions, or from overactivity of haemostatic mechanisms including both the platelets and the coagulation system.

The main therapeutic approach generated by the microvascular hypothesis has been the development of vasodilator products notably prostaglandin (PG) E_1 in Japan [13-15]. This appears to be moderately successful but is still in an early stage of development. Its main drawback is that it has to be administered by injection and causes a number of side effects so may not be appropriate for long term use.

GAMMA-LINOLENIC ACID, GLA: AN ENTIRELY NEW APPROACH

The use of gamma-linolenic acid (gamolenic acid, GLA) has evolved from observations originally made in Argentina 25 years ago on animals with diabetes. Brenner and his colleagues were investigating the metabolism of linoleic acid in diabetes and reported that it was abnormal [16].

Linoleic acid is the main essential fatty acid (EFA) in the diet. It is a vitamin-like essential nutrient which must be eaten because it cannot be made within the body [17]. But like several essential nutrients, linoleic acid itself has only limited roles. In order to be fully utilized within the body it must be metabolised within the organism along the pathway shown in figure 1.

Figure 1. An outline of essential fatty acid metabolism showing the step which is impaired in diabetes mellitus.

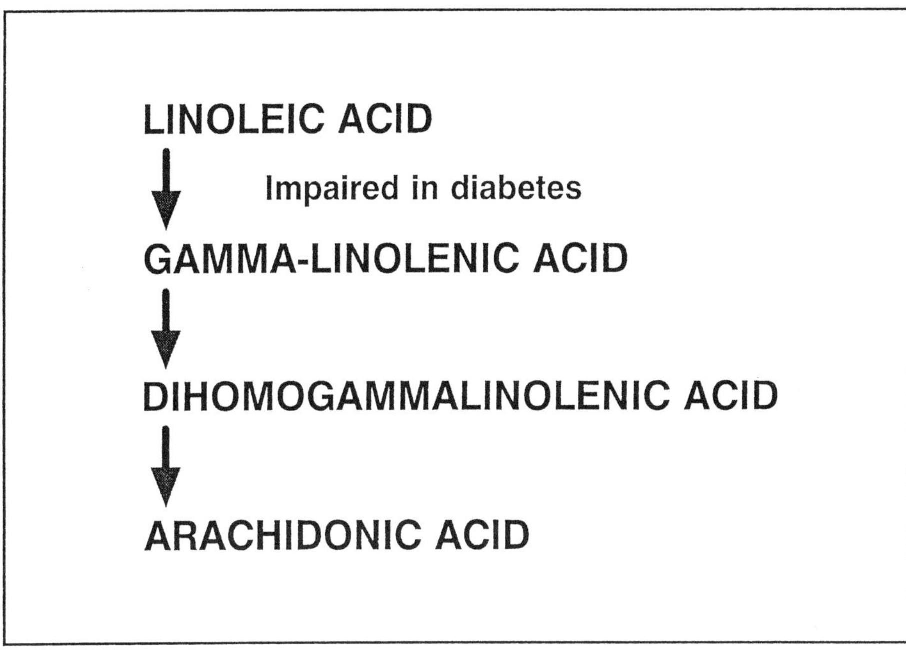

The first step, which Brenner found to be rate-limiting is the delta-6-desaturation of linoleic acid to GLA. GLA is then rapidly converted to dihomogammalinolenic acid (DGLA) which in turn is converted relatively slowly to arachidonic acid. Both DGLA and arachidonic acid can be metabolised to a range of short-lived compounds known as eicosanoids which are involved in the second by second regulation of all tissues, including the components of the microcirculation and the platelets. The eicosanoids include prostaglandins, leukotrienes and hydroxy-fatty acids.

The eicosanoids produced from DGLA are particularly desirable, while those derived from arachidonic acid are a mixture of pro-inflammatory, pro-thrombotic and vasoconstrictor substances and of other metabolites such as prostacyclin which have exactly the opposite effects. An adequate level of DGLA seems to be the key to the physiological regulation of the system. DGLA gives rise to two main metabolites, PGE_1 and 15-OH-DGLA [18]. PGE_1 has a wide range of desirable actions, including vasodilatation, inhibition of platelet aggregation, inhibition of inflammation and control of excessive phospholipase A_2 activity. Excess phospholipase activity leads to breakdown of membranes and release of large amounts of arachidonic acid: the release of arachidonic acid damages the membrane and leads to excessive production of harmful metabolites.

15-OH-DGLA, derived from DGLA, also limits the formation of harmful metabolites from arachidonic acid [18-19]. In particular it inhibits the 5- and 12- lipoxygenase enzymes which produce leukotrienes and other pro-inflammatory and pro-thrombotic substances. Thus in the presence of adequate amounts of DGLA, arachidonic acid is conserved within membranes where it plays an essential structural role and is prevented from being converted to excessive amounts of harmful metabolites.

We now know that in diabetes there is a major block in the EFA metabolite pathway at the first step, delta-6-desaturation. As a result there is restricted conversion of dietary linoleic acid to GLA and beyond. This can be shown directly in diabetic animals by measuring the activity of the enzyme in the liver, or indirectly in diabetic humans by measuring the ratios of linoleic acid to its metabolites, a high ratio indicating reduced delta-6-desaturation activity. There are now many papers in the literature from many different groups which describe a reduced rate of conversion of linoleic acid to GLA in diabetes [16,19-26].

This reduced flow of metabolites down the EFA pathway is likely to have many important adverse consequences, some of which are obviously of importance in diabetes. These include:

1. Lack of adequate amounts of EFAs such as DGLA and arachidonic acid for normal membrane structure. EFAs are very important in neural membranes. Since the EFAs are major fluidizing components of membranes their absence is likely to lead to stiffer red blood cells and an increased blood viscosity. Stiff red cells and elevated blood viscosity have been described in diabetes [27].

2. Lack of adequate amounts of vasodilator and anti-aggregatory eicosanoids such as PGE_1 and prostacyclin. These are likely to result in a tendency to constriction of the microvessels and to intra-vascular aggregation.

3. Lack of adequate control of arachidonic acid metabolism by DGLA. As a result arachidonic acid is likely to be lost from membranes and converted to pro-thromobotic, vasoconstrictor and pro-inflammatory metabolites. The loss of arachidonic acid will damage membrane structure and lead to its depletion from key components of the second messenger system such as phosphatidyl-inositol and diacly-glycerol [28]. Low arachidonic acid levels in nerve diacyl-glycerol have been described in diabetes [28].

These are important changes in membrane structure and in second messenger systems resulting from inadequate GLA formulation and its consequences. it is evident that they could play major roles not only in diabetic neuropathy but also in other complications of diabetes. The concept immediately suggests two possible approaches to managing EFA metabolism in diabetes:

1. The administration of very large amounts of linoleic acid in an attempt to overcome the block and increase the flow to GLA and beyond.

2. The by-passing of the block by the provision of linoleic acid and metabolites beyond the rate-limiting step [30,31]. This was actually tried by Brenner as long ago as 1968. He showed that testicular atrophy in diabetic rats could be prevented by treatment with arachidonic acid [29]. However, he did not follow up this promising approach and nothing more was done until the recent development of the idea of using GLA

Investigators in France proposed that GLA might be useful in managing the cardiovascular complications of diabetes [25] while Horrobin suggested that diabetic neuropathy might be the complication most likely to respond [30,31]. This suggestion was based on the known importance of EFAs and their metabolites in neuronal membranes and in the control of the microcirculation.

SOURCE OF GLA

GLA is a normal intermediate in human metabolism. Within the body it is very rapidly converted to DGLA. GLA and DGLA are found in small amounts of some foods, notably organ meats.

They are found in relatively large amounts in human breast milk and a fully breast fed baby consumes of the order of 20-40 mg of GLA + DGLA per kg per day [19].

For practical purposes, the main source of GLA for clinical use is the seed oil of the evening primrose (Oneothera spp). This is an exceptionally simple oil in which almost all the non-GLA fatty acids present are the generally desirable linoleic and oleic acids. Unfortunately, but as it to be expected, wild varieties of the plant lead to seed oils of widely varying compositions, inappropriate for medical use.

As a result of an intensive plant selection and breeding programme, Scotia Pharmaceuticals Ltd. has developed EF4, a type of evening primrose oil (SC115) with constant composition which delivers 40 mg of GLA per capsule. EF4 has been subjected to complete animal toxicology evaluations, including full carcinogenicity studies in two species. It is manufactured to pharmaceutical standards.

ANIMAL STUDIES

Julu conducted the first animal studies on EF4 in diabetic neuropathy [32,33]. Julu has now carried out a long series of studies on the effects of EF4 in rats made diabetic by streptozotocin. The main conclusions of Julu's work are as follows [32,33] (fig 2).

1. When administered at the time of initiation of diabetes, EF4 could prevent slowing of conduction velocity in both sensory and motor large and small myelinated nerves.

2. When administered later, once neuropathy had become established, EF4 could reverse neuropathy.

3. The neuropathy response was not associated with or attributable to any improvements in the underlying diabetes. Neither blood glucose nor glycosylated haemoglobin levels were improved by EF4.

These animal observations by Julu have now been confirmed and extended by several other groups. Tomlinson et al also found that EF4 could prevent the development of slowed motor nerve conduction in diabetic animals [34,35]. However EF4 did not correct sorbitol of fructose levels, did not elevate depleted myo-inositol and did not normalise axonal transport of substance P.

Since nerve conduction was normal in spite of elevated sorbitol, depleted inositol and disturbed axonal transport, this study casts serious doubts on the ideas that these phenomena are in any way central to the phenomenon of neuropathy. The observations suggest that the neuropathy may relate to changes in phospholipid structure of the neuronal membrane and/or to abnormal neuronal microvascular function.

Low levels of arachidonic acid have been found in neuronal phospholipids from diabetic animals with neuropathy [28].

Further light on possible mechanisms was indicated by studies of Cameron and Cotter in Aberdeen [36]. Like Julu and Tomlinson they demonstrated that EF4 could prevent reductions in conduction velocity in sciatic motor and saphenous sensory nerves [45]. Linoleic acid had no such effect, supporting the view that the neuropathy is related to a deficit not of linoleic acid itself but of linoleic acid metabolities. A characteristic feature of diabetic neuropathy is the resistance of diabetic nerves to ischaemic conduction block. This phenomenon is frequently cited as evidence in favour of the microvascular hypothesis. In crude and over-simplified terms, it is assumed that the resistance to ischaemia is evidence that the nerve has become "used" to a reduced availability of oxygen. Cameron and Cotter found that EF4 restored conduction velocity and also restored normal sensitivity to ischaemia in diabetic nerves [36].

The Aberdeen group are also interested in the changes in muscle function, notably the greatly increased fatiguability, in diabetes. They found that EF4 could reduce the mucsle abnormalities, especially the fatiguability of the soleus.

PRELIMINARY CLINICAL STUDY

The animal results of Julu led Jamal and Carmichael to initiate a pilot, randomized, double-blind, placebo-controlled study in diabetic neuropathy [37]. Diabetic patients of either type with neuropathy were randomly assigned to receive GLA in the form of EF4 capsules or placebo capsules for a period of 6 months. They were given 320 mg of GLA per day and assessed at the beginning and end of the trial for motor nerve conduction velocity, sensory nerve action potential amplitude, compound muscle action potential and hot and cold thermal thresholds in both upper and lower limbs. They were also subjected to a structured neurological examination of sensory function and reflexes. Plasma phospholipid fatty acid compositions were measured.

Of the 10 neurophysiological parameters, all improved in the EF4 group while all deteriorated, albeit often only to a small degree, in the placebo group. The difference between the EF4 and placebo groups was statistically significant for all but the 2 cold thresholds. Symptoms also improved significantly in the EF4 group.

Both groups of patients had plasma phospholipid DGLA and arachidonic acid levels significantly below the normal range.

Both DGLA and arachidonic acid rose significantly in the EF4 group but not in the placebo group. There were no significant changes in HbA_{1c} in either group.

The results of this study are therefore consistent with those of the animal investigators. Administration of EF4 was able to reverse existing neurological damage without any effect on control of glucose metabolism.

MULTICENTRE TRIAL OF EF4

The results of the animal and preliminary human investigators led to a multicentre study being set up in seven centres, six in the UK and one in Finland (table1) [38].

Table 1. The Centres and Lead Investigators Involved in the Multicentre Trial.

Centre	Lead Investigator
Glasgow University Medical School UK	A Weir
King's College Hospital Medical School, UK	P Watkins
St Bartholomew's Hospital Medical School, UK	E Gale
Guy's Hospital Medical School, UK	H Keen
North Staffordshire Royal Infirmary, UK	J Scarpello
Royal Free Hospital Medical School, UK	P K Thomas
Rehabilitation Research Centre, Turku, Finland	J-P Halonen

Table 2. Summary of the Design of the Multicentre Trial

Seven Centres involved

Patients randomised to active or placebio for 1 year.

All patients on active for a 2nd year

Dose 12 x 500mg EF4 capsules each containing 40mg GLA, or placebo/day

Measurements at 0, 3, 6, 12, 18 and 24 months:

- Motor nerve conduction velocity (MNCV), compound muscle action potential (CMAP) and sensory nerve action potential (SNAP) in arm and leg
- hot and cold thresholds at ankle and wrist
- structured neurological examination of arm and leg
- sensation, muscle strength, reflexes of arm and leg

111 patients were entered into a randomized, double-blind, placebo-controlled parallel study for one year (table 2). The dose was 480 mg of GLA/day given as 6 EF4 capsules each

morning and evening. There was provision for all patients who wished to do so to continue for a second year. Unknown to the patients, but known to the doctors, all patients in the second year were subjected to active treatment. Assessments were made at baseline, 3, 6 and 12 months in the first year and at 18 and 24 months in those patients who continued for a second year. 54 patients were assigned to EF4 and 57 to placebo. 2 patients on EF4 and 9 on placebo dropped out before the first evaluation. Thus 52 patients on EF4 and 48 on placebo had at least one evaluation while 44 in the EF4 group and 40 in the placebo group completed the full study.

At each assessment point each patient was tested for motor nerve conduction velocity (MNCV), compound muscle action potential amplitude (CMAP), sensory nerve action potential amplitude (SNAP) and hot and cold thresholds in both upper and lower limbs.

Table 3. Changes in Neurophysiological Parameters in Response to EF4 (Multicentre Trial)

Summary of the results of the multicentre double-blind, placebo-controlled trial of EF4 in diabetic neuropathy. Patients were treated with EF4 or placebo for 12 months, following which all patients received EF4 on a single blind basis. This figure shows the result of the first phase of the trial. 100 patients were assessed, 52 in the EF4 group and 48 in the placebo group. The figure shows the mean changes from baseline in the neurophysiological parameters, a plus sign indicating improvement and a minus sign indicating deterioration. The significances on the differences between the EF4 and the placebo responses are shown.

Motor Nerve Conduction Velocity (m/s)	**EFA (n=52)**	**Placebo (n=48)**	**p<**
Arm	+ 2.37	- 2.14	0.01
Leg	+ 2.23	- 1.86	0.01
Compound action potential (nV)			
Arm	+ 1.44	- 1.13	0.01
Leg	+ 1.22	- 0.62	0.01
Sensory nerve action potential (uV)			
Arm	+ 2.41	- 1.28	0.001
Leg	+ 1.68	- 0.96	0.02
Thermal threshold - hot (°C)			
Wrist	+ 0.84	- 0.39	0.01
Ankle	+ 0.54	- 0.15	NS
Thermal throshold - cold (°C)			
Wrist	+ 0.82	- 0.29	0.01
Ankle	+ 0.79	- 0.42	NS

At the same time an experienced neurologist conducted a detailed and structured neurological examination of sensory function, tendon reflexes and muscle weakness in both upper and lower limbs. HbA_{1c}, haematology, urea, electrolytes and liver enzymes were measured at each visit.

The results of the 10 neurophysiological assessments are shown in Table 3 [38]. All 10 parameters were improved with EF4, 8 significantly so. All 10 deteriorated modestly on placebo, 4 significantly so. The effect of EF4 was significantly better than that of placebo for 8 of the 10 parameters.

Table 4. Changes in Clinical Neurological Parameters in Diabetc Neuropathy in Response to EF4

The results of the clinical neurological assessments in the multicentre trial. The scores are based on standardised scores in a structured neurological examination. The significance of the differences between the change on EF4 and the change on placebo are shown (Mann-Whitney U test).

Muscle weakness ($x\ 10^2$)	**EF4 (n=52)**	**Placebo (n=48)**	**p<**
Arm	+ 4.9	- 7.4	0.01
Leg	+ 5.4	- 9.2	NS
Tendon reflexes (10^2)			
Arm	+ 2.9	-12.0	0.02
Leg	+17.7	+ 0.5	0.05
Sensation (10^2)			
Arm	+ 6.9	-7.3	0.02
Leg	+ 15.0	- 8.4	0.01

The results of the neurological assessments were similar (table 4). All 6 improved on EF4 while 5 of the 6 deteriorated on placebo. The effect of EF4 was always better than that of placebo, significantly so in 5 of the 6 cases.

The improvements on EF4 treatment and deterioration on placebo were progressive over the 12 month period. Results in the patients who have now completed 24 months treatment show that improvement continues over a period of at least 2 years. This is not surprising given the slow rate of neuronal regeneration. In those patients switching from placebo treatment in the first year to EF4 in the second, the first year deterioration was consistently followed by second year improvement.

Neither age, sex, diabetes type, age of onset nor duration of diabetes had any significant impact on results. For MNCV, females did slightly better than males, long term diabetics slightly better than short term ones, and non-insulin dependant diabetics slightly better than insulin-dependant ones, but in no case did the difference between the groups approach statistical significance.

The major parameter which influenced response was the HbA_{1c} level. For the 10 neurophysiological parameters and the 6 clinical ones, when the starting HbA_{1c} level was 10% or less EF4 was always significantly better than placebo. When that starting level was above 10%, EF4 was always better than placebo but the differences were never significant. The interaction between clinical response and starting HbA_{1c} concentration was assessed further by looking at the relationship between the two in individual patients. Results were similar for all parameters. In the EF4 treated patients there was a clear negative relationship, the lower the HbA_{1c} level in the patient, the better being the improvement. The relationship also held for the various centres, the lower the mean HbA_{1c} level in the centre, the better being the improvement.

During the trial HbA_{1c} rose slightly in both EF4 and placebo groups with no significant differences between the two. There was therefore no evidence that treatment was either improving or causing deterioration in the underlying control of diabetics.

CONCLUSION

Thus the multicentre trial provided further confirmation of the results of the animal studies and the preliminary human trial. EF4 is effective in reversing clinical and neurophysiological features of diabetic neuropathy without producing any improvement or indeed any deterioration in diabetic control.

REFERENCES

1. Pirart J. Diabetes mellitus and its degenerative complications: a prospective study of 4400 patients observed between 1947 and 1973. Diabetes Care 1978; 1 (3): 168-183.

2. Dyck PJ, Thomas PK, Asbury AK et al (eds). Diabetic Neuropathy. Saunders, Philadelphia, 1987.

3. Andreani D, Crepaldi G, Di Mario U & Pozzo G (eds). Diabetic Complications: Early Diagnosis and Treatment. John Wiley, Chichester, 1987.

4. Maser RE, Pfeifer MA, Dorman JS, Kuller LH, Becker DJ, Orchard TJ. Diabetic autonomic neuropathy and cardiovascular risk. Arch Intern Med 1990; 150(6): 1218-1222.

5. American Diabetes Association. Report and recommendations of the San Antonio conference on diabetic neuropathy. Muscle and Nerve. 1988; 11: 661-667.

6. Graf RJ, Halter JB, Pfeifer MA et al. Glycemic control and nerve conduction abnormalities in non-insulin-dependent diabetic subjects. Ann Intern Med 1981; 94(5) : 307-311.

7. Cameron NE, Leonard MB, Ross IS, Whiting PH. The effects of sorbinil on peripheral nerve conduction velocity, plyol concentrations and morphology in the streptozotocin diabetic rat. Diabetologia 1986; 29(3): 168-174.

8. Gillon KRW, Hawthorne JN, Tomlinson DR. Mto-inositol and sorbitol metabolism in relation to peripheral nerve function in experimental diabetes in the rat: the effect of aldose reductase inhibition. Diabetologia 1983; 25(4): 365 371.

9. Guy RJC, Gilbey SG, Sheehy M, Asselman P, Watkins PJ. Diabetic neuropathy in the upper limb and the effect of twelve months sorbinil treatment. Diabetologia 1988; 31: 214-220.

10. Boulton AJM, Levin S, Comstock J. A multicentre trial of the aldose-reductase inhibitor, tolrestat, in patients with symptomatic diabetic neuropathy. Diabetologia 1990; 33: 431-437.

11. Florkowski CM, Rowe BR, Nightingale S, Harvey TC & Barnett AH. Clinical and neurophysiological studies of aldose reductase inhibitor ponalrestat in chronic symptomatic diabetic peripheral neuropathy. Diabetes 1991; 40:129-133.

12. Jamal GA. Pathogenesis of diabetic neuropathy: the role of the n-6 essential fatty acids and their eicosanoid derivatives. Diabetic Med 1990; 7:574-579.

13. Yasuda H, Sonobe M, Yamashita M et al. Effect of prostaglandin E_1 analogue TFC 612 on diabetic neuropathy in streptoztocin-induced diabetic rats. Diabetes 1989; 38:832-838.

14. Itoh H, Horie H, Namba M et al. Therapeutic effect of Prostaglandin E_1 (lipo-PGE_1, PGE_1-CD) on diabetic neuropathy. J Japan Diab Soc 1986; 29 (suppl 1):88-90.

15. Hoshi K, Mizushima Y, Kiyokawa S, Yanagawa A. Prostaglandin E_1 incorporated in lipid microspheres in the treatment of peripheral vascular diseases and diabetic neuropathy. Drugs Exptl Clin Res 1986; 12(8):681-685.

16. Mercuri O, Peluffo RO, Brenner RR. Depression of microsomal desaturation of linoleic to gamma-linolenic acid in the alloxan diabetic rat. Biochim Biophys Act 1966; 116:409-411.

17. Rivers JPW, Frankel TL. Essential fatty acid deficiency. Br Med Bull 1981; 37(1): 59-64.

18. Miller CC, McCreedy CA, Jones AD, Ziboh VA. Oxidative metabolism of dihomogammalinolenic acid by guinea pig epidermis: evidence of generation of anti-inflammatory products. Prostaglandins 1988; 35(6): 917-938.

19. Horrobin DF. Gamma-linolenic acid. Rev Contemporary Pharmacotherapy 1990; 1(1):1-41.

20. Faas FH, Carter WJ. Altered fatty acid desaturation and microsomal fatty acid composition in streptozotocin diabetic rat. Lipids 1980; 15(11):953-961.

21. Holman RT, Johnson SB, Gerrard JM et al. Arachidonic acid deficiency in streptozotocin-induced diabetes. Proc Nat Acad Sci USA 1983; 80:2375-2379.

22. Huang Y-S, Fujii K, Takahashi R et al. Effect of diabetes on the metabolism of n-3 and n-6 fatty acids in rats. IRCS J Med Sci 1985; 13:1145-1146.

23. Poisson J-P. Comparative in vivo and in vitro study of the influence of experimental diabetes on rat liver linoleic acid delta 6- and delta 5-desaturation. Enzyme 1985; 34: 1-14.

24. Arisaka M, Arisaka O, Fukuda Y, Yamashiro Y. Prostaglandin metabolism in children with diabetes mellitus. I. Plasma prostaglandin E2, F2 , TXB2 and serum fatty acid levels. J Paed Gastroenterol Nutr 1986; 5: 878-882.

25. Chaintreuil J, Monnier L, Colette et al. Effects of dietary gamma-linolenate supplementation on serum lipids and platelet function in insulin-dependent diabetic patients. Human Nutr: Clin Nutr 1984; 38C: 121-130.

26. Tilvis RS & Miettinen TA. Fatty acid composition of serum lipids, erythrocytes and platelets in insulin-dependent diabetic women. J Clin Endocr Metab 1985; 61(4): 741-745.

27. Simpson LO. Altered blood rheology in the pathogenesis of diabetic and other neuropathies. Muscle Nerve 1988; 11(7): 725-744.

28. Zhu X, Eichberg J. 1,2-diacylglycerol content and its archidonyl-containing molecular species are reduced in sciatic nerve from streptoztozocin-induced diabetic rats. J Neurochem 1990; 55(3): 1087-1090.

29. Brenner RR, Peluffo RO, Mercuri O, Restelli MA. Effect of arachidonic acid in the alloxan diabetic rat. Am J Physiol 1968; 215(1): 63-70. [B 30. Horrobin DF. The roles of essential fatty acids in the development of diabetic neuropathy and other complications of diabetes mellitus. Prostaglandins Leukot Essential Fatty Acids Reviews 1988: 31: 181-197.

31. Horrobin DF Essential fatty acids, psychiatric disorders and neuropathies In: Omega-6 Essential fatty Acids: Pathophysiology and Roles in Clinical Medicine. Horrobin DF, ed. New York: Wiley-Liss, 1990: 305-319.

32. Julu POO. Gamma-linolenic acid: a novel remedy for diabetic neuropathy in experimental animals. In. Omega-6 Essential Fatty Acids: Pathophysiology and Roles in Clinical Medicine. Ed Horrobin DF. New York: Wiley, 1990; pp465-476.

33. Julu POO. Essential fatty acids prevent slowed nerve conduction in streptozotocin diabetic rats. J Diabetic Complications 1988; 2(4): 185-188.

34. Tomlinson DR, Robinson JP, Compton AM. The effects of gamma-linolenic acid treatment on motor nerve conduction velocity and axonal transport of substance P in diabetic rats. In: Omega-6 Essential Fatty Acids: Pathophysiology and Roles in Clinical Medicine. Ed Horrobin DF. New York: Wiley, 1990 pp 457-463.

35. Tomlinson DR, Robinson JP, Compton AM, Keen P. Essential fatty acid treatment - effects on nerve conduction, polyol pathway and axonal transport in streptozotocin diabetic rats. Diabetologia 1989; 32: 655-659.

36. Cameron NE, Cotter MA, Robertson S. Essential fatty acid diet supplementation. Effects on perioheral nerve and skeletal muscle function and capillarization in streptotozocin-induced diabetic rats. Diabetes 1991; 40(5): 532-539.

37. Jamal GA, Carmichael H. The effect of gamma-linolenic acid on human diabetic peripheral neuropathy: a double-blind placebo-controlled trial. Diabetic Med 1990; 7: 319-323.

38. Keen H, Allawi J, Payan J et al. Treatment of diabetic neuropathy with gamm-linolenic acid. Submitted for publication.

AAS 37
Prostaglandins in the
Cardiovascular System

EFFECT OF N-3 FATTY ACIDS ON EICOSANOID FORMATION: IMPLICATIONS FOR PLATELET THROMBOTIC FUNCTIONS

G. Hornstra(1), M.A.H. Feijge (2) and J.W.M. Heemskerk(1, 2)

Departments of Human Biology (1) and Biochemistry (2), Limburg University, P.O. Box 616, 6200 MD Maastricht, The Netherlands.

The rapid production of most eicosanoids (prostaglandins, thromboxanes, leukotrienes) and hydroxy fatty acids in response to a variety of stimuli is an enzymatic process. Consequently, the amount of products formed depends on the available amounts of the C_{20} precursor fatty acids dihomo-γ-linolenic acid, 20:3(n-6), arachidonic acid, 20:4(n-6), and timnodonic acid, 20:5(n-3), mainly stored in the membrane phospholipids. These fatty acids are taken up as such from the diet or are synthesized from dietary linoleic acid, 18:2(n-6), γ-linolenic acid, 18:3(n-6), or α-linolenic acid, 18:3(n-3). These latter ultimate eicosanoid precursors, however, can also give rise to the formation of other longer-chain, more-unsaturated fatty acids which, by competing with the C_{20} precursor fatty acids for the cyclo-oxygenase and lipoxygenase enzymes, may affect enzymatic eicosanoid synthesis. As a result, stimulated eicosanoid formation may not only depend on the precursor content in the cell membranes, but may theoretically be influenced by the entire polyunsaturated fatty acid profile of membrane phospholipids. Extensive animal studies, however, have demonstrated that the amounts of the *direct* precursor fatty acids in membrane phospholipids of blood platelets is by far the most important determinant of their eicosanoid formation upon stimulation (Hornstra, 1985). This also seems to hold for man: replacement of arachidonic acid by timnodonic acid in platelet phospholipids as a result of fish consumption caused a considerable reduction in the stimulated formation of arachidonic acid-derived thromboxane B_2 (TxB_2), 12-hydroxyheptadecatrienoic acid (HHT), and 12-hydroxyeicosatetraenoic acid (HETE). At the same time, the formation of the analogous products from timnodonic acid (TxB_3, HHTE and HEPE) was significantly enhanced. Since timnodonic acid is a relatively poor substrate for the enzymes involved in eicosanoid formation, the increased formation of the timnodonate-derived products does not make up for the reduced production of the eicosanoids from arachidonic acid. Consequently, fish(oil) consumption is associated with a net reduction in eicosanoid formation (Hornstra et al., 1990a).

In the studies mentioned, product formation was measured in citrated platelet-rich plasma, activated with a relatively high dose of collagen. When aggregation was triggered in citrated whole blood, using a much more gentle way of triggering (as judged from the resulting degree of aggregation), a comparable trend was obtained for TxB_2 formation, but the fish effect was not significant anymore. Since the diet-induced differences in TxB_2-formation were found to be strongly correlated with the changes observed for platelet aggregation, it can be concluded that the amount of fish consumed in the study was obviously too small to cause significant effects. This conclusion was supported by the observation that the fish effect was strongly influenced by dietary compliance: the better the volunteers complied to the dietary regimen, the greater was the reduction of TxB_2 formation in the fish group (Hornstra et al. 1990b).

In experimental animals, fish oil consumption has been shown to change the fatty acid profile of vascular phospholipids in a similar way as observed for platelet phospholipids. For both rat and rabbit, the well known replacement of arachidonic acid by timnodonic acid was clearly seen in the vascular tissue, and this resulted in a reduced formation of prostacyclin (PGI_2) upon mechanical stimulation. Interestingly, we were unable to demonstrate any formation of PGI_3 (Hornstra et al., 1981). The response of human vascular phospholipid fatty acids on fish(oil) consumption has not been investigated, but there are no reasons to believe that the fatty acid changes would be different from that in experimental animals. Consequently, an increase is expected in the formation of PGI_3 concomitant with a decreased PGI_2 formation. Indeed, in human urine the amount of a major metabolite of PGI_3 has been reported to increase but, in contrast to the expectations, the urinary excretion of a major PGI_2 metabolite was increased as well (Fischer & Weber, 1984) or at least remained unaltered (von Schacky et al., 1985; Knapp et al., 1986). This has been taken as evidence that the total production of prostacyclin in man increases upon fish(oil) consumption. In our mackerel study we obtained comparable results: PGI_3 formation increased as judged from the urinary excretion of its major metabolite, and PGI_2 either remained stable or even increased. In this latter case we noted a strong relationship between the excretion of both series of metabolites (Hornstra et al., 1990b). This has been observed by others also (Fischer et al. 1986) and it indicates that either a common factor is involved in the higher formation of both PGI_2 and PGI_3 upon fish consumption, or that the enhanced production of PGI_2 is an analytical artefact.

There is no doubt, that fish(oil) consumption causes a reduction in the formation of platelet thromboxanes and, consequently, in platelet aggregation. Animal studies, however, strongly indicate that the TxA_2-sensitivity of blood platelets is higher, the lower their content of arachidonic acid and, consequently, their formation of thromboxanes. Thus we demonstrated in platelet-rich rat plasma that the slope of the relationship between collagen-stimulated TxA_2-formation (as reflected by the formation of HHT) and the aggregation response is steeper, the lower the diet-induced arachidonic acid content of these platelets and, consequently, their endogenous TxA_2-production (Fig. 1). In order to

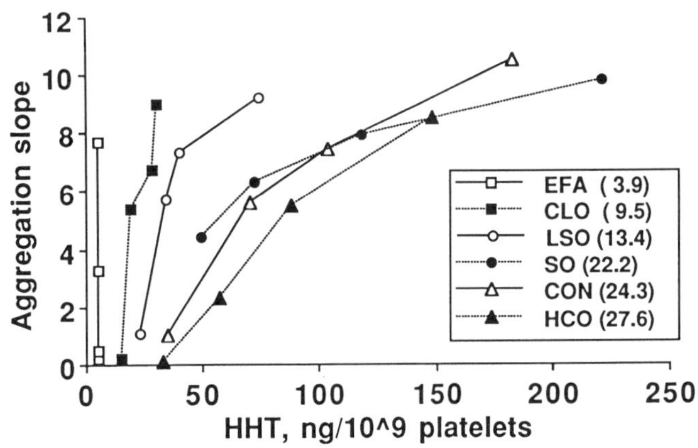

Fig. 1 Relationship between collagen-induced HHT formation (ng/10^9 platelets) and aggregation velocity (slope) of platelets obtained from rats fed different dietary fatty acids (50 energy % of fat). Each point represents the mean of 6 determinations carried out in platelet-rich plasma pools, each obtained from 4 animals. Abbreviations: EFA, essential fatty acid-deficient diet; CLO, cod-liver oil; LSO, linseed oil; SO, sunflowerseed oil; CON: low-fat control group (5 en% SO); HCO, hydrogenated coconut oil diet. Numbers in parentheses indicate the arachidonic content (% of total fatty acids) of platelet phospholipids.

explain this effect further studies were carried out with washed platelets, which had been treated with indomethacin to prevent the formation of endogenous thromboxanes upon platelet stimulation. As a replacement of endogenous TxA_2, various amounts of the TxA_2-mimicking agent U46619 were added together with collagen, and again it was found that the resulting aggregation was higher, the lower the TxA_2 producing potency of the platelets. Platelets from fish oil-fed rats, low in arachidonic acid, gave a higher degree of aggregation than platelets from animals fed sunflowerseed oil (rich in linoleic acid) or hydrogenated coconut oil (rich in saturated fatty acids) (Heemskerk et al., 1991a). This diet-induced difference in TxA_2-sensitivity was unlikely to be due to differences in the interaction of U46619 with the platelet membrane: number and affinity of PGH_2/TxA_2-receptors present on platelets from animals fed different dietary fats were not significantly affected as judged from binding studies with U46619, as well as with the high affinity TxA_2 antagonist, SQ 29548 (Heemskerk et al., 1991a). Consequently, the dietary fat effect on the TxA_2-sensitivity of blood platelets is unlikely to be caused by changes in TxA_2-receptor properties. An early event in the stimulus-response reaction of platelets is the activation of phospholipase C, resulting in the formation of inositol phosphates and diacyl glycerol. Stimulation of indomethacin-treated platelets from rats fed different diets with either thrombin or the TxA_2-mimicking agent U46619 resulted in inositol phosphate formations that were proportional to the degree of platelet aggregation: fish oil platelets produced more inositol phosphates than platelets of animals fed hydrogenated coconut oil, whereas platelets of sunflowerseed oil-treated rats took an intermediate position (Heemskerk et al., 1991a). Therefore, it is likely that the dietary fat effect is located in a very early phase of stimulus-response coupling. For instance, it may involve the activity of GTP-binding proteins.

Platelet aggregation and secretion requires an increase in cytosolic free Ca^{2+}. This Ca^{2+} rise is known to be the result of two processes. Free Ca^{2+} can be released from intracellular stores, a process initiated by inositol 1,4,5-trisphosphate (IP_3) that is formed by the action of phospholipase C on phosphatidyl inositol 4,5-biphosphate. Additionally, extracellular Ca^{2+} can enter the cytosol by the activation of receptor-mediated cation channels in the plasma membrane. As described above, the phospholipase C activity of activated rat platelets, and consequently IP_3 production, was found to be modulated by the type of dietary fat. Recently, we have demonstrated that rat platelets are relatively deficient in intracellular Ca^{2+} stores (Heemskerk et al., 1991b). Therefore, the contribution of the IP_3-mediated Ca^{2+}-response to increase the cytosolic Ca^{2+} can be expected to be very limited indeed. This raises the question whether the receptor-mediated Ca^{2+} entry pathway would also be influenced by the dietary fat type. This possibility is supported by our observation (Table I) that the activation response of rat platelets strongly depends on the presence of extracellular Ca^{2+}. Furthermore, the dietary fish(oil) effect on collagen-induced platelet aggregation appeared to be modified by the extracellular Ca^{2+} concentration (Fig. 2). Therefore, it is feasible that the effect of dietary lipids on the aggregability of rat platelets is also mediated by a modulation of the trans-membranal calcium flux into the platelets. This is currently under investigation.

Table I: Effect of extracellular Ca^{2+} concentration $[Ca^{2+}]_e$ on the serotonin secretion of activated rat platelets. Washed, $[^{14}C]$serotonin-loaded platelets were activated for 5 min at the indicated conditions.

Agonist	$[Ca^{2+}]_e$ (µM)	Serotonin secretion (% of total)
Thrombin (2 nM)	10	7.9
	50	30.0
	500	74.9
Collagen (10 µg/ml)	10	6.7
	50	38.5
	500	51.5

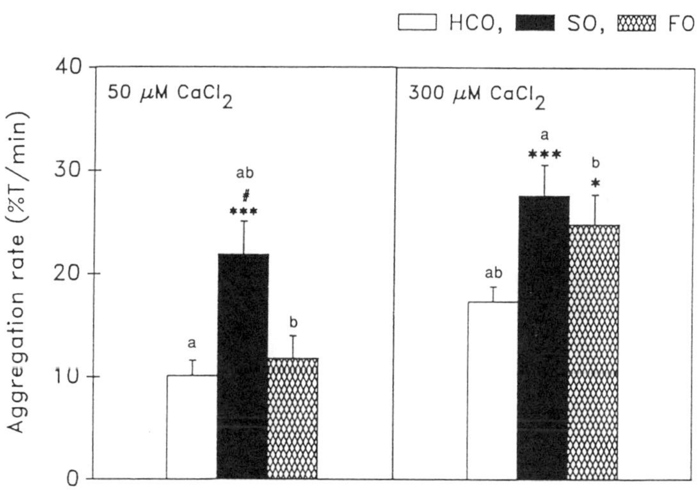

Fig. 2 Influence of extracellular Ca^{2+} concentration on collagen-induced aggregation of dietary fat-modulated platelets. Data are mean values ± SE (n = 6-8). Abbreviations for diet types: HCO, hydrogenated coconut oil; SO, sunflowerseed oil; FO, fish oil diet. Bars with the same superscript differ significantly from each other.

REFERENCES

Fischer, S. and Weber, P.C.: Prostaglandin I_3 is formed in vivo in man after dietary eicosapentaenoic acid. Nature 307: 165-168 (1984)

Fischer, S., Weber, P.C. and Dyerberg, J.: The prostacyclin/thromboxane balance is favourably shifted in Greenland Eskimos. Prostaglandins 32: 235-240 (1986)

Heemskerk, J.W.M., Feijge, M.A.H., and Hornstra, G.: Dietary fat modifies thromboxane A_2-induced stimulation of rat platelets. Biochem. J., 278: 399-404 (1991a)

Heemskerk, J.W.M., Feijge, M.A.H., Rietman, E., and Hornstra, G.: Rat platelets are deficient in internal Ca^{2+} release and require influx of extracellular Ca^{2+} for activation. FEBS Lett. 284: 223-226 (1991b)

Hornstra, G.: Regulation of eicosanoid production by fatty acid availability. Adv. Inflamm. Res. 10: 1-6 (1985)

Hornstra, G., Christ-Hazelhof, E., Haddeman, E., Hoor, F. ten, and Nugteren, D.H.: Fish oil feeding lowers thromboxane- and prostacyclin production by rat platelets and aorta and does not result in the formation of prostaglandin I_3. Prostaglandins 21: 727-738 (1981)

Hornstra, G., Houwelingen, A.C. van, Kivits, G.A.A., Fischer, S. and Uedelhoven, W.: Influence of dietary fish on eicosanoid metabolism in man. Prostaglandins, 40: 311-329 (1990a)

Hornstra, G., Houwelingen, A.C. van, Kivits, G.A.A., Fischer,S., and Uedelhoven, W.: Dietary fish and prostanoid formation in man. Adv. Prost. Thromb. Leukotr. Res. 21: 225-228 (1990b)

Knapp, H.R., Rielly, I.A.G., Alessandrini, P. and FitzGerald, G.A.: In vivo indexes of platelet and vascular function during fish-oil administration in patients with atherosclerosis. New Engl. J. Med. 314: 937-942 (1986)

Schacky, C. von, Fischer, S. and Weber, P.C.: Long-term effects of dietary marine ω-3 fatty acids upon plasma and cellular lipids, platelet function, and eicosanoid formation in humans. J. Clin. Invest. 76: 1626-1631 (1985)

AAS 37
Prostaglandins in the
Cardiovascular System

INFLUENCE OF OMEGA-3 FATTY ACIDS ON THE PROSTAGLANDIN-METABOLISM IN HEALTHY VOLUNTEERS AND PATIENTS SUFFERING FROM PVD

A. Gazsó[1], D. Horrobin[2], H. Sinzinger[1]

[1]Wilhelm Auerswald-Atherosclerosis Research Group Vienna, Nadlergasse 1, A-1090 Vienna;
[2]Efamol Research Institute, Nova Scotia, Canada

1. INTRODUCTION

Greenland Eskimos show a remarkebly low incidence of ischemic heart disease leading to the speculation that part of the apparent protective effect against atherosclerosis they have may be attributed to changes in haemostatic variables and platelet function [1,2,3].

2. MATERIAL AND METHODS

2.0. Study design

- It was a placebo controlled, double blind study, which was designed open ended for patients and limited to 6 weeks for volunteers.
- 18 healthy volunteers (6 female, 12 male, 29 mean age) were monitored during a 6-week period of modified fatty acid intake.
- 19 patients (4 female, 15 male, 63 mean age) suffering from peripheral vascular disease (PVD) stage II were divided into 3 similar groups as described below.
- The tests were made before entry and after 3 and 6 weeks for volunteers and after 3 weeks and each 3 months for patients.

2.1. Laboratory follow up

- Radiothinlayer chromatography (RTLC) of platelets by means of ^{14}C-arachidonic acid and incubation for 5 minutes at 37°C
- Malondialdehyde assay (MDA) of thrombin activated platelets measured after reaction with thiobarbituric acid.
- Platelet aggregation and sensitivity according to the method of Born (1963) using 100 μl 10 μmol ADP/600 μl platelet rich plasma (PRP).
- Various concentrations (0.125 - 1ng/600 μl PRP) were added as an inhibitor 1 minute before the induction of aggregation. Results are expressed as ID_{50}.
- Serum thromboxane B_2 after incubation for 60 minutes at 37°C and determination by means of a radioimmuno-assay.

2.2. Fatty acid content of capsules

- Capsules are filled with 500 mg oil each (filling weight 513 ± 7.5mg). Therefore, the consumption of 12 capsules per day leads to the intake of extra 200kJ.
- The contents of the three types of capsules are as follows:
  Efamol-marine capsules (group I in this trial) contain 400mg evening primrose oil plus 100mg fish oil containing 18 mg eicosapentaenoic acid (EPA, 20:5n-3), whereas *Efamol* capsules (group III) contain 42 mg gamma-linolenic acid (GLA, 18:3n-6) plus 360 mg linoleic acid only. 10 mg D-α-tocopherylacetate (vitamin E) are added to each capsule as an antioxidant. *Olive oil* was used as a placebo substance (500mg per capsule, group II)

2.3. Volunteers and patients

Volunteers and patients were divided into 3 groups (roman I-III) according to the three types of capsules. The daily intake in these 3 groups was as follows: **group I**: 220 mg eicosapentaenoic acid (EPA), 140 mg docosahexaenoic acid (DHA), 390 mg gamma-linolenic acid (GLA) and 3480 mg linoleic acid, **group II**: 6g olive oil, **group III**: 6 g evening primrose oil containing 520 mg GLA and 4320 mg linoleic acid.

3. RESULTS

3.1. VOLUNTEERS

3.1.1. Conversion of arachidonic acid by platelets

Daily intake of fatty acids in group I resulted in a significant ($p < 0.01$) increase of unconverted AA (fig.1). AA conversion of the other 2 groups was slightly (but not significantly) inhibited. Corresponding to the decrease in AA conversion, platelet TXB_2 formation was reduced in group I, but the decline in AA conversion mainly resulted in a raised 12-HETE formation. In volunteers' groups I and II 12-HETE formation decreased due to the enhanced TXB_2 and HHT synthesis (fig.2).

3.1.2. MDA-formation (fig.3)

MDA-formation decreased in all the three groups after 6 weeks, group I showing the most pronounced effect. There was an increase in MDA-formation after 3 weeks only in group II, possibly related to a rise in the content of non-essential fatty acids (placebo) of platelet membranes.

3.1.3. Serum-TXB_2 formation (fig.4)

Serum thromboxane levels decreased significantly in both active groups by 28% (in group I) and 52% (group III) respectively. There was no significant change of this parameter in the placebo group.

3.1.4. Platelet aggregation and sensitivity (fig.5)

ID_{50} decreased significantly only in group I (EPA+GLA), although a drop was also noticed in group III (GLA). However, this effect vanished after 6 weeks. Platelet sensitivity was not affected in group II, as expected in a placebo group.

3.2. PATIENTS

3.2.1. Radiothinlayer chromatography

In groups I (EPA + GLA) and III (GLA) a slight but insignificant decrease in TXB_2-formation could be observed, which was not connected to a decrease in AA-conversion, which dropped consistently, but to an increase of 12-HETE-formation (fig.6).

The increase of TXB_2-formation in patients' group II (placebo) after 3 weeks was rather striking, but this effect vanished completely after 3 months. No other changes could be detected (fig7).

3.2.2. MDA-formation (fig.8)

The changes in MDA-formation were similar to those in the corresponding volunteers' groups. A decrease in MDA-formation occured in all 3 groups, but MDA-levels returned nearly to their prevalue in group II (6% decrease).

After 3 months only groups I and III showed a stable decrease in MDA-formation of about 22% and 19%, respectively.

3.2.3. Serum-TXB_2 formation (fig.9)

Serum-TXB_2 levels decreased in all three groups, dropping by 50% in group I and to one fourth of the prevalues in group III, respectively. The change in group II was not significant.

3.2.4. Platelet sensitivity (fig.10)

ID_{50} values decreased in group I (35%) and group III (49%) after 3 months. The distinct effect in group II after 3 weeks vanished after 3 months.

4. DISCUSSION

Ω-3 fatty acid intake results in a generalized depression of prostanoids of the 2-series, as indicated by lower platelet MDA-formation and the diminished AA-conversion [4,5,6]. This generalized depression is likely to be connected with a change in the fatty acid composition of tissue phospholipids and the free fatty acid pool [7,8]. This can explain the distinct effects of changing of the dietary intake of fatty acids on the tissue eicosanoid patterns and also the beneficial influences on atherosclerotic cardiovascular [9,10,11] and chronic inflammatory diseases [12,13].

However, Eskimos have high levels of dihomogamma-linolenic acid (DGLA, 20:3n-6), an n-6 fatty acid which is a precursor of PGE_1, and 15-OH-DGLA (15-OH-dihomogamma-linolenic acid, 15-OH-20:3n-6) which also has desirable cardiovascular and anti-inflammatory effects.

The reported health benefits in Eskimos may be attributable to the combined effects of 20:3n-6 and 20:5n-3. We have attempted to imitate the Eskimo picture by giving low amounts of 18:3n-6, the immediate 20:3n-6 precursor, as well as 20:5n-3.

The main result of this study is the effect of extremely low doses of EPA and GLA on platelet aggregation. This suggests that there may be a synergistic effect of n-6 and n-3 fatty acids at low doses which is greater than the effect of high doses of n-3 fatty acids alone.

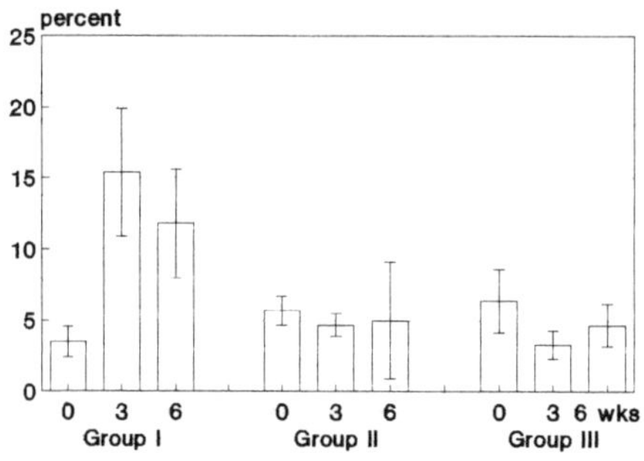

fig.1: AA-conversion in volunteers
(mean +/- SEM, n=7/5/6)

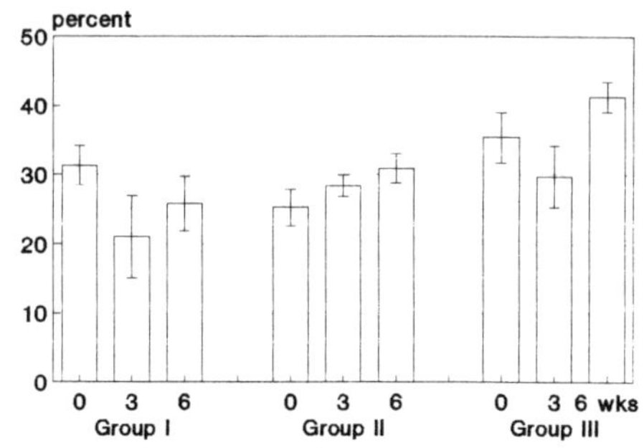

fig.2: TXB2-formation in volunteers
(mean +/- SEM, n=7/5/6)

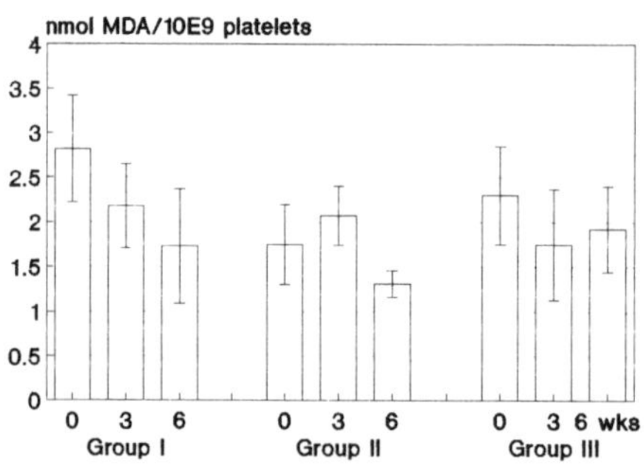

fig.3: MDA-formation in volunteers
(mean +/- SEM, n=7/5/6)

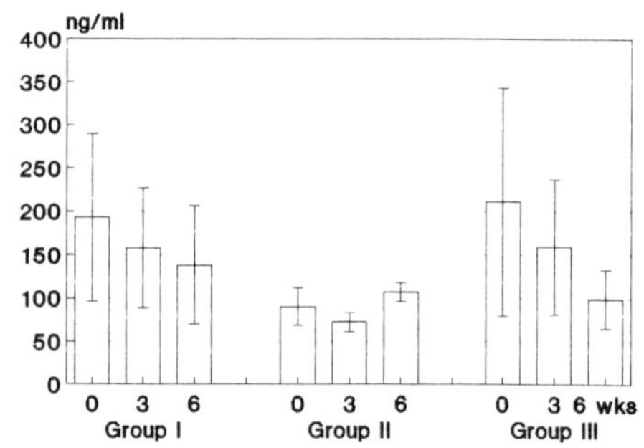

fig.4: Serum-TXB2-formation in volunteers (mean +/- SEM, n=7/5/6)

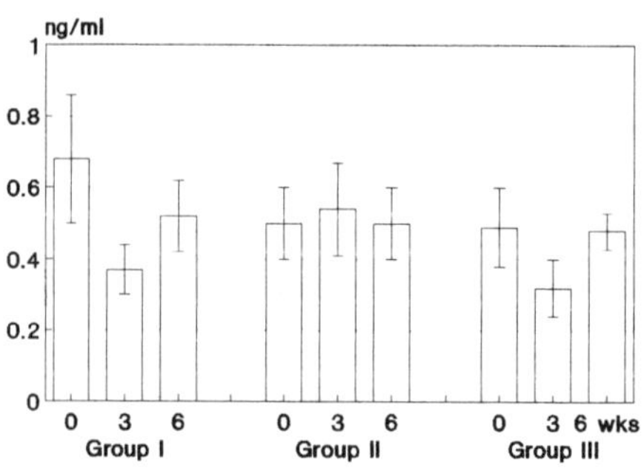

fig.5: sensitivity to PGI2 (volunteers)
(mean +/- SEM, n=7/5/6)

RESULTS

VOLUNTEERS

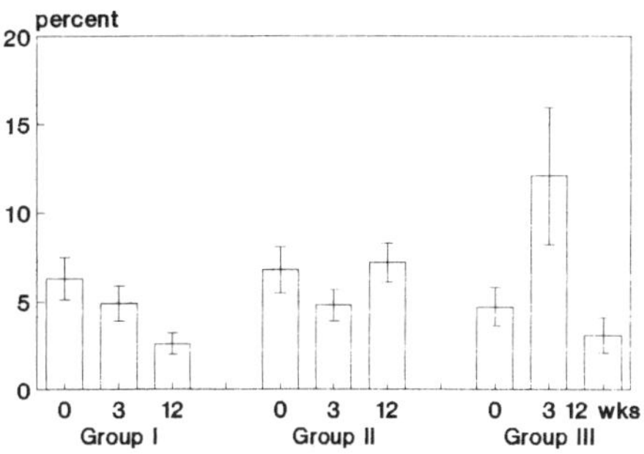

fig.6: AA-conversion in patients
(mean +/- SEM, n=9/6/4)

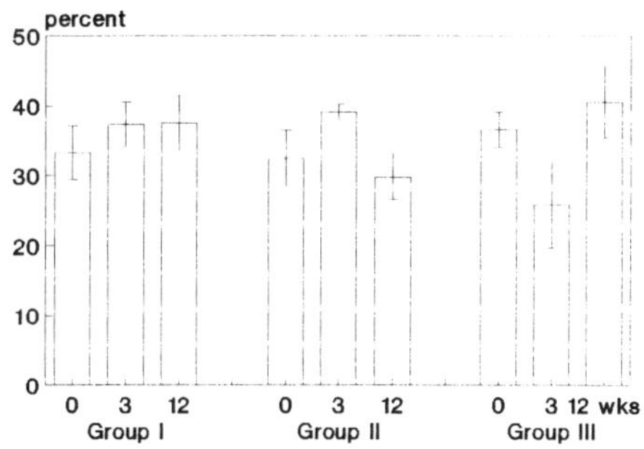

fig.7: TXB2-formation in patients
(mean +/- SEM, n=9/6/4)

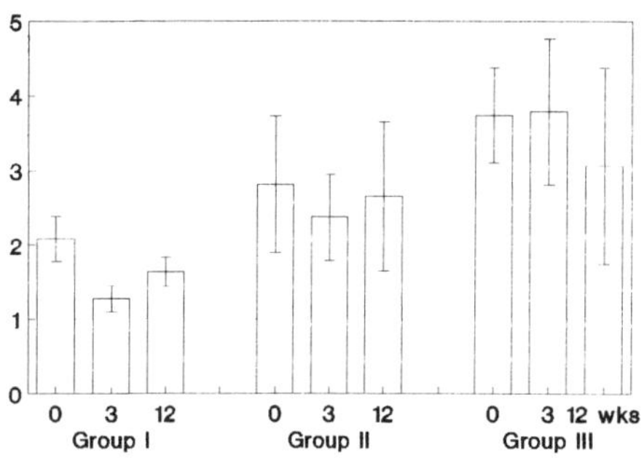

fig.8: MDA-formation in patients
(mean +/- SEM, n=9/6/4)

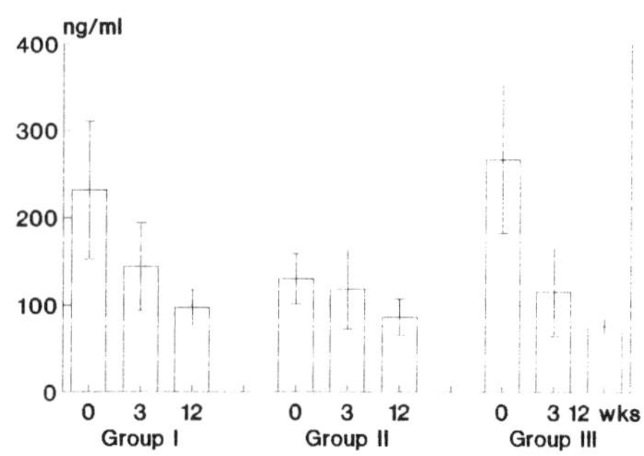

fig.9: Serum-TXB2-formation (patients)
(mean +/- SEM, n=9/6/4)

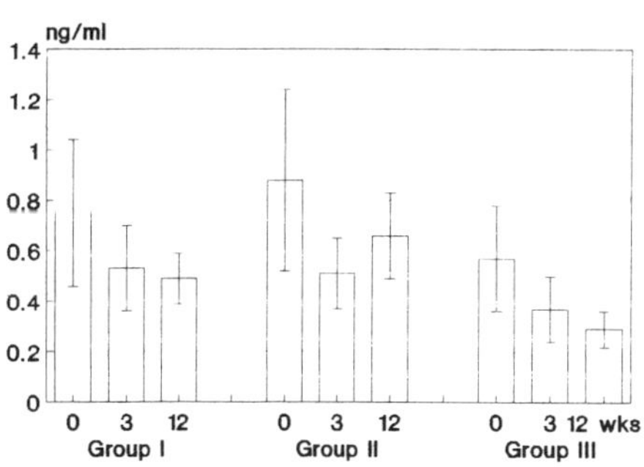

fig.10: sensitivity to PGI2 (patients)
(mean +/- SEM, n=9/6/4)

RESULTS

PATIENTS

5. REFERENCES

1.Bang HO, Dyerberg J, Sinclair HM, The bleeding tendency in Greenland Eskimos, Dan Med Bull 27: 202, 1980.

2.Dyerberg J, Bang HO, Haemostatic function and platelet polyunsaturated fatty acids in Eskimos, Lancet ii: 433, 1979.

3.Dyerberg J, Linoleate-derived polyunsaturated fatty acids and prevention of atherosclerosis, Nutr Rev, 44: 125, 1986.

4.Fischer S, Weber PC, Thromboxane A_3 (TXA_3) is formed in human platelets after dietary eicosapentaenoic acid (20:5w3), Biochim Biophys Res Commun 116: 1091, 1983.

5.Fischer S, Weber PC, Dyerberg J, The prostacyclin-/thromboxane balance is favourably shifted in Greenland Eskimos, Prostaglandins 32: 235, 1986.

6.Fischer S, Weber PC, Prostaglandin I_3 is formed in vivo in man after dietary eicosapentaenoic acid, Nature 307: 165, 1984.

7.Lands WEM, Kulmacz RJ, The regulation of the biosynthesis of prostaglandins and leukotrienes, Prog Lipid Res 25: 105, 1986.

8.Harris WS, Fish oils and plasma lipid and lipoprotein metabolism in humans: a critical review, J Lipid Res 30: 785, 1989.

9.Knapp HR, Reilly IAG, Alessandrini P, Fitzgerald GA, In vivo indexes of platelet and vascular function during fish-oil administration in patients with atherosclerosis, N Engl J Med 314: 937, 1986.

10.Kromhout D, Bosschieter EB, de Lezenne Coulander C, The inverse relation between fish consumption and 20-year mortality from coronary heart disease, N Engl J Med 312: 1205, 1985.

11.Norell SE, Ahlbom A, Feychting M, Pedersen NL, Fish consumption and mortality from coronary heart disease, Br Med J 293: 426, 1986.

12.Vilaseca J, Salas A, Guarner F, Rodríguez R, Martínez M, Malagelada J-R: Dietary fish oil reduces progression of chronic inflammatory lesions in a rat model of granulomatous colitis. Gut, 5: 539-544, 1990

13.Karmali RA, Marsh J, Fuchs C, Effect of omega-3 fatty acids on growth of a rat mammary tumor, JNCI, 73: 457-61, 1985.

AAS 37
Prostaglandins in the
Cardiovascular System

RECEPTOR BINDING PROPERTIES OF THE NEW AND SPECIFIC THROMBOXANE RECEPTOR ANTAGONIST BAY U 3405

Harald Darius, Jutta Michael-Hepp, and Jürgen Meyer

Department of Medicine II, Johannes Gutenberg - University,
Langenbeckstrasse 1, 6500 Mainz 1, Germany

SUMMARY

Human platelet membranes were used to characterize the receptor binding properties of the specific thromboxane receptor antagonist ^{3}H-SQ 29548 and the displacement of ^{3}H-SQ 29548 from its binding site by the new thromboxane receptor antagonist Bay u 3405. The specific binding of ^{3}H-SQ 29548 was saturable with an association rate constant of 1 x 10^{-11} mol^{-1}min^{-1} and a dissociation rate constant of 0.032 min^{-1}. Nonspecific binding of ^{3}H-SQ 29548 was below 10%. When Scatchard plot analysis was performed on equilibrium saturation binding the k_D was 69 nmol/l and the B_{max} was calculated as 3.9 pmol/mg membrane protein. ^{3}H-SQ 29548 was dose dependently displaced from its binding site by addition of increasing concentrations of Bay u 3405 yielding an IC_{50} value of 68$\pm$12 nmol/l, being not significantly different from the IC_{50} of nonlabelled SQ 29548 (38$\pm$13 nmol/l). The results show that Bay u 3405 is a potent and specific thromboxane receptor antagonist, displacing ^{3}H-SQ 29548 from its binding site on human platelet membranes with IC_{50} values being not significantly different. These receptor binding properties and the long biological half life reported in vivo make Bay u 3405 a promissing compound for the treatment of human cardiavascular diseases.

INTRODUCTION

Thromboxane A_2 (TXA_2) is one of the arachidonic acid products synthetized by platelets in response to specific stimuli. Platelet activation, aggregate formation and release of vasoactive mediators is one of the crucial points in the sequelae of pathophysiologic events resulting in tissue damage and organ failure during myocardial ischemia and circulatory shock. Thus, effective antagonism of the vasoconstrictor, proaggregatory and cytolytic effects of TXA_2 is the therapeutic target stimulating research in the area of thromboxane synthesis inhibitors and receptor antagonists (Lefer & Darius, 1987).

Pinane thromboxane A_2 was the first receptor antagonist used for studying of the role of thromboxane as a mediator in shock and ischemia (Nicolaou et al., 1979; Schrör et al., 1980). Thereafter a number of thromboxane receptor antagonists has been synthetized, with SQ-29548 probably being the most potent and specific receptor antagonist used for experimental research until now (Darius et al., 1985). However, due to the long term toxicology of the compound it never was studied in humans in the clinical setting. Recently, Bay u 3405 was introduced as a new and specific receptor antagonist with potent platelet inhibitory effects in vivo and ex vivo (Seuter et al., 1989). In this study the receptor binding properties of SQ 29548 and the inhibitory effects of Bay u 3405 on SQ 29548 binding were investigated in human platelet membranes.

MATERIALS AND METHODS

Plasma membranes of human platelets were prepared from platelet-rich plasma by centrifugation at 1,000 x g for 25 min. The pellet was resuspended in ice-cold Tris buffer (50 mmol/l, pH 7.4) and homogenized with an ultra-turrax (24,000 rpm for 15 s). The suspension was centrifuged at 165,000 x g for 30 min. The resulting pellet was washed twice and resuspended in an assay buffer containing (conc. in mmol/l): NaCl 135; KCl 5.0; $CaCl_2$ 2; $MgCl_2$ 1, Tris-HCl 10, pH 7.4. Protein content was determined by the method of Peterson.

The binding experiments were performed by incubating aliquots of the membrane preparation in 250 μl of assay buffer with radioactive labelled ^{3}H-SQ 29548 and the other test compounds at 4° C for 40 min. Following the incubation the membranes were diluted with ice cold buffer and vacuum filtered through Whatman GF/B glassfiber filters. After washing filters were transfered into scintillation cocktail and radioactivity was determined in a LKB-Pharmacia Rack Beta Szintillation Counter. Nonspecific binding was determined in the presence of 100 μmol/l of the thromboxane antagonist BM 13505.

Results were calculated by Scatchard analyses and the inhibition of ^{3}H-SQ 29548 binding by Bay u 3405 was calculated from inhibition curves by a nonlinear, computer assisted least square method.

RESULTS

The kinetic of ^{3}H-SQ 29548 binding to the platelet membranes was studied by altering the time of incubation up to a period of 60 min. Total binding of ^{3}H-SQ 29549 reached equilibrium after 20 min. When expressed as percent of total binding the nonspecific binding was rather low and accounted for approximately 10 %. The observed rate constant for ^{3}H-SQ 29549 association (k_{ob}) of 0.133 min^{-1} was calculated. When equilibrium for ^{3}H-SQ 29549 binding was reached, addition of another thromboxane receptor antagonist e.g. BM 13505 in a concentration of 100 μmol/l resulted in displacement of the specifically bound ^{3}H-SQ 29549. From these data a dissociation rate constant (k_{-1}) of 0.032 min^{-1} was calculated. According to the equation $k_1 = (k_{ob} - k_{-1})/L$ the rate constant of association k_1 was 1 x 10^{-11} l mol^{-1}min^{-1}. The k_D was calculated from five experiment as 4.84 nmol/l by using the equation $k_D = k_{-1}/k_1$.

The steady state binding was measured by incubating platelet membranes with concentrations of ^{3}H-SQ 29549 ranging from 5 - 300 nmol/l. The specific binding showed saturation with increasing concentrations of ^{3}H-SQ 29549 (Fig. 1). In contrast, nonspecific bindng increased linearly and was not saturable. Scatchard analysis revealed a k_D of 69 nmol/l and a B_{max} of 3.9 pmol/mg (n=4)(Fig. 1, inset).

The specific binding of ^{3}H-SQ 29549 was dose dependently inhibited by the new thromboxane receptor antagonist Bay u 3405 (Fig. 2). The IC_{50} value was calculated being 68$\pm$12 nmol/l. The potency of Bay u 3405 to inhibit the binding of ^{3}H-SQ 29549 was not statistically different from non-labelled SQ 29548 (IC_{50} 38$\pm$13 nmol/l). However, the receptor antagonists SQ 28668, BM 13505 and the agonist U 46619 were significantly less potent with IC_{50} values of 302$\pm$52, 480$\pm$40 and 4550$\pm$1050 nmol/l, respectively.

DISCUSSION

The occupation of thromboxane receptors on human platelets is the precondition for the effective and selective inhibition of platelet functions. TXA_2 probably represents the most important physiologic positive feed back mechanism for the augmentation of a proaggregatory signal and the recruitment of a larger cohort of circulating platelets to form a thrombus, if a prothrombogenic stimulus is present. Thus, selective blockade of thromboxane receptors may result in a nonresponsiveness of the hemorrheologic system to prothrombogenic stimuli. In an ideal way, this effect should be accomplished without totally abolishing the physiological response to vessel injuries i.e. termination of a bleeding due to the rupture of smaller or larger blood vessels.

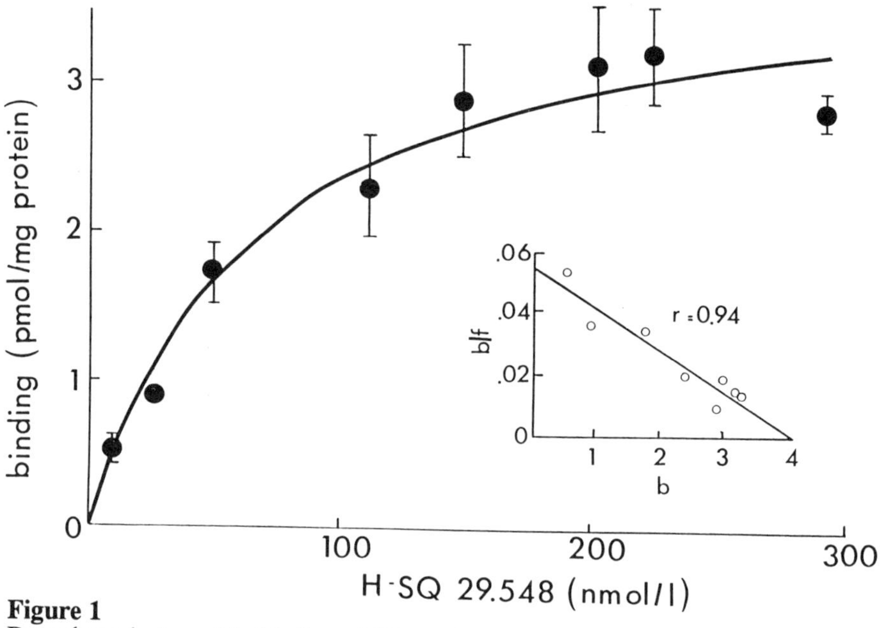

Figure 1
Dose dependent specific binding of ^{3}H-SQ 29548 to human platelet membranes incubated for 40 min at 4° C. The insert (Fig. 1b) represents the Scatchard analyses of the data giving the k_D as 69 nmol/l and the B_{max} as 3.9 pmol/mg protein.

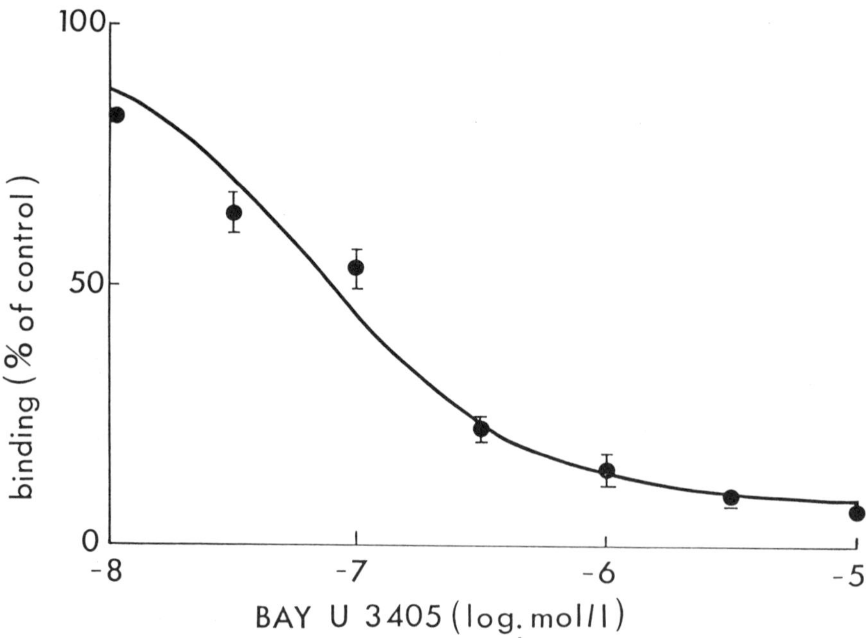

Figure 2
Displacement of ^{3}H-SQ 29548 from its specific binding sites on human platelet membranes by increasing concentrations of the new thromboxane receptor antagonist Bay u 3405. The IC_{50} value is 68±12 nmol/l.

The recently introduced thromboxane receptor antagonist Bay u 3405 binds with high affinity to human platelet membranes and displaces radioactively labelled ^{3}H-SQ 29549 from its binding sites. The IC_{50} value of 68 nmol/l is not statistically different from the IC_{50} of nonlabelled SQ 29548, suggesting equal potency of the two compounds. However, equal potency in receptor binding assays does not necessarily mean, that the two compounds exert an equally effective inhibition of platelet aggregation in vivo. The data presented with Bay u 3405 for its in vitro and ex vivo platelet inhibitory effects are quite encouraging. Seuter et al. (1989) published data showing that human platelet aggregation in vitro is inhibited in concentrations between 0.01 and 0.1 μg/ml. Additionally, platelet aggregation in rats measured ex vivo was dose dependently inhibited, with inhibitory effects being present as long as 16 hrs following intake of 100 μg/kg b.w.. In case these effects are confirmed in other models of in vivo platelet aggregation (Darius & Lefer, 1985) and the long term toxicity studies with Bay u 3405 do not prevent its use in humans, this compound may become an interesting research tool in human pathophysiology. Due to the long half life of Bay u 3405 in vivo this compound may even have a chance of becoming a standard regimen in patients with cardiovascular diseases associated with activated platelets and a higher risk of thrombotic or thrombembolic events.

REFERENCES

Darius H., Lefer, A.M. (1985) Anti-aggregatory effects of thromboxane receptor antagonists in vivo.
Thromb.Res. 40, 663-676.

Darius, H., Smith J.B., Lefer, A.M. (1985) Beneficial effects of a new potent and specific thromboxane receptor antagonist (SQ 29548) in vitro and in vivo.
J.Pharmacol.exp.Therap. 235, 274-281.

Lefer, A.M., Darius, H. (1987) A pharmacological approach to thromboxane receptor antagonism.
Fed.Proc. 46, 144-148.

Nicolaou, K.C., Magolda, R.L., Smith, J.B., Aharony, D., Smith, E.F., Lefer, A.M. (1979) Synthesis and biological properties of pinane-thromboxane A_2 (TXA_2). A selective inhibitor of coronary artery constriction, platelet aggregation and thromboxane formation. Proc.Natl.Acad.Sci. (USA) 70, 2566-2590.

Schrör, K., Smith, E.F.III, Bickerton, M., Smith, J.B., Nicolaou, K.C., Magolda, R., Lefer, A.M. (1980) Preservation of ischemic myocardium by pinane thromboxane A_2. Am.J.Physiol. 238, H87-H92.

Seuter, F., Perzborn, E., Rosentreter, U., Böshagen, H., Fiedler, V.B. (1989) Inhibition of platelet aggregation in vitro and ex vivo by the new thromboxane antagonist (3R)-3-(4-Fluorophenyl-sulfonamido)-1-2-3-4-tetrahydro-9-carbazolepropanoic acid.
Drug Res. 39, 1525-1527.

AAS 37
Prostaglandins in the
Cardiovascular System

STEREOSPECIFIC AND NON-STEREOESPECIFIC EFFECTS OF IBUPROFEN ON HUMAN PLATELET AND POLYMORPHONUCLEAR LEUKOCYTE FUNCTIONS.

M. Villanueva*, R. Heckenberger, M. Palmér, and K. Schrör

Institut für Pharmakologie, Heinrich-Heine-Universität Düsseldorf, Moorenstraße 5, D-4000 Düsseldorf 1, FRG

*): permanent address: Departamento De Fisiologia Y Farmacologia, Faculdad de Medicina, Universidad de Alcalá, 28871 Alcalá de Henares (Madrid), Spain

SUMMARY: This study compares biological activities of racemic ibuprofen (rac-IBU) and its S(+) and R(-) enantiomeres in human platelet and polymorphonuclear cells (PMN). Rac-IBU inhibited cyclooxygenase-related platelet functions (aggregation, thromboxane (TX) B_2 formation) in vitro, the S-(+) enantiomer being 40-100-times more active than the R-(-) form. rac-IBU also inhibited PMN functions (O_2^- generation, β-glucuronidase release). These effects in PMN were not stereospecific. The data suggest cyclooxygenase-independent actions of ibuprofen in human PMN which may contribute to its antiinflammatory effects in vivo.

INTRODUCTION

It is generally appreciated that non-steroidal antiinflammatory drugs (NSAID) reduce vascular symptoms of acute inflammation through inhibition of prostaglandin biosynthesis. However, there is evidence that NSAID may also exert antiinflammatory effects independent of cyclooxygenase inhibition, e.g. via inhibition of white cell function and cytokine release (Abramsson et al, 1985). Thus, the question arises whether it is necessary to accept all the unwanted side effects of prostaglandin synthase inhibition for clinical use of NSAID. For example, a recent clinical trial has shown that the therapeutic efficacy of rac-ibuprofen in patients suffering from osteoarthritis of the knee was the same, whether the drug was applied at a (low) analgesic or (higher) antiinflammatory dose (Bradley et al, 1991).

An interesting pharmacological approach to deal with this issue is to study enantioselectivity of effects of these substances on target cells. One major class of NSAID, the 2-arylpropionic acid derivatives, are chiral compounds, although in most cases marketed as racemic mixtures. Ibuprofen (IBU) belongs to this group. Consequently, the inhibition of the cyclooxygenase in vitro resides almost exclusively in the S-(+) enantiomer (Adams et al, 1976; Geisslinger et al, 1989).

This study compares the inhibitory effects of racemic IBU with its S(+) and R(-) stereoisomeres on human platelet and polymorphonuclear cell (PMN) function and eicosanoid generation.

MATERIALS AND METHODS

Preparation of platelets and PMN. Blood was taken by venipuncture from healthy donors who had not taken any medication within the last two weeks prior to the study. The blood was collected into acidic citrate/dextrose (Biostabil[R], 1/10; v/v). Platelet-rich plasma (PRP) was prepared by centrifugation at 300 x g and room temperature for 10 min. The PRP was also used to prepare washed platelets according to standard laboratory procedures. The platelets were finally dissolved in an isotonic buffer solution, supplemented with 50 µg/ml apyrase and 300 µg/ml fibrinogen. The platelet count was adjusted to 250,000 cells/µl. Aggregation and TX generation were measured in these washed platelet suspensions following the procedures described below.

PMN were prepared from the remaining sediment as previously described (Hecker et al, 1990). The cell count was adjusted to a final stock concentration of 5 x 10^7 cells/ml.

Measurement of platelet aggregation and thromboxane formation. Platelet aggregation was determined photometrically. After a 2 min incubation of 400 µl PRP with 90 µl Tris buffer (50 mM, pH 7.4) containing the compounds to be tested, collagen (2.5 µg/ml) was added and the changes in light transmission were recorded for 10 min at constant stirring of the samples at 1,200 rpm and 37°C. At 10 min, indomethacin (30 µM) (Luitpold Pharma, München, FRG) and EDTA (7.7 mM) (final concentrations) were added, the platelet pellet removed and the platelet-free supernatant used for radioimmunoassay of thromboxane (TX) B_2.

Stimulation of PMN and measurement of O_2^- and β-glucuronidase release. PMN (5 x 10^6 cells) were incubated in PBS, supplemented with Ca^{++} (1 mM) and Mg^{++} (1 mM) at 37°C in a total volume of 1.0 ml. After 10 min incubation with ibuprofen (Dolorgiet Pharma, St. Augustin, FRG) or the respective vehicles, the cells were stimulated by FMLP (30 nM). At time 20 min, the reaction was stopped by centrifugation at 12,000 x g at 4°C. Superoxide anion generation was determined spectrophotometrically in terms of superoxide dismutase (SOD, 300 IU/ml) inhibitable reduction of ferricytocrome C at 550 nm. The values were corrected for O_2-generation by unstimulated cells (usually 5-10 nmol O_2^- x 10^6/cells). β-glucuronidase was measured in cytochalasin B (5 µg/ml) treated PMN as previously described (Hecker et al, 1990).

Calculations and Statistics. The molar potency and IC_{50} values were calculated from individual concentration-response curves. The data are mean ± s.e. mean of n experiments. Statistical analysis was performed with the two-tailed t-test. P levels of $p < 0.05$ were considered significant.

RESULTS

Inhibition of platelet aggregation and platelet cyclooxygenase in presence and absence of plasma. All compounds inhibited platelet aggregation and thromboxane formation. In PRP, (S+)IBU was about 15 times more potent than the (R-) stereoisomere. This difference became considerably greater in washed platelets. This confirms the expected stereospecificity of action and the reduced effectivity of the compound by binding to plasma albumin.

Table I: Inhibitory effect of racemic IBU and its enantiomers on collagen (2.5 µg/ml) stimulated aggregation and thromboxane (TXB_2) formation in PRP and washed platelets (WP).

	PRP (IC_{50}, µM)		WP (IC_{50}, µM)	
	Aggregation	TXB_2	Aggregation	TXB_2
rac- IBU	134 ± 63	50 ± 27	1.3 ± 0.3	0.3 ± 0.1
S(+)-IBU	88 ± 44	26 ± 15	0.6 ± 0.4	0.2 ± 0.1
R(-)-IBU	1260 ± 670*	380 ± 60*	33.0 ± 6.80*	15.6 ± 1.2*

Data are mean ± SEM of 3-6 experiments in each group.
*): $p < 0.05$ (S-(+)-IBU or R(-)-IBU vs. rac-IBU)

Inhibition of superoxide anion generation and β-glucuronidase release in PMN. Stimulation with FMLP enhanced O_2- formation about 3-fold above control, amounting to 27.1 ± 1.2 nM $O_2^-/5 \times 10^6$ cells (n=20). rac-IBU caused a dose-dependent inhibition of FMLP-induced O_2^- generation which became significant at 100 µM ($p < 0.05$). No differences were obtained between rac-IBU and its stereoisomers (Table II). Indomethacin also inhibited FMLP-induced (data not shown).

Stimulation with FMLP increased β-glucuronidase more than sixfold above control (n=21). rac-IBU inhibited this effect in a dose-dependent way. The inhibition was significant at $\geq$ 300 µM ($p < 0.05$) (Table II). Indomethacin also inhibited FMLP-induced O_2^- formation and enzyme release (data not shown).

Table II: Inhibitory effect of racemic IBU and its enantiomers on FMLP (30 nM) stimulated O_2^- formation and β-glucuronidase release in human PMN.

	O_2^- (IC_{50}, mM)	β-glucuronidase (IC_{50}, mM)
rac- IBU	0.60 ± 0.13	0.44 ± 0.08
(S+)-IBU	0.50 ± 0.11	0.53 ± 0.12
(R-) IBU	0.43 ± 0.08	0.58 ± 0.09

Data are mean ± SEM of 4-9 experiments in each group.
No significant differences between the groups were found ($p > 0.05$).

Tissue concentration of ibuprofen. Table III demonstrates the IBU concentrations in the incubation media as compared to PMN. It is evident that the tissue concentration is similar or slightly higher than the concentration in the bath medium. Importantly, there is no interconversion between the enantiomers as seen from the equal distribution between the two isomers of rac-IBU.

Table III: Tissue (PMN) and supernatant concentrations of ibuprofen

Compound		concentration [µg/g or µg/ml] PMN	supernatant
S(+) - IBU		241 ± 12	216 ± 4
R(-) - IBU		219 ± 10	196 ± 2
rac - IBU	(S+)	136 ± 2	108 ± 4
	(R-)	131 ± 4	100 ± 3
	Σ	267	208

The data are mean ± SEM of n = 6 determinations. No significant differences were obtained between PMN and the incubation medium ($p > 0.05$)

DISCUSSION

There is currently much debate about the use of chiral compounds, i.e. the replacement of racemic mixtures by the active enatiomere (Lennard, 1991). This discussion is also relevant for ibuprofen (Williams, 1990). Indeed, in this study, the S(+) isomere is about twice as potent in inhibiting thromboxane formation and platelet function in comparison to the rac-compound. This raises the question whether the cyclooxygenase inhibitory activity of the S(+) isomere is not "diluted" by adding an inactive compound, eventually resulting in introducing "isomeric ballast and ...medicinal pollution of the patient" (Ariens, 1990).

This study demonstrates that the inhibition of PMN function is not a stereoselective effect of IBU. Although the concentrations of the compound were somewhat higher than thos required for inhibition of platelet cyclooxygenase, they were still in the level to be expected after therapeutic administration. We have also excluded any enantionselective interconversion of the isomeres in our assay which is well known to occur in vivo (Chen et al, 1991). Earlier studies by others had already shown that cyclooxygenase inhibition is not necessary for inhibition of PMN function (Abramson et al, 1985). Our results confirm this. Additionally we have found that IBU and its stereoisomers are equipotent inhibitors of leukotriene B_4 formation in human PMN at concentrations comparable to those which inibited PMN function (not shown). Thus, PMN inhibition by IBU appears not to require cyclooxygenase inhibition. In contrast, inhibition of prostaglandin formation by NSAID might even result in enhanced PMN-activation, because PGE-type compounds are potent inhibitors of PMN function (Hecker et al, 1990).

Certain NSAID, including IBU, in addition to their ability to inhibit the cyclo-oxygenase pathway are also able to inhibit the lipoxygenase pathway (Vanderhoek et al, 1984). Another attractive explanation for a prostaglandin-independent inhibition of PMN function by IBU is the interference with the heme-arachidonic acid interaction (Kennedy et al, 1990). Generation of oxygen free radicals is catalyzed by the heme-containing enzyme NADPH-oxidase. IBU interaction with the heme group of the NADPH-oxidase might cause inhibition of oxygen free radical formation. Since iron-chelating compounds possess anti-inflammatory activity (Sedgwick et al, 1984) it is tempting to speculate that IBU could exert its anti-inflammatory effects, at least in part, by preventing iron-mediated generation of oxidants and lipid peroxidation.

In conclusion, we have shown a significant PMN-inhibitory action of racemic ibuprofen which appears to be independent of its inhibitory effect on the cyclooxygenase. Since many of the clinical side effects of NSAID result from their inhibition of prostaglandin formation, a racemic compound or the R(-) isomere may be superior to the S(+) enantiomere because of less inhibition of prostaglandin-formation but still preserved antineutrophil activity (Wallace et al, 1990). Clinical studies are required to prove this hypothesis.

ACKNOWLEDGEMENTS

The authors are most grateful to Dolorgiet Pharma (St. Augustin, FRG) for kindly providing racemic ibuprofen and its isomeres and to Drs. G. Berner and E. Posselt from this company for kindly performing the determination of ibuprofen.

REFERENCES

Abramson, S., Korchak, H., Ludewig, R., Edelson, H., Haines, K., Levin, R.I., Herman, R., Rider, L., Kimmel, S., and Weissmann, G. (1985) Modes of action of aspirin-like drugs. Proc. Natl. Acad. Sci. (USA) 82, 7227-7231.

Adams, S.S., Bresloff, P., and Mason, C.G. (1976) Pharmacological differences between the optical isomers of ibuprofen; evidence for metabolic inversion of the (-)-isomere. J. Pharm. Pharmacol. 28, 256-265.

Ariens, E.J. (1990) Racemic therapeutics-Problems all along the line. In: Chirality in Drug Design and Synthesis, Academic Press London, pp. 29-43

Bradley, J.D., Brandt, K.D., Katz, B.P., Kalasinski, L.A., and Ryan, S.I. (1991) Comparison of an antiinflammatory dose of ibuprofen, an analgesic dose of ibuprofen, and acetaminophen in the treatment of patients with osteoarthritis of the knee. New Engl. J. Med. 325, 87-91.

Chen, C.-S., Shieh, W.-R., Lu, P.-H., Harriman, S. and Chen, C.-Y (1991) Metabolic stereoisomeric inversion of ibuprofen in mammals. Biochim. Biophys. Acta 1078, 411-417.

Evans, A.M., Nation, R.L., Sansom, L.N., Bochner, F., and Somogyi, A.A. (1991) Effect of racemic ibuprofen dose on the magnitude and duration of platelet cyclooxygenase inhibition: relationship between inhibition of thromboxane production and the plasma unbound concentration of S(+) ibuprofen. Br. J. Clin. Pharmacol. 31, 131-138.

Geisslinger, G., Stock, K.P., Bach, G.L., Loew, D., and Brune, K. (1989) Pharmacological differences between R(-) and S(+)-ibuprofen. Agents and Actions 27, 455-457.

Hecker, G., Ney, P., and Schrör, K. (1990) Cytotoxic enzyme release and oxygen centered radical formation in human neutrophils are selectively inhibited by E-type prostaglandins but not by PGI_2. Naunyn Schmiedeberg's Arch. Pharmacol. 341, 308-315.

Kennedy, T.P., Rao, N.V., Noah, W., Michael, J.R., Jafri, M.H., Gurtner, G.H., and Hoidal, J.R. (1990) Ibuprofen prevents oxidant lung injury and in vitro lipid peroxidation by chelating iron. J. Clin. Invest. 86, 1565-1573.

Ku, E.C., Lee, W., Kothari, H.V., Kimble, E.F., Liauw, L., and Tjan, J. (1985) The effects of diclofenac sodium on arachidonic acid metabolism. Semin. Arthritis Rheum. 15, 36-41.

Lennard, M.S. (1991) Clinical pharmacology through the looking glass: reflections on the racemate vs enantiomer debate. Br. J. Clin. Pharmacol. 31, 623-625.

Sedgwick, A.D., Blake, D.R., Winwood, P., Moore, R., Al-Duaij, A., and Willoughby, D.A. (1984) Studies into the effects of the iron chelator desferrioxamine on the inflammatory process. Eur. J. Rheumathol. Inflammation 7, 87-94.

Vanderhoek, J.Y., and Bailey, J.M. (1984) Activation of a 15-lipoxygenase/leukotriene pathway in human polymorphonuclear leukocytes by the anti-inflammatory agent ibuprofen. J. Biol. Chem. 259, 6752-6756.

Wallace, J.L., Keenan, C.M., and Granger, D.N. (1990) Gastric ulceration induced by nonsteroidal anti-inflammatory drugs is a neutrophil-dependent process. Am. J. Physiol. 259, G462-G467.

Williams, K.M. (1990) Enantiomers in arthritic disorders. Pharmacol. Ther. 46, 273-295.

AAS 37
Prostaglandins in the
Cardiovascular System

STUDY OF THE MECHANISM OF PROSTACYCLIN (PgI_2) ACTION ON MYOCARDIAL CONTRACTILITY

M. Pavlović, D. Petković, M. Cvetković, K. Zdjelar, V. Starčević and O.Bosnić

Department of Physiology, Medical Faculty, University of Belgrade, Yugoslavia

SUMMARY: The experiments done on the isolated right ventricle of rat heart suspended in the bath for isolated organs with oxygenated Tyrode's solution showed that PgI_2 ($2,3 \times 10^{-6}$ mmol) produced its positive inotropic effect indirectly by promoting both beta-adrenoreceptors and calcium entry through slow calcium channels because this effect could be blocked by propranolol ($2,3 \times 10^{-2}$ mmol - beta-adrenoreceptor blocker) or verapamil ($4,3 \times 10^{-3}$ mmol - slow calcium channel blocker).

INTRODUCTION

Prostacyclin (PgI_2- the main cyclooxygenase product of arachidonic acid) exerts many biological effects. Among them it is a potent vasodilating agent (Moncada et al., 1985, Schrör and Moncada, 1979), the most potent endogenous inhibitor of platelet aggregation (Moncada et al., 1978), protect myocardium against ischemia (Ogletree and Leffer, 1978) and may play a role in the physiological regulation of myocardial blood flow (Alfonso et al., 1974). PgI_2 also produces positive intropic influence on isolated rat atria (Sterin-Borda et al., 1980), right ventricle of the rat heart (Pavlović et al., 1990) and this effect required additional energy supply from glycogenolytic processes (Pavlović et al., 1991).

In this study we examined the possible mechanism of the positive intropic action of prostacyclin. We have supposed that it is indirect and dependent on calcium movement and beta-adrenergic receptor stimulation. For this purpose we used verapamil - slow calcium channel blocker and propranolol - beta-adrenoreceptor blocker.

MATERIALS AND METHODS

Experiments were done on the isolated right heart ventricles of Wister rats weighing 200-210 g. Immediately after preparation the ventricles were set on boot-like elactrodes and suspended in an isolated organ bath with Tyrode's solution. Contractions were induced by square wave impulses of 1 Hz frequency with the intensity twice higher than that of the treshold and recorded via an isometric transducer (7003) on a microdynamometer (7050, Ugo Basile). After a stabilization period of 30 minutes the investigated substances were added into the bath and contractions were recorded continously for the next 30 minutes.

The following substances were used: Prostacyclin (Flolan, Wellcome, UK), Propranolol (ICI, Macclesfield) and Verapamil (Knoll).

RESULTS

Fig. 1 shows control record of PgI_2 (2,6 x 10^{-6}mmol) action on the right ventricle of rat heart. It induced immediate significant increase of the amplitude of contractions which after about ten minutes returned to the basal level and stayed on it till the end of experiments (30 minutes).

Control record of the effects of propranolol (2,3 x 10^{-2}mmol) and verapamil (4,3 x 10^{-3}mmol) showed well known negative inotropic effect (not shown).

Fig. 2 shows record of simulatenous action of prostacyclin with either verapamil (A) or propranolol (B). It can be seen only slight insignificant increase in the very beginning of action which was followed by continous decline till the end of experiment.

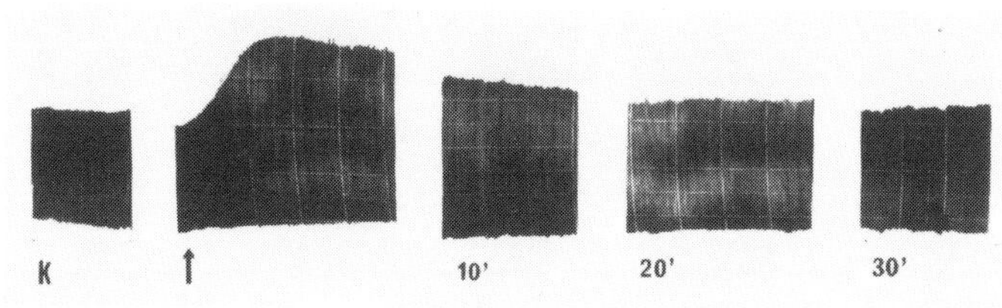

Fig. 1. Effect or prostacyclin (2,6 x 10^{-6} mmol) on the amplitude of contractions in isolated right ventricle of rat heart. K. control, arrow indicates application of prostacyclin.

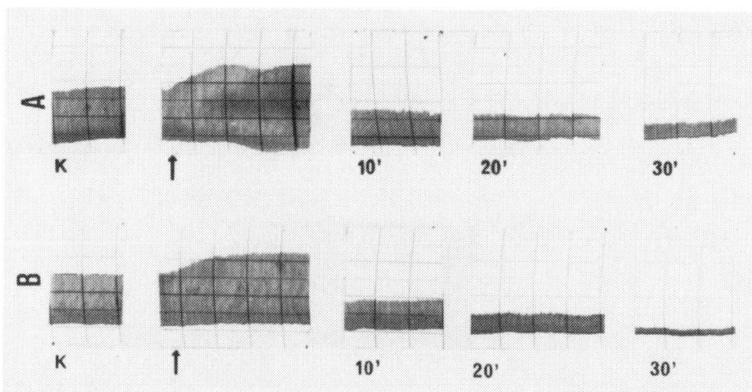

Fig. 2. Effects of simultaneous action of prostacyclin with verapamil (A) or propranolol (B) on the amplitude of contractions in isolated right ventricle of rat heart. K. control, arrow indicates simultaneous application of prostacyclin and verapamil (A) or propanolol (B).

Fig. 3 shows the effect or prostacyclin applied 5 minutes ofter preincubation of the heart preparation with either verapamil (A) or propranolol (B). Propranolol completely abolished the effect of prostacyclin, while 5 minutes preincubation with verapamil still caused slight prostacyclin positive effect. This effect of prostacyclin was also abolished when the heart preparation was preincubated with verapamil for 15 minutes.

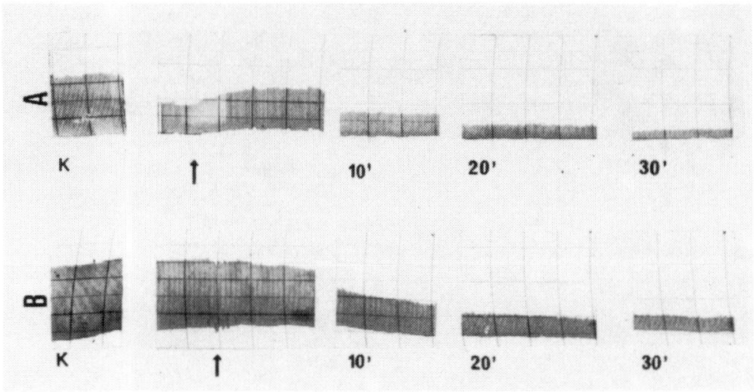

Fig. 3. Effect of prostacyclin on the amplitude of contractions in isolated right ventricle of rat heart after 5 minutes preincubation with verapamil (A) or propranolol (B). K. control, arrow indicates application of prostacyclin.

DISCUSSION

These results suggest that PgI_2 participates in regulation of myocardial contractility, but the mechanism of the inotropic effect of PgI_2 has not been extensively studied. In the perfused rat heart it was attributed to either norepinephrine release (Sterin-Borda et al., 1980), coronary vasodilatation (Raz et al., 1977) or modification of calcium movement in the heart cells (Vernimmen and Auclair, 1980). Our findings in the present work are in agreement with above statement and showed that PgI_2 produced its effect indirectly by promoting both, beta-adrenoreceptors and calcium entry through slow calcium channels because we were able to abolish the positive inotropic effect of PgI_2 showing that both pathways are involved in contractile process of the myocardium.

REFERENCES

Alfonso, S., Bandow, G.T., and Rowe, G.G. (1974) Indomethacin and prostaglandin hypothesis of coronary blood flow regulation. J. Physiol. 241, 299-308.

Moncada, S., Korbut, R., Bunting S., and Vane, J.R. (1978) Prostacyclin is a circulating hormone. Nature 273, 767-768.

Moncada, S., Flower, R.J., and Vane, J.R. (1985) Prostaglandins, Prostacyclin, Tromboxane A_2 and Leukotrienes. In: The Pharmacological Basis of Therapeutics (Gillman, A.G., Goodman, L.S., Rall, T.W., and Murad, F., eds), Macmillan Pub. Co. New York, p. 660.

Ogletree, M.L., and Leffer, A.M. (1978) Prostaglandin-induced preservation of the ischemic myocardium. Circ. Res. 42, 218-224.

Pavlović, M., Petković, D., Mujović, V., Bosnić, O., Cvetković, M., Zdjelar, K., and Macut, Dj. (1990) Influence of prostacyclin (PgI_2) on the content of glycogen in the myocardium. Abstract book, p.121. XLIV Congresso Nazionale della Societa Italiana di Anatomia, 24-26 Sept. Bologna, Italy.

Pavlović, M., Petković, D., Cvetković, M., Janković, V., Oklobdžija, M., Zdjelar, K., Macut, Dj., Bosnić, O., and Mujović, V., (1991) Glycogenolytic effect of prostacyclin (PgI_2) on the myocardium. Per. Biol. 93, 307-308.

Raz, A., Isakson, P.C., and Minkes, M.S. (1977) Characterization of a novel metabolic pathway of arachidonate in coronary vasodilatator. J. Biol. Chem. 252, 1123-1127.

Schrör, K., and Moncada, S. (1979) Effect of prostacyclin on coronary circulation, heart rate and myocardial contractile force in isolated hearts of guinea pig and rabbit - comparision with prostaglandin E_2. Prostaglandins, 17, 367-373.

Sterin-Borda, L., Canga, L., Borda, E.S., Gimeno, M.F., and Gimeno, A.L. (1980) Inotropic effect of prostacyclin (PgI_2) on isolated rat atria at different contraction frequencies. Naunyn-Schmiedeberg's Arch. Pharmacol. 313, 95-100.

Vernimmen, C., and Auclair, M.C. (1980) Transmembrane recording in monolayers of newborn rat heart cells. Biol. Cell, 37, 143-147.

AAS 37
Prostaglandins in the
Cardiovascular System

ANTITHROMBOTIC EFFECTS OF THE PROSTACYCLIN ANALOGUE NAXAPROSTENE AFTER ORAL AND INTRADUODENAL APPLICATION IN RABBIT CAROTID ARTERY THROMBOSIS

J. Schneider

Grünenthal GmbH, Department of Pharmacology, Zieglerstr. 6, W-5100 Aachen, FRG

SUMMARY: The antithrombotic efficacy of the prostacyclin analogue naxaprostene has been tested in rabbits with copper coil-induced carotid artery thrombosis. With oral pretreatment, 10 mg/kg naxaprostene prevented thrombotic arterial occlusion; with intraduodenal pretreatment the efficacy of naxaprostene was enhanced and 1 mg/kg was sufficient to exert an antithrombotic effect. The final average carotid blood flow at 180 min compared to the flow immediately before thrombus induction was 85 ± 25 % and 47 ± 18 % in animals treated with 10 mg/kg p.o. resp. 1 mg/kg i.d. naxaprostene. Parallel to the antithrombotic effect, naxaprostene inhibited ADP- and collagen-induced fall in circulating platelets. In anesthetized rabbits there was no dissociation between antithrombotic and hypotensive effects of naxaprostene.

INTRODUCTION

Platelet adhesion and aggregation are centrally involved in the development of arterial thrombosis. Drugs which interfere with platelet activation have an important role in the treatment of thrombotic disease. The prostacyclin analogue naxaprostene (CG 4305) (Flohé et al., 1983) may be a useful antithrombotic agent due to its platelet inhibiting activity. Its antithrombotic ability was tested in anesthetized rabbits where the insertion of a copper coil into a carotid artery evoked a strong thrombogenic stimulus. The efficacy of oral administration of naxaprostene to prevent the formation of fibrin- and platelets-containing occlusive thrombi was compared with the efficacy after intraduodenal administration. Inhibition of platelet aggregation as the proposed mechanism of prophylactic antithrombotic activity of naxaprostene has been evaluated by means of reduction of ADP- and collagen-induced thrombocytopenia.

MATERIAL AND METHODS

Male White New Zealand rabbits (ca. 2 kg b.w.t.) were anesthetized with thiopentone (25 mg/kg i.v.). The spontaneous breathing animals then inhaled a 40/60 vol.-% mixture of carbogen/N_2O. Myorelaxation was provided by proprionylpromazine (0.3 mg/kg + 0.3 mg/kg·hr i.v.). A polyethylene catheter was introduced into the abdominal aorta and connected to a Statham pressure transducer to measure arterial blood pressure. The right common carotid artery was prepared and dissected free from connective tissue; an electromagnetic flow probe (Hellige, Freiburg, FRG) was placed around the artery to measure carotid blood flow. For insertion of the thrombogenic copper coil, the blood flow was transiently interrupted by two clamps about 3 and 5 cm proximal to the flow probe. The artery was longitudinally incised between these two clamps and a copper coil (1 cm in length and 1 mm internal diameter) was inserted into the lumen of the carotid artery. The copper coil was fixed by two circular sutures and the clamps were released. This procedure lasted less than 2 minutes. The blood flow was monitored up to 180 min after insertion of the thrombogenic copper coil. At 180 min ADP (100 µg/kg·min for 2.5 min) and at 195 min collagen (25 µg/kg·min for 5 min) were infused to decrease the number of circulating platelets. The platelets were counted (Sysmex microcell counter, Toa medical electronics, Kobe, Japan) in blood samples drawn before and 1 resp. 5 min during ADP- or collagen infusions.

Naxaprostene was suspended in carboxymethylcellulose (CMC) plus Tween and given orally or intraduodenally 30 min before the insertion of the copper coil.

RESULTS

In 6 vehicle (CMC/Tween)-treated control animals the carotid arteries totally occluded at 9 ± 1 (7 - 11) min after insertion of the thrombogenic copper coil. Treatment with 1 mg/kg p.o. naxaprostene (n = 6) did not prevent the carotid thrombosis (complete occlusion after 13 ± 2 min). With 10 mg/kg p.o. naxaprostene, in 5 of 6 animals thrombotic occlusion was prevented; the patency rate at 180 min thus was 83 %. When given via the intraduodenal (i.d.) route, 1 mg/kg naxaprostene was sufficient to inhibit arterial occlusion in 4 of 5 animals (80 % patency rate) (Fig. 1).

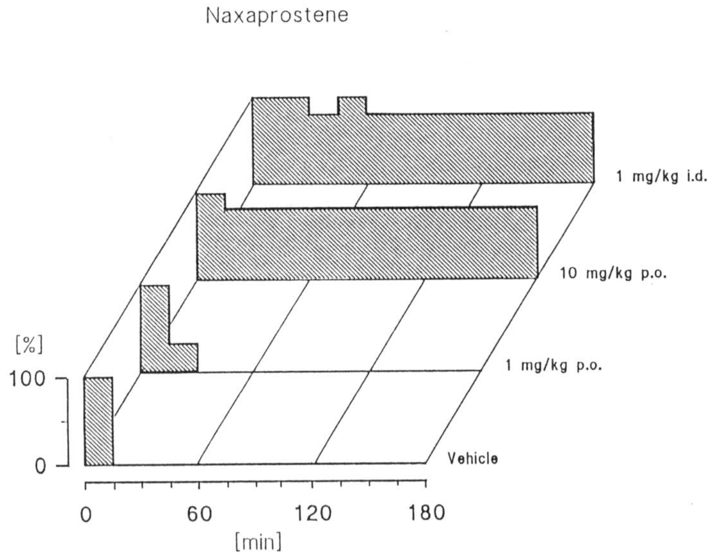

Figure 1: Effect of naxaprostene on patency rate of rabbit carotid arteries after insertion (time = 0 min) of a thrombogenic copper coil. n = 5 - 6 animals per group.

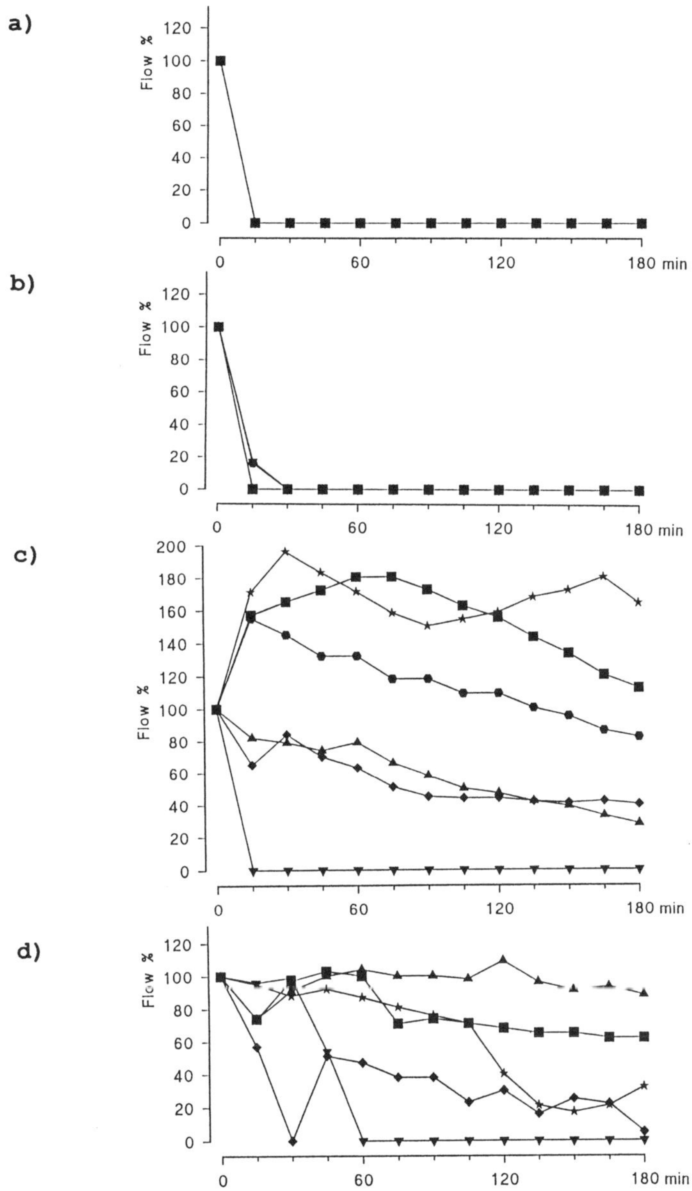

Figure 2a - d: Individual flow patterns in carotid arteries after insertion of a copper coil. Flow as % of value obtained immediately after insertion of the copper coil. Rabbits were pretreated with vehicle (a), 1 mg/kg p.o. (b), 10 mg/kg p.o. (c) and 1 mg/kg i.d. (d) naxaprostene.

The flow rate at 180 min as percentage of the flow immediately after the insertion of the copper coil was 85 ± 25 % in 5/6 rabbits in which complete occlusion had been prevented by 10 mg/kg p.o. naxaprostene; in 4/5 rabbits in which the carotid occlusion had been prevented by 1 mg/kg i.d. naxaprostene, the final flow rate was 47 ± 18 %. The individual flow patterns for the four different treatment groups are shown in Fig. 2a - d.

At 180 and 195 min after insertion of the copper coil, i.e. 210 and 225 min after applications of naxaprostene or vehicle, inhibition of ADP- and collagen-induced thrombocytopenia has been investigated (Table I).

Table I: Inhibition (%) by naxaprostene vs vehicle of ADP- and collagen-induced thrombocytopenia (means ± s.e.m.)

Naxaprostene	%-inhibition of fall in circulating platelets induced by ADP	Collagen
1 mg/kg p.o.	17 ± 11	39 ± 9
10 mg/kg p.o.	69 ± 11*	59 ± 4*
1 mg/kg i.d.	40 ± 17	50 ± 15

* $p < 0.05$ vs vehicle (Mann-Whitney test)

The mean arterial blood pressure of the anesthetized rabbits was reduced by naxaprostene (Table II).

Table II: Change of mean arterial blood pressure (MABP) after p.o.- or i.d.-administration of naxaprostene in anesthetized rabbits (30 min p.appl. vs prevalues).

Change in MABP	CMC	Naxaprostene 1 mg/kg p.o.	10 mg/kg p.o.	1 mg/kg i.d.
Δ mm Hg (means ± s.e.m.)	+7 ± 3	+5 ± 7	-25 ± 9*	-24 ± 2*

* $p < 0.05$ vs prevalue (paired t-test)

DISCUSSION

The insertion of a copper coil into carotid arteries of rabbits induced a strong thrombogenic stimulus with a rapid and complete arterial occlusion in all vehicle controls. Histological examination (not shown here) showed that these mixed thrombi consisted of fibrin and platelet aggregates. The prophylactic application of the prostacyclin analogue naxaprostene, given orally or intraduodenally 30 min before the insertion of the copper coil, protected against the arterial thrombotic occlusion. Inhibition of platelet aggregation by naxaprostene (Flohé et al., 1983) is suggested as the mechanism of this antithrombotic effect. This interpretation is strongly supported by the reduction of ADP- and collagen-induced thrombocytopenia by naxaprostene that was evaluated parallel to its antithrombotic activity.

Although naxaprostene has a higher chemical and metabolic stability than the natural prostacyclin (Flohé et al. 1983), is has been characterized pharmacologically only after parenteral administration (Schneider and Friderichs, 1985). This is the first report on the oral efficacy of naxaprostene. After oral application, a relative high dose of 10 mg/kg produced a significant antithrombotic effect. The availability of naxaprostene was enhanced after intraduodenal administration when 1 mg/kg was sufficient to protect against thrombotic occlusion. The effect of 1 mg/kg i.d., however, was less than the effect of 10.0 mg/kg p.o.; the factor of the relative higher efficacy of intraduodenal versus peroral application of naxaprostene is thus smaller than 10. The antithrombotic effect of naxaprostene, given orally or intraduodenally, lasted at least for the experimental period of 180 min.

General anesthesia increases the hypotensive activity of naxaprostene (Schneider and Friderichs, 1985); thus, in anesthetized rabbits there was no dissociation between antithrombotic and hypotensive effects of naxaprostene.

REFERENCES

Flohé, L., Böhlke, H., Frankus, E., Kim, S.-M.A., Lintz, W., Loschen, G., Michel, G., Müller, B., Schneider, J., Seipp, U., Vollenberg, W., Wilsmann, K. (1983), Arzneim.Forsch./ Drug Res. 33, 1240 - 1248

Schneider, J. Friderichs, E. (1985). In: Prostaglandins and Other Eicosanoids in the Cardiovascular System (K. Schrör, Ed), Karger, Basel, pp. 279-285

AAS 37
Prostaglandins in the
Cardiovascular System

INCREASE IN ENDOGENOUS FIBRINOLYSIS AND PLATELET ACTIVITY DURING EXERCISE IN YOUNG VOLUNTEERS

Brixi Beisiegel, Norbert Treese, Gerd Hafner,
Jürgen Meyer and Harald Darius

II. Medizinische Klinik
(Direktor: Prof. Dr. J. Meyer)
Klinisch-Pharmakologisches Labor
Johannes Gutenberg - Universität,
Mainz, FRG

SUMMARY

The influence of physical exercise and intake of oral contraceptives on endogenous fibrinolytic activity and platelet aggregation behaviour was studied in young healthy women and compared to an age matched group of male volunteers. Physical exercise beyond the anaerobic threshold significantly increased the activity of tissue-plasminogen activator (t-PA) in male and female volunteers from initial values of 1.6±0.1 and 1.8±0.2 IU/ml to 5.5±1.0 and 5.3±0.9 IU/ml ($P<0.01$), respectively. In women taking low-dose estrogen oral contraceptives t-PA increased from 1.5±0.2 to 3.8±0.5 ($P<0.01$). There were no major alterations in plasminogen activator inhibitor - I (PAI-I) plasma activities. Platelet activity during exercise was significantly enhanced in male test persons indicated by a significant decrease in the ED_{50} values for ADP. In contrast, in women ED_{50} values were basically unaltered, irrespective of the intake of oral contraceptives.

There are marked gender differences in activation of the endogenous fibrinolytic system and platelet sensitivity in response to physical exercise. These alterations suggest a prethrombotic potential in women, augmented by the intake of oral contraceptives.

INTRODUCTION

Acute venous and arterial thromboses may occur following strenuous physical exercise in previously healthy young individuals. In addition to female gender the intake of oral contraceptives (OC) is another known risk factor for acute thromboses in young women (Ciavatti etal, 1982). To study gender differences of the coagulation system, endogenous fibrinolytic activity and platelet aggregation healthy male and female volunteers were tested under control conditions (initial value) and spiroergometric exercise beyond the anaerobic threshold. Additionally, the influence of low-dose estrogen oral contraceptives was evaluated in the female study population.

MATERIALS AND METHODS

Twelve male and sixteen female healthy volunteers (18-35 years) were studied for their endogenous fibrinolytic activity and platelet aggregation behaviour. The female group subdivided into a group of 10 women without intake of low-dose estrogen oral contraceptives (-OC), 6 women did take contraceptives (+OC). All volunteers were non-smokers, without a known history of coagulation or platelet disorders. None of them had previously experienced a thrombotic event. The physical exercise testing was done at 10:00 a.m., by bicycle spiroergometry with continuous measurement of O_2 uptake, CO_2 output, heart rate, blood pressure, and ECG. The exercise level increased steadily by 20 Watts/min for women and by 30 Watts/min for men. The first blood sample was withdrawn at 9:00 a.m. after a 20 minute resting period in supine position. The second blood sample was taken immediately after the volunteers had exceeded the anaerobic threshold.

The following parameters were measured:

- ED_{50} for ADP (1-30 μM)- induced platelet aggregation in platelet-rich plasma using a turbidometric system
- IC_{50} for iloprost inhibition of ADP (10μM)-induced aggregation
- Tissue-plasminogen activator plasma activity measured photometrically with COA Set t-PA (KabiVitrum Diagnostica, Mölndal, Sweden) in acidified plasma (Chandler etal, 1989).
- Plasminogen activator inhibitor plasma activity measured photometrically with COASET PAI (KabiVitrum Diagnostica)
- Plasma lactate levels measured in capillary blood by an electrochemical method using a platinium electrode in a YSI 23L Analyzer (Yellow Springs Instrument, Ohio).

RESULTS

Platelet aggregation studies revealed marked differences in the initial ED_{50} values for ADP before exercise (Fig.1). While men had an ED_{50} value of 3.9±0.6 μM and women without contraceptives 2.9±0.6, women with oral contraceptives showed an increased susceptability towards aggregatory stimuli with an ADP ED_{50} of 1.3±0.3 μM. During exercise in men platelets became more activated and the ED_{50} value decreased to 3.0±0.6 μM. In contrast, platelet susceptability towards ADP was unaltered in women, irrespective of the intake of OC (Fig. 1).

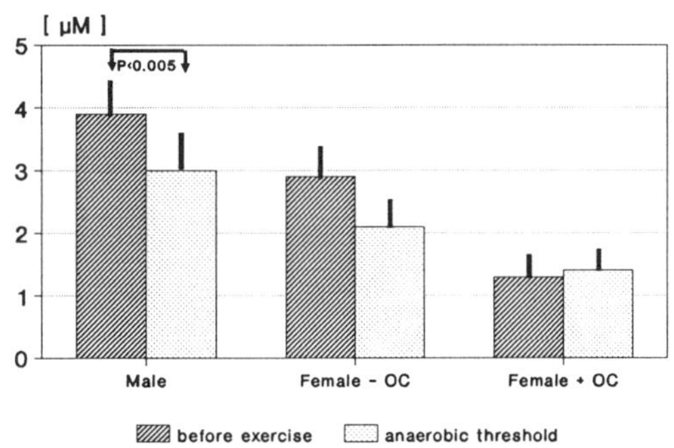

Figure 1
ED_{50}-values for ADP-induced platelet aggregation, before and after exceeding the anaerobic threshold during spiroergometric exercise in male (n=12) and female volunteers without intake of low-dose estrogen oral contraceptives (-OC; n=10) and with contraceptives (+OC ;n=6).

The results obtained in ADP-induced aggregation were confirmed for iloprost as an inhibitor of ADP (10μM)-induced aggregation.

The IC50 value for iloprost inhibition of platelet aggregation was significantly increased in men during exercise (Fig. 2). In contrast, there were no significant alterations in both groups of female volunteers (Fig. 2).

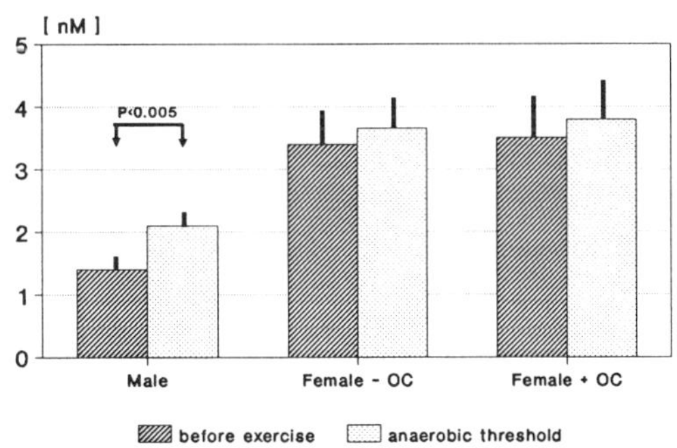

Figure 2
Inhibitory concentration (IC_{50}) for Iloprost as inhibitor of ADP (10μM)-induced platelet aggegation. The IC_{50}-value for Iloprost is significantly increased in men during exercise. There are no significant alterations in both female groups.

Plasma t-PA activity before initiation of exercise was not significantly different between the three groups of volunteers. In response to exercise beyond the individual anaerobic threshold in men plasma activity of t-PA was significantly increased from 1.6±0.1 to 5.5±1.0 IU/ml. In women the t-PA activity in plasma increased significantly too, however the increase was less pronounced in women with intake of contraceptives (Fig. 3).

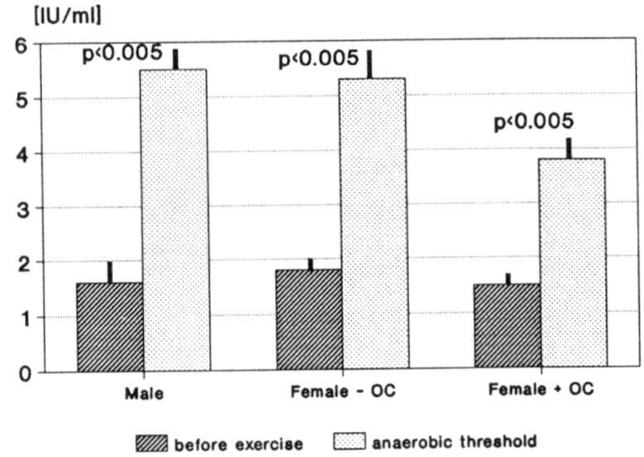

Figure 3
Plasma t-PA activity under control conditions and exercise values. There is a significant increase in plasma t-PA activity during exercise beyond the individual anaerobic threshold in men and both female test groups with and without intake of oral contraceptives.

The mean values for the activity of PAI-I in plasma ranged from 16 to 22 AU/ml and were not significantly altered in all test groups during exercise.

The mean values for the initial plasma lactate levels ranged from 0.5 to 1.1 mmol/l for the three groups studied and were significantly increased during exercise in all individuals studied (Fig. 4). Lactate levels in men were markedly higher compared to the female study population. Both female groups exerted an identical increase in lactate production during exercise (Fig. 4).

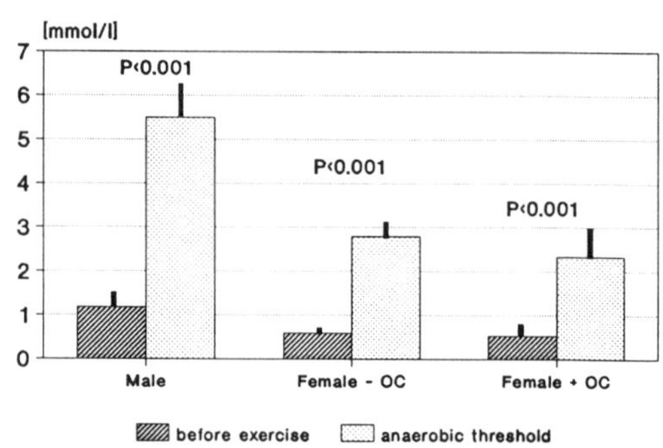

Figure 4
Plasma lactate levels during exercise. All three groups exerted a significant increas e in plasma lactate when compared to initial values before start of exercise.

The exercise parameters are depicted in table 1. The level of exercise at the anaerobic threshold was not significantly different between the male and female study population.

Although the maximum exercise levels were markedly higher in men, the duration of exercise was also identical, because the steepness of increase in exercise levels was 30 Watts/min in men and 20 Watts/min in females. There were no differences in heart rate, blood pressure or exercise parameters between the two female groups (Table 1).

Parameter	Males		Females - OC		Females + OC	
	i.v.	exer.	i.v.	exer.	i.v.	exer.
heart rate [beats/min]	75 ± 11	175 ± 13	81 ± 14	180 ± 9	68 ± 7	176 ± 10
ABP syst. [mm Hg]	129 ± 11	201 ± 19	110 ± 6	187 ± 13	120 ± 14	178 ± 12
ABP diast. [mm Hg]	80 ± 7	88 ± 15	74 ± 7	84 ± 11	76 ± 5	80 ± 7
VO_2 max [ml/kg/min]		33 ± 6		37 ± 8		37 ± 6
VO2 anaerobic [ml/kg/min]		20 ± 5		29 ± 7		26 ± 9
max.exercise [Watts]		203 ± 35		179 ± 8		178 ± 13
exer.anaerobic [Watts]		144 ± 41		138 ± 17		127 ± 30
exer.duration* [min]		7.8 ± 1.7		9.2 ± 0.4		9.0 ± 0.3

*: increase in exercise levels 30 Watts/min for males, 20 Watts/min for females
i.v. = initial value before exercise
exer. = maximal exercise

Table 1
Exercise parameters in men and women with (+OC) and without intake of oral contraceptives (-OC).
ABP = arterial blood pressure
VO_2max = maximal oxygen consumption
VO_2anaerobic = oxygen consumption at the anaerobic threshold

CONCLUSION

The risk of developing an acute thrombotic event is rather low in young healthy volunteers, who do not present any clinical signs of advanced atherosclerotic disease. However, in this low risk population women are more likely to develop a thrombotic event than men, especially if oral contraceptives are taken. This increased risk is not characterized by altered basic parameters for platelet aggregation behaviour, coagulation parameters or endogenous fibrinolysis. Therefore, in this study physical exercise was utilized to stimulate platelets to aggregate and endothelial cells to release t-PA in humans (Uno etal, 1989). The spiroergometric exercise test is an objective method to measure the exercise level and the adaptive capacity of the cardiopulmonary system independent of the individual training state (Wasserman etal, 1987). Spiroergometric exercise levels were identical in the two female study groups while men were capable of exerting a higher exercise level, when measured as exercise at the anaerobic threshold.

In all three groups tested there was a marked activation of the fibrinolytic sytem under exercise conditions. The study showed a significant increase in plasma t-PA activity under exercise conditions in men and women. However, the increase in women with intake of oral contraceptives is somewhat lower, although still statistically significant different from the initial values. The plasma levels of the physiological and functional antagonist of t-PA i.e. PAI-I were not altered by exercise in any of our volunteers, indicating the key role of endothelial cell stimulation for the increase in plasma t-PA activity. One of the factors which may act as mediators for the release of t-PA by endothelial cells may be the endothelial cell derived relaxing factor (EDRF). Recently, Grodzinska etal (1990) demonstrated that the nitrovasodilator molsidomine was able to stimulate endogenous t-PA release in healthy male volunteers.

Platelet susceptability to proaggregatory stimuli was measured by ADP dose response curves. There is no difference in the ED_{50} values for ADP in men and women without intake of oral contraceptives. Platelets in men became significantly more activated under exercise conditions as demonstrated by a decrease in the ED_{50} value ($P<0.05$), when compared to the two groups of women. In both female groups there was no significant alteration in ADP ED_{50} under exercise conditions. However, women with intake of oral contraceptives showed a lower ED_{50} for ADP, indicating an increased platelet susceptability under control conditions and following stimulation by exercise.

The results obtained with ADP were supported by the experiments performed in order to test platelet susceptability towards anti-aggregatory endothelial cell mediators. The IC_{50} values for the chemically stable PGI_2 analog iloprost were 1.5 ± 0.2 nM in men, being significantly lower when compared to 3.4 ± 0.2 and 3.5 ± 0.2 nM in women without and with contraceptives.

The study demonstrates a significant gender difference in platelet aggregation behaviour and activation of the endogenous fibrinolytic system under resting conditions and during physiological exercise. Women taking oral contraceptives seem to exert a higher platelet susceptability towards proaggregatory stimuli, a lower sensitivity towards antiaggregatory endothelial mediators and a diminished increase in plasma t-PA activity during exercise. These findings are coherent with the higher risk to develop a thrombotic event in this population.

REFERENCES

Chandler, W.L., Schmer, G., and Stratton, J.R. (1989) Optimum conditions for the stabilization and measurement of tissue plasminogen activator activity in human plasma J.Lab.Clin.Med. 113, 362-371.

Ciavatti, M.M., Davenas, E., Blache, D., Monnier, M. A., and Renaud, S. (1982) Biosynthesis of platelet lipids in relation to aggregation in women using oral contraceptives. Contraception 25, 629-638.

Grodzinska, L., Hafner, G., and Darius, H. (1990) Effect of Molsidomine on t-PA and PAI Activity in Man: A Double Blind, Placebo Controlled Study. Thromb.Haemost. 64, 486.

Uno, M., Tsuji, H., Watanabe, M., Sawada, S., Toyoda, T., and Nakagawa, M. (1989) Detection of Impaired Fibrinolytic Activity in Coronary Artery Disease- Electrophoretic and Immuno-Blotting Analysis of Tissue Plasminogen Activator. Jap. Circ. J. 53, 229- 236.

Wassermann, K., Hansen, J.E., Due, D.Y., Whipp B.J. (1987) Principles of exercise testing and interpretation. Lea & Febiger, Philadelphia.

AAS 37
Prostaglandins in the
Cardiovascular System

ASSOCIATION BETWEEN TOTAL CHOLESTEROL AND THROMBOXANE B_2 LEVELS IN OFFSPRING OF PARENTS SUFFERING FROM PREMATURE CORONARY ARTERY DISEASE

K. Mihai[1], J.Pető[2], A. Makáry[2], S. Tímár[3]

[1]Department of Pediatrics, [2]Experimental pathology, Department of Pathology, and [3]Department of Cardiology, County Hospital, Kecskemét, Hungary

SUMMARY

Relationship between plasma thromboxane B_2 concentration and serum total cholesterol level was studied in 129 healthy 3 to 18 years old children, 77 girls and 52 boys, without any family history of premature coronary artery disease and in 181 offspring, 105 girls and 76 boys, of parents suffering from acute myocardial infarction before the age of 45. It was identified an enhancement in serum total cholesterol level of endangered children, and an elevated release of thromboxane A_2 in affected girls. A significant negative correlation was found between serum total cholesterol concentration and plasma thromboxane B_2 level in healthy girls. However, there was no correlation between serum total cholesterol level and plasma thromboxane B_2 concenration in the children whose parents had premature coronary artery disease. It appears, from our results, that this in an alteration of thromboxane A_2 release of platelets in children of families with high risk of cardiovascular diseases.

INTRODUCTION

Coronary artery disease is the leading cause of death in Hungary. There is evidence that atherosclerosis begins in early childhood and advences into later life. For primary prevention it is therefore need to study the occurence of cardiovascular risk factors in childhood and adolescence.

Thromboxane A_2 and prostacyclin are the main eicosanoids formed in the cardiovascular system. Experimental and clinical studies have suggested that both hypercholesterolaemia and distrubances in the regulation of prostacyclin and biosynthesis of thromboxane A_2 might play an important role in the development of athero-sclerosis and in the pathogenesis of coronary artery disease syndromes. (Ross & Glomset, 1976; Nidorf et al, 1989; Patrono et al., 1990).

The present study was undertaken to determine whether the serum total cholesterol and plasma thromboxane A_2 concentration alteres in offspring of parents who have had an acute myocardial infarction before the age of 45.

MATERIALS AND METHODS

129 healthy 3 to 18 years old children, 77 girls and 52 boys, without any family history of cardiovascular diseases, as controls and 181 offspring, 105 girls and 76 boys, of parents suffering from premature coronary artery disease were investigated. Blood samples were collected by vanipuncture after fasting overnight at 7 a.m. after 15 minute quiet bed-rest. The children were abstinent. None of them was a smoker. They had no medication before the start of the study. Hormonal contraceptives had not been taken. Serum total cholesterol were determined by using an enziymatic test (SERA-PAK, Reanal, Hungary). Thromboxane A_2 was analysed as its hydrolitic product from plasma containing Na_2--ethylene- diamine- tetraacetate and indomethacin. Before radio-

immunoassay measurement (^{125}I-thromboxane B_2 RIA kit, Amersham, England, and Izinta, Hungary) plasmas were extracted on C_{18}-phase (Mihai et al., 1991).
Data were entered into a Dbase program and analysed by using the IBM computer. Results are expressed as means $\pm$ SD for cholesterol, and mean$\pm$SEM for thromboxane B_2.Atherogenic index was calculated according to Klimov's formula. Statistical differences were assessed by Student's _t_ test. Linear regression models were applied to determine the association between examined parameters, and the significance by using the _F_ table.

RESULTS

As seen in Table I. serum total cholesterol levels were significantly higher in affected children than in controls. Plasma thromboxane B^2 concentration was elevated in daughters, and atherogenic index in sons of parents with acute myocardial infarction compared to these concentrations of control healthy children.

TABLE I. EXAMINED PARAMETERS IN OFFSPRING OF PARENTS WITH PREMATURE MYOCARDIAL INFARCTION AND CONTROLS

		CONTROL CHILDREN		ENDANGERED CHILDREN	
		GIRLS	BOYS	GIRLS	BOYS
	n	77	52	105	76
SERUM TOTAL CHOLESTEROL					
(mmol/l)	$\bar{x}$	4.00	3.66	4.69^{xx}	4.19^{xx}
	SD	0.66	0.58	1.26	0.96
PLASMA THROMBOXANE B_2					
(pg/ml)	$\bar{x}$	196	275	322^{x}	254
	SEM	12.76	16.78	54.36	29.48
ATHEROGENIC INDEX					
	$\bar{x}$	2.75	2.38	3.42	2.88^{xx}
	SD	0.94	0.87	1.68	1.07

SIGNIFICANT DIFFERENCE COMPARED TO CONTROL x $p < 0.05$ xx $p < 0.001$

A significant negative correlation was found between serum

total cholesterol level and thromboxane B_2 production in healthy girls (Fig.1). No statistically significant association was identified these parameters in offspring of parents suffering from premature coronary artery disease (Fig.2). There was no difference in platelet count among all the groups.

FIG.1.

Correlation between serum total cholesterol and plasma thromboxane B_2 in healthy children

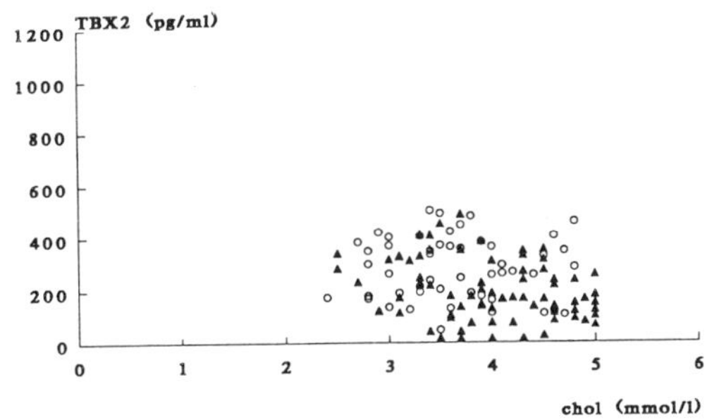

○ boys
n = 52
Y = 25.3274 x + 182.487
F = 0.749

▲ girls
n = 77
Y = - 54.1035 x + 413.592
F = 8.391
$p < 0.025$

FIG.2.

Correlation between serum total cholesterol and plasma thromboxane B_2 in offspring of parents suffering from premature myocardial infarction

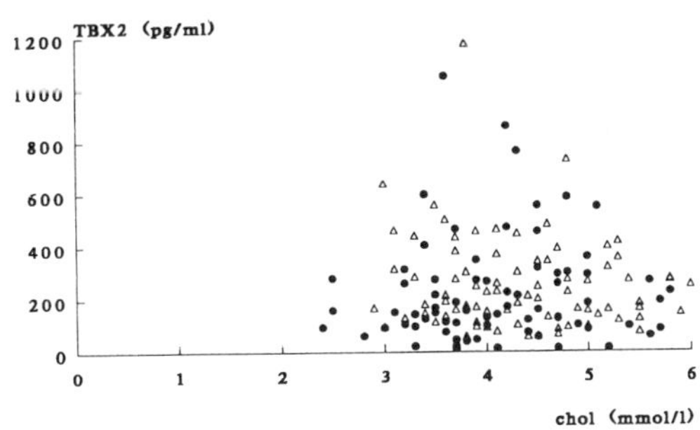

● boys
n = 76
Y = 2.2911 x + 245.129
F = 0.0048

△ girls
n = 105
Y = 56.4840 x + 57.405
F = 1.6985

DISCUSSION

The role of platelets in the pathogenesis of atherosclerosis is well accepted (Sinzinger et al.,1990). It has been suggested that platelet aggregation and release of platelet-derivated substances in damaged, and atherosclerotic coronary arteries may be important in the pathogenesis of coronary artery disease syndromes (Mustard & Packham,1969). Hypercholesterolaemia may promote the atherosclerotic process not only by the accumulation of cholesterol in vascular tissue, but also due to alteration of thromboxane A_2 and prostacyclin pruduction (Carvalho et al., 1974; Stuart et al., 1980; Pfister et al. , 1988). Increased formation rates of thromboxane A_2 have been demonstrated in patients with various type of angina pectoris and with acute myocardial infarction (Walinsky et al.,1984; Fitzgerald et al., 1986; Ohmori et al., 1987; Pomerantz et al., 1989).
We have shown an enhancement in serum total cholesterol of endangered children, and from alteration of atherogenic index, a decrease in the protective HDL -cholesterol level in sons of parents suffering from premature coronary ertery disease, and an elevated release of thromboxane B_2 in affected girls. We have found a significant negative association between serum total cholesterol and thromboxane B_2 levels in healthy girls. It was identified statistically significant correlation neither between serum total cholesterol and plasma thromboxane B_2 concentrations nor atherogenic index and thromboxane B_2 level in children whose parents have had an early acute myocardial infarction.

CONCLUSION

The results of this study suggest the appearance of alteration in thromboxane A_2 release from platelets in offspring of parents suffering from premature coronary artery disease. Further examinations necessary to know the exact cause of this mechanism.

ACKONOWLEDGMENTS

We thank Éva Kolthay, Isotope Laboratory, for radioimmunoassay measurements.

REFERENCES

Carvalho, A.C.A., Colman, R.W., Lees, R.S. (1974) Platelet function in hyperlipoproteinemia
N.Engl. J.Med. 290, 434-438.

Fitzgerald, D.J.,Roy,L.,Catella,F.,FitzGerald,G.A. (1986) Platelet activation in unstable coronary disease
N.Engl.J.Med. 315, 983-989.

Mihai,K.,Pető,J.,Kolthay,É.,Makáry,A. (1991) Prostacyclin and thromboxane levels in children of parents suffering from early ischemic heart disease
Acta Paediatr.Hung. 31, 113-118

Mustart, J.F.,Packham,M.A. (1969) Platelet function and myocardial infarction
Circulation Suppl. 40, 20-30.

Nidorf,S.M.,Strum,M.,Strophair,J.,Kendrew,Ph.J.,Taylor,R.R. (1989) Whole blood aggregation, thromboxane release and the lyso derivate of platelet activating factor in myocardial infarction and unstable angina
Cardiol.Res. 23, 273-278

Ohmori,M.,Kuzuya,T.,Kodama,K.,Nanto,Sh.,Kamada,T.,Tada,M.(1987) Thromboxane A_2 as an enhancing factor of coronary vasospasticity in variant angina
Jap. Circulation J. 51, 495 - 502

Patrono,C.,Ciabbatoni,G.,Davi,G. (1990) Thromboxane biosynthesis in cardiovascular diseases
Stroke 21 (suppl IV), IV-130-IV-133

Pfister,S.L.,Schmitz,J.M.,Willerson,J.,Campbell,WB. (1988) Characterization of arachidonic acid metabolism in Watanabe

heritable hyperlipidemic (WHHL) and New Zeland white (NZW) rabbit aortas
Prostaglandins 36, 515-532

Pomerantz,K.B., Hajjar,D.P. (1989) Eicosanoids in regulation of arterial smooth muscle cell phenotype, proliferative capacity, and cholesterol metabolism
Arteriosclerosis 9, 413 - 429

Ross,R.,Glomset,J.A. (1976) The pathogenesis of atherosclerosis
New Engl.J.Med. 295, 469-420

Sinzinger,H., Virgolini,I.,Fitscha,P. (1990) Platelet kinetics in patients with atherosclerosis
Thromb.Research 57, 507-516

Stuart,M.J.,Gerrard,J.M.,White,J.G.(1980) Effect of cholesterol of production of thromboxane B_2 by platelets in vitro
N.Engl.J.Med. 302, 6-10

Walinsky,P.,Smith,B.J.,Lefer A.M., Lebenthal,M.,Urban,P. Greenspon ,A.,Goldberg, Sh. (1984) Thromboxane A_2 in acute myodardial infarction
Am.Heart.J. 108, 868-872

AAS 37
Prostaglandins in the
Cardiovascular System

PLATELET PGI_2-RECEPTOR BEHAVIOUR CHANGE AFTER TREATMENT WITH ACETYLSALICYLIC ACID IN HEALTHY VOLUNTEERS

Th. Böhm, Irene Virgolini and H. Sinzinger

Wilhelm Auerswald Atherosclerosis Research Group (ASF) Vienna, Austria.

SUMMARY: After treatment of human platelet membrane fractions with different concentrations of acetylsalicylic acid (ASA) the Iloprost binding capacity (B_{max}) and also the dissociation constant (K_d) of the high-affinity PGI_2-receptor increased significantly ($p<0.01$, low-affinity receptor only an increase of B_{max}, $p<0.01$), whereas only a significant ($p<0.05$) increase of the K_d of the high-affinity receptor was observed for intact platelets.

INTRODUCTION

Recently, Dutta-Roy & Sinha (1987) have shown that the receptor protein for prostaglandin (PG) I_2 at the platelet membrane exhibits a molecular mass of 190 kD, composed of two non-identical subunits with molecular masses of 85 and 95 kD, respectively. The interaction with the receptor protein is rapid, saturable, reversible and specific for PGI_2 and PGE_1 (Dutta-Roy & Sinha, 1987; Schäfer et al., 1979). Scatchard analysis of the purified receptor revealed two binding sites, a high-affinity (K_d=9.8 nM), and a low-affinity one (K_d=0.7 µM).

Down- or up-regulation of receptors, changes in the affinity of a ligand to the receptor protein, sensitization and de-sensitization of the second messenger pathway are basic modes for PG-receptor-expression. The underlying mechanisms are an extensive stimulation by PGs, leading to continuous high second messenger levels, and as a self-protective process to down-regulation of membrane receptor density and desensitization (Gorman et al., 1980; Robertson et al., 1980; Blair et al., 1982). On the other hand, reduced stimulation through inhibition of PG-biosynthesis by ASA results in an increase of receptor density (Rice et al., 1980) and sensitivity of platelets to antiaggregatory PGs (Sinzinger et al., 1984).

A dose of 40 or only 20 mg a day has been recommended to be optimal for inhibition of thromboxane (TX)-biosynthesis without interfering with PGI_2-production by vascular endothelial cells (Patrignani et al., 1982; Patrono et al., 1980).

MATERIALS AND METHODS

BLOOD SAMPLING; Twenty healthy volunteers (18-24 a) served as blood donors. None had taken aspirin or other drugs interfering with platelet function or PG-biosynthesis. For all tests Aspisol (BAYER AG, Leverkusen, Germany) was used and diluted to adequate concentrations with assay buffer (50 mmol/l Tris-HCl, pH 7.5, containing 5 mmol/l $MgCl_2$). A dose range of 10 to 10000 mg/5 l blood was tested.

PLATELET PREPARATION

1.MEMBRANE FRACTIONS: One hundred and fifty ml blood were drawn without venous occlusion into polypropylene syringes by venipuncture. Blood was anticoagulated 1:9 with sodium citrate (3,8% wv). The whole blood volume was divided into 3 parts, adequate ASA concentrations were added to 2 portions, the third one served as control. After incubation for 20 min at 37°C platelet rich plasma (PRP, 150g, 22°C) was further centrifuged at 5000g for 10 min. The resulting pellet was resuspended in buffer (25 mmol/l Tris-HCl, pH 7.5, containing 1 mmol/l $MgCl_2$ and 0.25 mmol/l sucrose), homogenized by ultraturrax and ultrasound, and centrifuged at 150g for 5 min. The resulting supernatant was centrifuged twice at 40000g for 10 min, the second time in sucrose–free buffer. The platelet membrane fraction was finally taken up in assay buffer.

2.INTACT PLATELETS: PRP was twice centrifuged at 700g for 20 min at 22°C. The pellet was resuspended in assay buffer plus 10% ACD-stabilisator (2.2% sodium citrate, 0.73% acid. citric., 2.45% glucose) to prevent platelets from aggregation. Washed platelets were adjusted to a final concentration of 2.10^5 platelets/µl.

3.BINDING STUDIES: Binding of Iloprost to human platelets was performed as previously described (Sinzinger et al., 1987).

4.RADIOTHINLAYER CHROMATOGRAPHY (RTLC): Prostaglandin biosynthesis was investigated as described in Sinzinger et al. (1989).

RESULTS

PERCENTAGE CALCULATION OF EACH EXPERIMENT: with membrane fractions in terms of differences between ASA treatment and control showed, that the K_d of the high-affinity receptor state increased from 1=100 % of control to 2.4±1.1 ($p < 0.01$) and the B_{max} raised to 1.8±0.6 ($p < 0.01$), whereas low-affinity receptor showed only an increased B_{max} (1.46±0.3, $p < 0.01$) (Fig.1).

Fig.1 Comparison of K_d and B_{max} of control and ASA experiments. All ASA experiments are expressed in % of control values. The values indicate the means ± SD for n=22; ● = $p < 0.01$, □ = $p < 0.05$, ○ = not significant; C = control, B = B_{max}

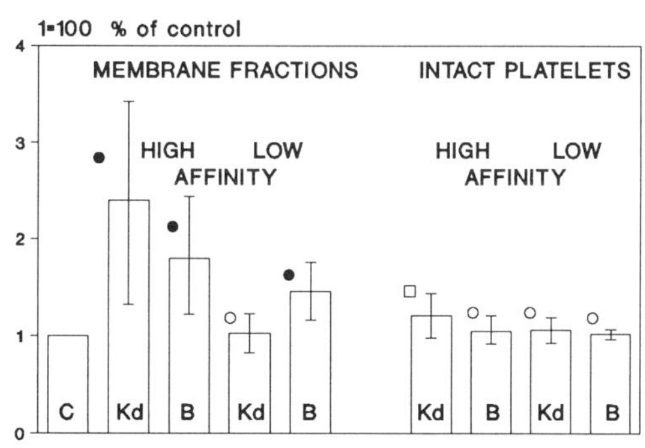

In the series with intact platelets even percentage calculation of each assay did not demonstrate differences between control and ASA incubations, only the K_d of the high-affinity binding sites increased significantly (1.2± 0.2, $p<0.05$) (Fig.1).

TREATMENT WITH DIFFERENT CONCENTRATIONS OF ASA: The most effective ASA doses were 10 mg up to 100 mg ASA/5 L whole blood (Fig.2) The K_d of the low-affinity receptor of membrane fractions was not elevated in any of the regimens used. Nevertheless, the B_{max} raised from 1 (control) to 1.5 beginning with 10 mg and maintained this value up to 10000 mg (Fig.2).

Fig.2 The values indicate the mean for 1<n<6. (▽) high affinity K_d; (○) low affinity K_d; (●) high affinity B_{max}; (□) low affinity B_{max}

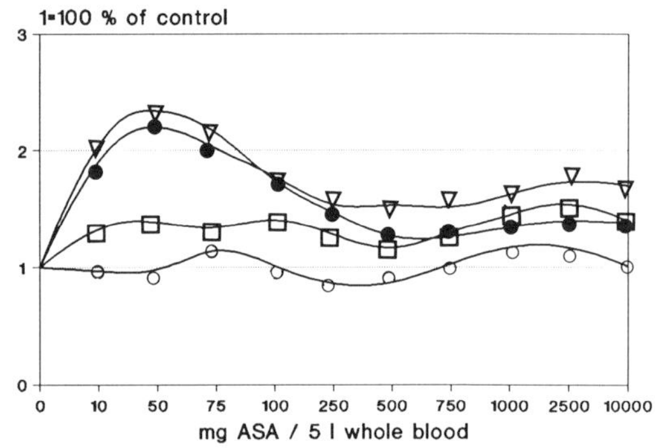

The experiments with intact platelets revealed only an increased K_d of the high-affinity receptor without influence on other parameters of the PGI_2-receptor (Fig.1). However, 10 mg to 100 mg were most effective, similar to membrane fraction behaviour (data not shown).

PROSTANOID BIOSYNTHESIS BY PLATELETS UNDER ASA INFLUENCE

Exogenously added ^{14}C-arachidonic acid (AA) to intact platelets was converted to detectable amounts of TXB_2, HHT, 12-HETE, PGE_2 and PGD_2.

Fig.3 % conversion of ^{14}C-AA to TXB_2, HHT, 12-HETE in the absence and presence of ASA. The values indicate the mean for 1<n<5; (△) TXB_2; (□) HHT; (○) 12-HETE;

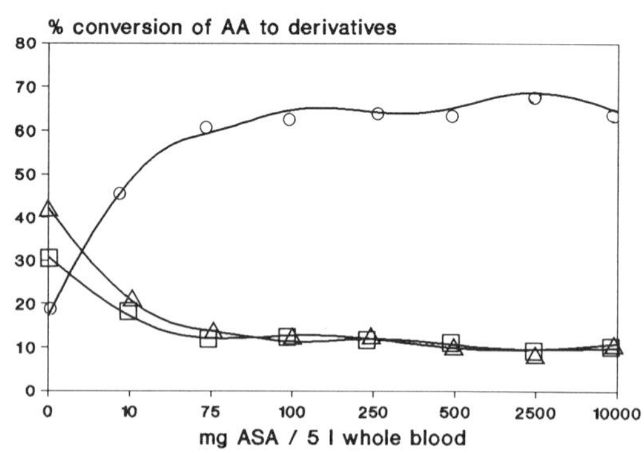

The values of % conversion of TXB_2, HHT, 12-HETE and the AA-residue after incubation with different ASA concentrations are shown in Fig.3 and Table 1.

Table 1 Effect of ASA on % conversion of ^{14}C-AA

	control (n=15)	ASA-concentration 10 mg (n=8)	100 mg (n=5)
TXB_2	42.1 ± 7.8	15.9 ± 6.6	10.3 ± 0.7
HHT	30.8 ± 0.9	14.4 ± 4.9	10.9 ± 2.2
12-HETE	17.2 ± 8.9	56.2 ± 4.9	66.6 ± 4.1
AA-residue	3.6 ± 2.1	7.3 ± 2.8	6.9 ± 1.9

DISCUSSION

In this study we demonstrate, that ASA altered high-affinity receptors of membrane fractions in comparison to control experiments in two different ways, which perhaps are resulting in the same benefit, namely to sensitize platelets to anti-aggregatory PGs.

The first effect was an increase in receptor density, allowing increased binding of Iloprost, perhaps resulting in higher cAMP-levels. An increased sensitivity (a positive indication for higher cAMP levels) to antiaggregatory PGs was demonstrated after daily ingestion of different ASA doses. This improved sensitivity was observed even with 1 mg per day and did not change from 20 up to 1000 mg (Sinzinger et al., 1989). One reason for an altered sensitivity could be an increased binding activity.

On the other hand, ASA decreases receptor affinity for binding, perhaps resulting in lower amounts of ligand occupying more receptor molecules per time unit, leading to higher second messenger levels in the "surrounding" platelets.

To summarize, ASA increases high-affinity receptor density, but decreases the affinity for ligand binding. These two events are perhaps consistent in terms of inhibiton of platelet aggregation and secretion by ASA.

Firstly, more binding sites are accompanied by increased adenylat-cyclase activity, when we assume that the measured enhanced sensitivity (Sinzinger et al., 1989) is caused by increased binding sites.

Secondly, according to experiments with frog-erythrocytes (Lefkowitz et al., 1977), decreased affinity may also lead to higher cAMP-levels and more platelets per time unit are involved through rapid dissociation of the ligand from the receptor.

The current data establish the low dose of 20 mg ASA daily to be appropiate in terms of improving platelet sensitivity and receptor behaviour. There was no difference between 10 and 10000 mg, on the contrary it appears that the influence on B_{max} and K_d is most effective in a range between 10 and 100 mg.

The effect of ASA on Iloprost binding to intact platelets is limited to affinity decrease of the high-affinity binding class. In a concentration range between 10 and 250 mg ASA the alterations appear more pronouncedly similar to membrane fractions, without alteration of B_{max} as well as of the high- and low-affinity receptor site. Nevertheless, this change can also result in increased AC-activity (see above).

Even RTLC results support the claim of 20 mg ASA to be optimal. TXB_2-conversion drops from control values of approximately 40% to 16% under 10 mg treatment and reaches a plateau of about 10% after a single dose of 100 mg (Fig.3).

In conclusion, the data demonstrate an influence of ASA on human platelet PGI_2-receptor activity, which was more pronounced after a single treatment of 10 to 100 mg than after higher doses, but the mode of action of ASA in this case remains to be elucidated. It could be a secondary effect following cyclooxygenase inhibition, or caused by disruption of normal signaling events and protein-protein interactions within the membrane or by blocking G-protein-dependent processes (Abramson and Weissmann, 1989).

REFERENCES

Abramson, S. B. and Weissman, G. (1989) The mechanism of nonsteroidal antiinflammatory drugs. Arthritis Rheum. 32, 1-9.

Blair, I. A., Leigh, P. J., MacDermot, J. (1982) Desensitization of prostacyclin receptors in a neuronal hybrid cell line. Br. J. Pharmacol. 77, 121-127.

Dutta-Roy, A. K., Sinha, A. K..(1987) Purification and properties of prostaglandin E_1 / prostacyclin receptor of human platelets. J. Biol. Chem. 262, 12685-12690.

Gorman, R. R., Hopkins, N. K. (1980) Agonist specific desensitization of PGI_2-stimulated cyclic AMP accumulation by PGE in human foreskin fibroblasts. Prostaglandins 19, 2-16.

Lefkowitz, R. J., Mullikin, D., Wood, C. L., Gore, T. B., and Mukherjee, C. (1977) Regulation of prostaglandin receptors by prostaglandins and guanine nucleotides in frog erythrocytes. J. Biol. Chem. 252, 5295-5303.

Patrignani, P., Filabozzi, P., Patrono, C. (1982) Selective cumulative inhibition of platelet thromboxane production by low-dose aspirin in healthy subjects. J. Clin. Invest. 69, 1366-1372.

Patrono, C., Ciabattoni, E., Pugliese, F., Pinca, E., Castrucci, G., De Salvo, A., Sotta, M. A., Peskar, B. A. (1980) Low-dose aspirin and inhibition of thromboxane B_2-production in healthy subjects. Thromb. Res. 17, 317-327.

Rice, M. G., McRae, J. R., Storm, D. R., Robertson, R. P. (1980) Up regulation of hepatic prostaglandin E receptors in vivo induced by prostaglandin synthesis inhibitors. Am.J. Physiol. 241, 291-297.

Robertson, R. P., Westcott, K. R., Storm, D. R., Rice, M. G. (1980) Down regulation in vivo of PGE receptors and adenylate cyclase stimulation. Am. J. Physiol. 239, 75-82.

Schäfer, A. I., Cooper, B., O'Hara, D., Handin, R.I. (1979) Identification of platelet receptor for prostaglandin I_2 and D_2. J. Biol. Chem. 254, 2914-2917.

Sinzinger, H., O'Grady, J., Fitscha, P., Kaliman, J. (1984) Extremely-low-dose aspirin (one milligram per day) renders human platelets more sensitive to antiaggregatory prostaglandins. N. Engl. J. Med. 18, 1052 1059.

Sinzinger, H., Steurer, G., Fitscha, P., Kraupp, O. (1987) The intrainfusion rebound platelet activation during continuous prostaglandin I2 infusion occurs at the receptor level. In:Prostaglandins in Clinical Research (H. Sinzinger and K. Schrör, eds), Alan, R. Liss, Inc., New York, 1987, pp 19-23.

Sinzinger, H., Virgolini, I., Peskar, B. A. (1989) Response of thromboxane A_2, malondialdehyde and platelet sensitivity to 3 weeks low-dose Aspirin (ASA) in healthy volunteers. Thromb. Res. 53, 261-269.

AAS 37
Prostaglandins in the
Cardiovascular System

IMPAIRED PGI2-STABILIZATION IN SEPTIC SHOCK PATIENTS

Andrea Podolsky, A. Vichytil, J.Pidlich, H.Sinzinger
2nd Department of Internal Medicine, University of Vienna, Wilhelm-Auerswald Atherosclerosis Research Group (ASF) Vienna, Austria.

SUMMARY: Lipids, lipoproteins, apolipoproteins and prostacyclin-half-life (PGI2-T/2) in vitro were determined in patients, who suffered from severe circulatory shock. Extremely lowered lipids, lipoproteins and apolipoproteins and an extremely shortened PGI2-T/2 were found, in these patients. These findings support the data of Yui and Aoyama that apolipoproteins may be an important coregulator of the biological half-life of PGI2 and thereby contribute to hemostatic dyregulation seen in these patients.

INTRODUCTION:

The stability of prostaglandin I2 (prostacyclin, PGI2) has been claimed to play an important regulatory role in haemostatic balancing (Lefer,1990). Pathological instability has been found on basis of a defect (Sinzinger et al.,1985) as well as in thrombotic thrombocytopenic purpura (Chen et al., 1981; Wu et al., 1982) and in myocardial infarction (Sinzinger et al., 1987). Recently, it has been shown, that binding to apolipoprotein A1 (APO A1) may determine its biological half life (Yui et al.,1988; Aoyama et al., 1990). We thus approached a clinical condition being associated with extremly low lipid- and apolipoprotein-values, i.e. sepsis and circulatory shock (Alvarez and Ramos, 1986; Cross et al., 1990), to measure the biological half-life of prostacyclin (PGI2-T/2).

MATERIAL AND METHODS:

Patients: Blood was collected from seven patients (4 males, 3 females, age 60 ± 4,7 years; mean±SEM) with severe septic shock admitted to the intensive care unit. Six of them died within the same day the blood was taken, one female patient survived.

Lipoprotein analysis: Determination of lipoproteins has been done according to the Lipid Research Clinic-method with minor modification using an ultracentrifuge and polyanion precipitation. In each fraction cholesterol and triglycerides have been determined by means of full enzymatic methods using Boehringer (Mannheim, Germany) reagents. Quality control has been performed using control sera Seronorm and Seronorm Lipid (Merck, Darmstadt, Germany). A coefficient of variation between 2,4 % and 3,5 % has been obtained.

Plasma preparation: 4,5 ml blood anticoagulated with 0,5 ml of 3,8 % sodium citrate were drawn from a central venous catheter. After a sedimentation plasma was separated twice by centrifugation under at least 1000 g for 10 minutes to avoid cellular contamination. The supernatant cellular free compartment was drawn into Eppendorf vials and stored at -20°C for the determination.

Assay: The inhibitory capacity of biologically active PGI2 on ADP-(1μM, 100 μl) induced platelet aggregation after incubation in patients plasma for various time intervals was used for quantitation of PGI2-T/2. Blood from healthy volunteers was used for the assay. Platelet-rich plasma (PRP) was obtained by centrifugation at 150 g for 5 minutes. Platelet-poor plasma (PPP) was achieved by a further centrifugation step at 1000 g for 10 minutes. PRP and PPP were adjusted afterwards to a constant final platelet count of $250 x 10^3/\mu l$. Different concentrations (1,2,4,8 or 16 ng, respectively) of PGI2 (The Upjohn Company, Kalamazoo, Michigan, USA) were incubated in 600 μl PPP at various time intervals (at least 3 tests 10 seconds - 20 minutes) at 37°C. Thereafter, 100 μl of this PPP (containing the PGI2 partially degraded to biologically inactive derivatives) were added to the adjusted PRP derived from the patients. The final volume in the cuvette amounted to 800 μl. From the various samples the decay curve was drawn and the T/2 calculated (in seconds). Control of the added PGI2 was performed by means of a specific radioimmunassay (RIA) for the stable derivative 6-oxo-PGF1α in unextracted samples using the double-antibody technique.

Statistical methods: The values are given as Mean ± SEM, the correlation has been calculated. Analysis for significance has been done using Student`s t-test.

RESULTS:

Table I summarizes the values for serum lipids, lipoproteins, apolipoproteins and PGI2-T/2 obtained from all patients. Patients 1.-5. suffered from a long-lasting sepsis (duration more than 2 weeks at the time of blood sampling), they were in circulatory shock and died within a few hours after blood was withdrawn. Patient 7 was in a circulatory shock secondary to sepsis for more than two weeks, too, when blood was taken, but she recovered. Patient 6 was in acute circulatory shock when she was admitted to the intensive care unit with a severe pulmonary embolism. Blood was taken immediately, but the patient died within the same day.

Table I: Serum lipids, lipoproteins, apolipoproteins and prostacyclin-half-life of the patients compared to normal values.

	sex/age	TC (mg/dl)	TG (mg/dl)	HDL-C (mg/dl)	LDL-C (mg/dl)	APO A1 (mg/dl)	APO B (mg/dl)	PGI2-T/2 (seconds)	
normal values		(100-200)	(<150)	(35-70)	(<130)	(102-215)	(59-155)	(600-900)	
1. F.J.	m/58	66,1	134,4	5,8	33,7	23,4	38,5	84	d
2. M.G.	m/75	67,6	100,2	15,9	36,9	50,1	46,1	127	d
3. S.P.	m/67	77,9	156,8	13,2	38,3	30,7	44,6	119	d
4. Z.L.	m/77	55,0	334,0	8,0	15,0	20,1	54,8	44	d
5. K.S.	f/55	117,0	---	8,8	63,2	20,1	109,0	26	d
6. P.M.	f/48	134,0	304,0	30,0	98,0	95,0	85,6	186	d
7. P.J.	f/46	371,0	383,0	30,0	293,7	133,0	261,0	551	s

m = male, f = female. d = died within the day the blood was taken, s = survived.

In all the patients who died (1.-6.), APO A1 (39,9±12; Mean±SEM; p<0,0003) was decreased and PGI2-T/2 (97,7±24; Mean±SEM; p<0,0001) was extremely reduced, compared to normal values, whereas it was nearly normal in the surviving patient (7). Both total-cholesterol (TC) and apolipoprotein B (APO B) were lowered in the male septic patients (1.-4.),however, it was normal in the two female patients who died (5.,6.) and elevated in the single female patient (7) who survived . All the septic patients who died (1.-5.), showed severe reduction of HDL-cholesterol (HDL-C) and very low levels of LDL-cholesterol (LDL-C) (males lower than the female patient 5), whereas patient 6 with pulmonary embolism and patient 7 who recovered from sepsis had nearly normal HDL-C-levels and normal (6) or increased (7) LDL-cholesterol (LDL-C)-levels, respectively Triglycerides (TG) were increased in nearly all patients, except in patients 1 and 2.

A really good correlation was seen between TC and PGI_2-T/2 (r=0,9) (Fig. 1.), APO A1 and PGI_2-T/2 (r=0,85) (Fig. 3) and LDL-C and PGI_2-T/2 (r=0,97) (Fig. 4). The correlation was not so strong between HDL-C and PGI2-T/2 (r=0,62) (Fig. 2) and APO B and PGI2-T/2 (r=0,69) (Fig. 5), respectively.

Fig. 1: Correlation TC - PGI2-T/2; r = 0,9

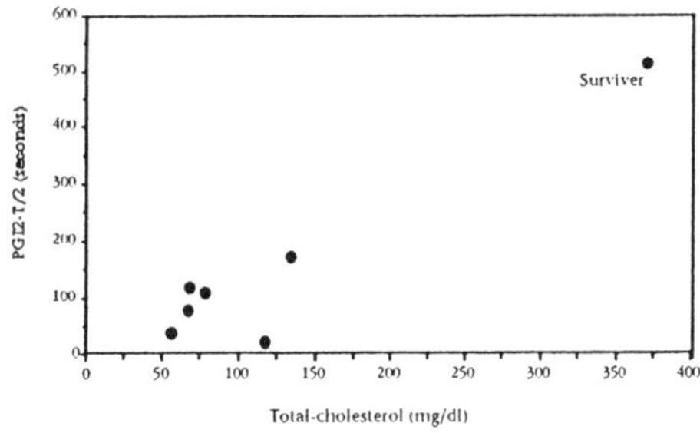

Fig. 2: Correlation HDL-C - PGI2-T/2; r = 0,62

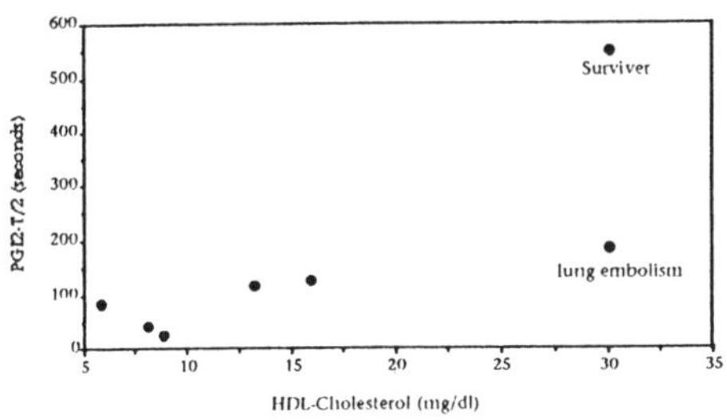

Fig. 3: Correlation APO A1 - PGI2-T/2; r = 0,85

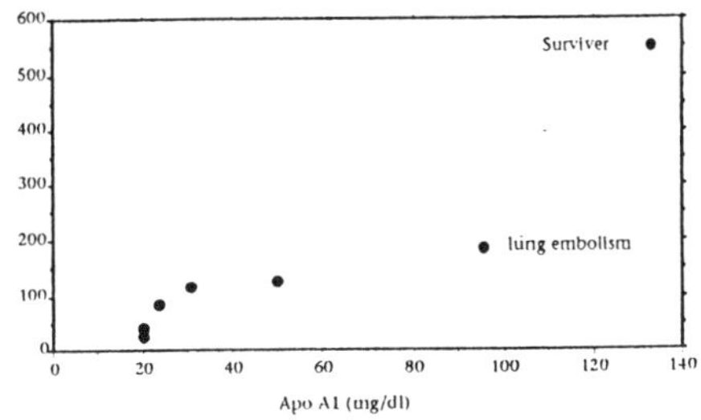

Fig 4: Correlation LDL-C - PGI2-T/2 r = 0,97

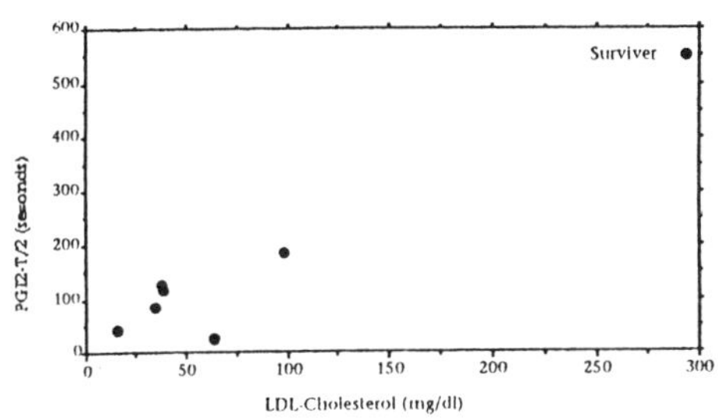

Fig. 5: Correlation Apo B - PGI2-T/2; r = 0,69

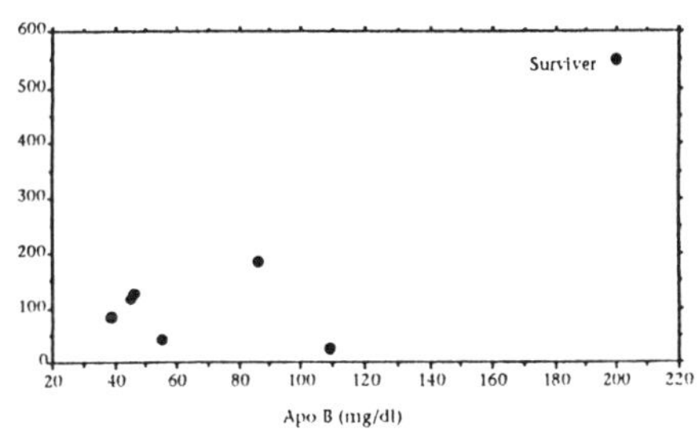

DISCUSSION:

The main finding of our study was, that patients, who suffered from severe sepsis for a long time (2-5 weeks) had an extremely shortened biological half-life of PGI2, corresponding to extremely lowered levels of HDL-C, TC, LDL-C and APO A1, before they died. Patient 6, who was in circulatory shock for just some hours before she died, due to pulmonary embolism, did not show such extremely decreased values of TC, lipoproteins and APO A1, whereas the PGI2-T/2 was shortened, too. Patient 7, however, who recovered from severe sepsis after a long period of time (nearly six weeks) did not show similar alterations in both, the lipid profile and the PGI2-T/2.

Not many data are available, but sepsis has been shown before as a clinical condition being associated with lowered TC, HDL-C, APO A and APO B and increased TG (Alvarez and Ramos, 1986). These changes were similar to those, we could see in our septic patients. Alvarez and Ramos did not find a relationship between the lipid-abnormalities, neither to the type of underlying illness, nor to the clinical situation, nor to the etiological infecting agent. But to a certain degree the alterations in serum lipids tend to normalize with general discovery. They supposed that the decrease of HDL-C in sepsis could be caused by escaping of lipoproteins to the extravascular space, together with other serum proteins, due to a general increase in capillary permeability, because of general inflammatory processes. , Hypoalbuminemia, however, was not a constant findig in our patients. Recently, Cross et al. (1990) found abnormal cholesterol esterification and abnormal cholesterol metabolism in patients with adult respiratory distress syndrom (ARDS). Whether or not their patients got intralipid infusions or total parenteral nutrition, they showed lipid abnormalities similar to those of patients, not receiving them. May be, hepatobiliary dysfunction is the reason for decrease in cholesterol ester formation, but this is not known at present.

Decreased stability of PGI2 has been reported on basis of a defect (Sinzinger et al., 1985), in thrombotic thrombocytopenic purpura (Chen et al., 1981), in certain disease stages of diabetes (Sinzinger et al., 1985), in acute myocardial infarction (Sinzinger et al., 1987) and unstable angina pectoris (Aoyama et al., 1990). Recently, Yui et al. (Yui et al., 1988) identified the hitherto-unknown "prostacyclin stabilizing factor" as APO A1. The same group showed that the APO A1 level and PGI2-T/2 are markedly lower in patients with unstable angina pectoris or acute myocardial infarction (Aoyama et al., 1990).

In our patients a really good correlation was seen between TC and PGI2-T/2, LDL-C and PGI2-T/2 and APO A1 and PGI2-T/2 but, interestingly, not, between HDL-C and PGI2-T/2. It may well be the shortened PGI2-T/2 in end-stage sepsis and circulatory shock is due to a severe polyorganic failure together with severe catabolic condition. The mechanism, however, is far from being understood and data from a larger number of patients dying of circulatory shock secondary to sepsis or other reasons would be of interest.

REFERENCES:

Alvarez C., Ramos A.: Lipids, lipoproteins and apoproteins in serum during infection. Clin.Chem.1986;32:142-145.

Aoyama T., Yui Y., Morishita H., Kawai C.: Prostaglandin I2 half-life regulated by high density lipoprotein is decreased in acute myocardial infarction and unstable angina pectoris. Circulation 1990;81:1784-1791.

Chen Y.C.: Enhanced plasmatic degradation of prostacyclin in thrombotic thrombocytopenic purpura. Lancet 1981;i:372-375.

Chen Y.C., McLeod B., Hall E.R., Wu K.K.:Accelerated prostacyclin degradation in thrombotic thrombocytopenic purpura. Lancet 1981;ii:267-269.

Cross E.C., Forte T., Stocker R., Louie S., Yamamoto Y., Ames B.N., Frei B.: Oxidative stress and abnormal cholesterol metabolism in patients with adult respiratory distress syndrome. J.Lab.Clin.Med.1990;115:369-404.

Lefer A.M.: Prostacyclin, high density lipoproteins and myocardial ischemia. Circulation 1990;81:2013-2015.

Sinzinger H.,Fitscha P., Peskar B.A.: Defekte im Prostaglandinsystem. V. Vererbte (?) Störung des Prostacyclinabbaues im Plasma (Defekt Wien-Döbling). Wien Klin Wochenschr 1985;97:726-729.

Sinzinger H., Kaliman J, Fitscha P., Peskar B.A.: Beschleunigter Abbau von Prostacyclin im diabetischen Plasma - ein weiterer Faktor der Störung des Hämostasegleichgewichtes ? Wien Klin Wochenschr 1985;97:693.

Sinzinger H., Fitscha P., Tiso B.: Decreased stability of prostacyclin after myocardial infarction. Lancet 1987;ii:106.

Wu K.K., Hall E.R., Papp A.C.: Prostacyclin stabilizing factor deficiency in thrombotic thrombocytopenic purpura. Lancet 1982;i:460-461.

Wu K.K., Hall E.R., Rossi E.C., Papp A.C.: Serum prostacyclin binding defects in thrombotic thrombocytopenic purpura. J.Clin.Invest.1985;75:168-174.

Yui Y., Aoyama T., Morishita H., Takahashi M., Takatsu Y., Kawai C.: Serum prostacyclin stabilizing factor is identical to apolipoprotein A1 (Apo A1). A novel function of Apo A1. J.Clin. Invest.1988;82:803-807.

AAS 37
Prostaglandins in the
Cardiovascular System

ASSOCIATION BETWEEN TOTAL CHOLESTEROL AND PLASMA THROMBOXANE B_2 IN HUMAN ADULTS

J. Pető, K. Mihai, I. Joó[x], A. Makáry

Department of Pathology, Department of Pediatrics, County Hospital, Kecskemét, [x]Central Laboratory, Town Hospital, Kiskunfélegyháza, Hungary

SUMMARY: Apparently healthy adults were examined for their lipid and thromboxane parameters. The correlation between the levels of total cholesterol in serum and thromboxane B_2 /TXB_2/ in plasma was strong mainly in men ($p < 0.01$). However, the association between atherogenic index /AI/ and TXB_2 levels tended to be higher in women. The authors suggest that, in healthy adults, elevated cholesterol levels coexist with abnormalities in thromboxane metabolism.

INTRODUCTION

It is established that platelets play an important role in the pathogenesis of atherosclerosis. A number of recent studies suggest that hypercholesterolaemia is associated with platelet activation (Carvalho et al., 1974, Stuart et al., 1980).
As a part of our screening examinations, we have determined serum total cholesterol and plasma TXB_2 levels in healthy Hungarian adults. Differences of cholesterol-thromboxane relationship in males and females are shown.

MATERIALS AND METHODS

78 apparently healthy adults (41 females and 37 males, 19-74 years, mean 36.5±17.6 years) without any clinical symptoms of atherosclerosis were investigated for their cholesterol and TXB_2 levels. None of the controls were taken any medication since at least two weeks prior to investigation. Blood was collected by venepuncture after fasting overnight. Total cholesterol and HDL-cholesterol levels in serum were measured by enzymatic method (Sera-Pak, Reanal, Budapest). TXB_2 levels were measured from plasma containing 7.4×10^{-3} M EDTA and 2.8×10^{-6} M indomethacin. Acidified plasma was extracted on C18-reverse phase, and then the TXB_2 content was determined by radioimmunoassay using commercial kits (Institute of Isotopes, Budapest), detailed elsewhere (Pető et al., 1991).

Atherogenic index was calculated according to Klimov's formula: AI = (TC - HDL-C) / HDL-C. Statistical differences were assessed by Student's t-test. Correlation coefficients and equations were calculated by linear regression analysis.

RESULTS

Half of the volunteers were normocholestorolaemic, while the others (32 persons, 41 %) had cholesterol levels higher than 6.0 mmol/l. According to total cholesterol and AI, mean levels were lower in women, but the differences were not statistically significant (Table I). There were positive correlations between cholesterol and TXB_2 in both sexes (Fig.1). The relationship between AI and TXB_2 levels was strong only in females (Fig.2).

Table I. Concentrations (mean$\pm$SEM) of total cholesterol and TXB_2, and AI-es in males and females

	n	T-Ch (mmol/l)	TXB_2 (pg/ml)	AI
Males	37	6.2 ± 0.3 ^{xx}	265 ± 36	5.3 ± 0.4
Females	41	5.5 ± 0.3 ^{x}	276 ± 27	3.8 ± 0.3 ^{xx}
All	78	5.9 ± 0.2 ^{xx}	271 ± 22	4.5 ± 0.3 ^{xx}

Significant correlation with TXB_2 levels: ^{x} $p<0.05$, ^{xx} $p<0.01$

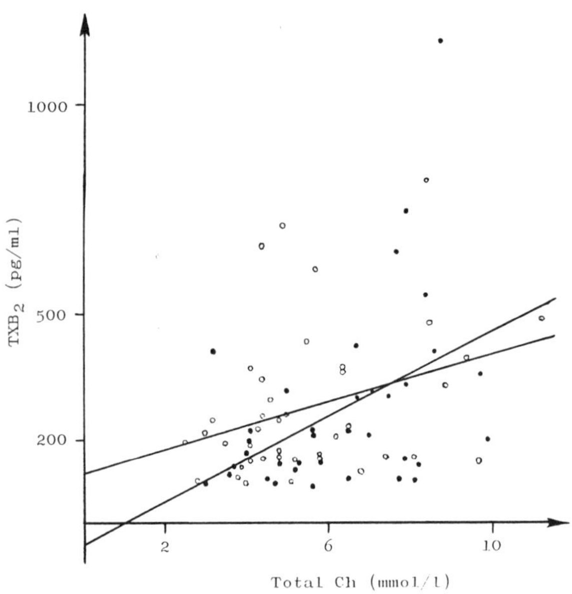

Fig.1. Correlation between total cholesterol and TXB_2 in healthy men (close circles) and women (open circles). Regression equations are: $y= 50.8\cdot x-51.7$, $r=0.438$, $p<0.01$ for males and $y= 28.1\cdot x+120.5$, $r=0.325$, $p<0.05$ for females.

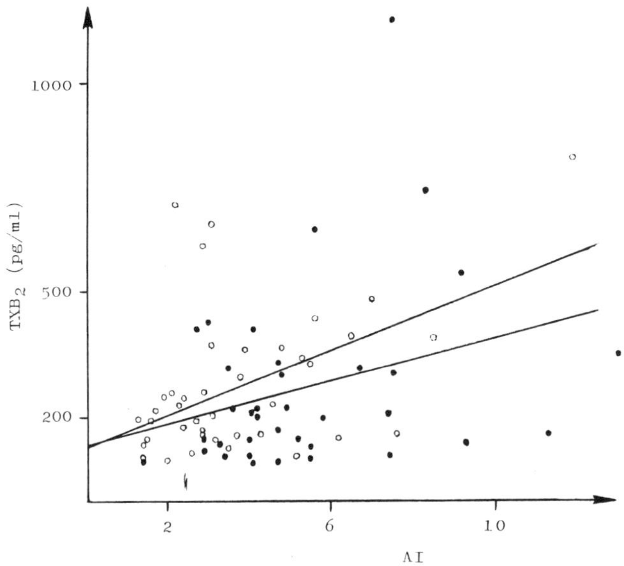

Fig.2. Correlation between AI and TXB_2 in men (closed circles) and women (open circles) / y= 25.4+129.6 , r= 0.294 for males and y= 38.7+127.1, r= 0.482, $p < 0.01$ for females/.

DISCUSSION

Although lipids have received most attention in relation to atherosclerosis, vessel wall injury, and as a consequence, platelet activation also has a role in the development of this process (Carvalho et al., 1974, Packham and Mustard, 1986). We have shown a strong positive correlation between the levels of total cholesterol and the metabolite of potent thrombocyte aggregator TXA_2. The relationship was stronger in men (Table I, Fig.1). However, the association between AI and TXB_2 levels proved to be higher in females (Fig.2).

These results are in accordance with studies suggesting association between blood lipids and prostaglandin metabolism (Stuart et al., 1980, Förster and Beitz, 1982). The higher correlation of AI and TXB_2, probably emphasizing the role of the protective HDL-cholesterol in women, needs further investigation.

CONCLUSION: The results show the appearance of disturbances in thromboxane metabolism with elevated cholesterol levels and/or atherogenic index in healthy human adults.

REFERENCES

Carvalho, A.C.A., Colman, R.W., Lees, R.S. (1974) Platelet function in hyperlipoproteinemia. N. Engl. J. Med. 290, 434-438.

Förster, W., Beitz, J. (1982) Regulation of the prostacyclin synthetase activity by lipids. Pharmacol. Res. Commun. 14, 227-240.

Packham, M.A., Mustard, J.F. (1986) The role of platelets in the development and complications of atherosclerosis. Semin. in Hematol. 1, 8-26.

Pető, J., Mihai, K., Makáry, A. (1991) Low level of prostacyclin as a risk of ischaemic heart disease. Int. J. Cardiol. 30, 237-239.

Stuart, M.J., Gerrard, J.M., White, J.G. (1980) Effect of cholesterol on production of thromboxane B_2 by platelets in vitro. N. Engl. J. Med. 302, 6-10.

AAS 37
Prostaglandins in the
Cardiovascular System

EFFECTS OF 9, 12, 15-OCTADECATRIEN-6-YNOIC ACID ON THE METABOLISM OF ARACHIDONIC ACID IN PLATELETS AND ON THE PLATELET AGGREGATION

M. Guichardant*, M. Michel, C. Borel, L. Fay, G. Crozier, D. Magnolato and P.A. Finot.
* to whom correspondence should be addressed
Nestec Ltd, Nestle Research Centre, Vers-chez-les-Blanc,
Post office Box 44 CH1000 Lausanne 26 Switzerland.

SUMMARY: An acetylenic fatty acid: 9,12,15-octadecatrien-6-ynoic acid (dicranin), extracted from Dicranum Scoparium was preincubated with platelets stimulated by exogenous arachidonic acid (20:4 n-6). Dicranin (10^{-4} M) weakly inhibited the cyclooxygenase activity as assessed by measurement of 12-hydroxy-heptadecatrienoic acid (HHT) In contrast, the 12-hydroxy-eicosatetraenoic acid (12-HETE) synthesized by the 12-lipoxygenase was strongly increased by about 650%. The same effects were observed with 10^{-6} M of dicranin but to a lesser extent.
The main platelet hydroxylated dicranin metabolite determined by GC-MS was a 13-hydroxy derivative
Platelet aggregation induced either by thrombin or by arachidonic acid or by U46619, an structural PGH_2 analogue was inhibited by 10^{-4} M of dicranin

INTRODUCTION

When platelets are aggregated by some of these agents, polyunsaturated fatty acids (PUFAs) are liberated from membrane phospholipids and metabolized via cyclooxygenase and/or lipoxygenase (1-3)
Some acetylenic analogues of PUFA(s) have already been investigated: 5,8,11-eicosatriynoic acid (ETY), 4,7,10,13-eicosatetraynoic and 5,8,11,14-heneicosatetraynoic acids (4-6). These acetylenic acids have specific inhibitory effect on lipoxygenase and a weak effect on cyclooxygenase. 5,8,11,14-eicosatetraynoic acid (ETYA) (7) inhibits both cyclooxygenase and lipoxygenase.

In these studies we used an acetylenic fatty acid which is found in several moss species (8, 9, 10) and have been extracted in our laboratory from the moss Dicranum Scoparium. This compound, which we have called "dicranin" is a 9,12,15-octadecatrien-6-ynoic acid and its effects on platelet aggregation and on cyclooxygenase and lipoxygenase activity is described.

MATERIALS AND METHODS

Reagents: 5,8,11,14-eicosatetraenoic acid (20:4 n-6) (arachidonic acid), 6,9,12,15-octadecatetraenoic acid (18:4 n-3) (stearidonic acid), thrombin were provided by Sigma Chemical Company (St Louis, MO, USA). [$1-^{14}C$] 5,8,11,14-20:4 was provided by Dupont-NEN products (Zürich, Switzerland). 12-OH-5,8,10-17:3 (HHT), 12-OH-5,8,11,14-20:4 (12-HETE) and 5,8,11,14-eicosatetra- ynoic acid (ETYA) were purchased from Cayman Chemical, (Ann Arbor, Mi, USA). Nova-Pak C18 4 μm column was obtained from Millipore AG, (Volketswil, Switzerland). α-Bromo-2,3,4,5,6-pentafluorotoluene and N,O-Bis-(trimethylsilyl)-trifluoroacetamide were from Fluka, (Buchs, Switzerland). The 13-hydroxy derivative of 18:2 (13-HODE) used as internal standard for the monohydroxylated fatty acid analysis was produced according to the method of Funk et al.(11).

Preparation of Dicranin: Dicranin was extracted and using CH_2Cl_2 from Dicranum Scoparium and purified by RP-HPLC as described elswhere (12).

Preparation of platelet suspension: Human platelet suspension was prepared according to the technique previously described (13).
For each assay, 5 ml of platelet suspension (300,000 platelets/mm^3) were preincubated with 10^{-4} M or 10^{-6} M of dicranin in ethanol or with ethanol alone for 10 min. They were then stimulated by 10 μM of arachidonic acid labelled with 3700 KBq of [1-^{14}C] 5,8,11,14-20:4.

Platelet aggregation studies: Aggregations were performed according to the technique of Born (14) using human thrombin, arachidonic acid or U46619, a structural analogue of PGH_2 as inducers. Platelets were preincubated with 10^{-4} M or 10^{-6} M of dicranin or with 10^{-6} M of its 13-OH-metabolite for 0, 10 or 20 min.

Monohydroxylated fatty acid analysis: Lipid extracts were separated on silica gel TLC plates with hexane/ diethyl ether/ acetic acid (60/40/1 by vol).The radioactive monohydroxylated fatty acids extracted with diethyl ether were analyzed by reversed-phase high performance chromatography (RP-HPLC) analysis. The eluent (methanol/water (pH 3 with acetic acid) (73/27 by vol)) was pumped at a flow rate of 1 ml/min. Monohydroxylated fatty acids, detected at λ = 234 nm were quantified by using the response of the internal standard(13-HODE).

Derivatization of the monohydroxylated fatty acids: Hydroxylated fatty acids were derivatized as pentafluorobenzyl esters hydrogenated or not and their hydroxy groups were derivatized to trimethylsilyl ether according to the technique previously described (15).

GC-MS of monohydroxylated fatty acids: A Hewlett Packard gas chromatograph was interfaced with a Finnigan MAT 8430/SS300 mass spectrometer (Finnigan MAT, Bremen, Germany). The column was a 30 m DB5 fused silica capillary column (J&W Sci) and helium was used as carrier gas. The oven temperature set at 160° C during 1 min was then raised to 250° C at 30° C/min, then to 310° C at 5° C/min. The temperature remained at 310° C for 2 min. Electron impact mass spectra were obtained with an electron impact source at 180 °C. The ionization energy was 70 eV and a mass range from 40 to 800 was scanned.

RESULTS

Monohydroxylated fatty acids synthesized: The platelets were preincubated or not with 10^{-4} and 10^{-6} M of dicranin and then stimulated by 10^{-5} M of 20:4 n-6 for 10 min. HHT and 12-HETE produced by the cyclooxygenase and the lipoxygenase, respectively were both isolated and quantified by HPLC (Fig.1) as described in "Methods".

Studies with exogenous radiolabelled arachidonic acid confirm that 12-HETE synthesis was markedly increased when platelets were preincubated with 10^{-4} M of dicranin. This molecule did not affect the cyclooxygenase end-product formation as shown by the HHT radioactivity which was unchanged with the dicranin (table I).

TABLE-I

Synthesis of HHT and 12-HETE from labelled arachidonic acid (20 μM) added to platelets. Results are expressed in percentage of the total radioactivity in the different lipid classes separated by TLC using the following solvent mixture: hexane/diethyl ether/acetic acid (60/40/1 by vol) as eluant.

	control	DICRANIN 10^{-4} M	DICRANIN 10^{-6} M
initial spot	11.61 ± 1.49	12.32 ± 0.85	11.71 ± 1.98
12-HHT	9.73 ± 1.33	9.92 ± 1.00	8.30 ± 1.49
12-HETE	6.66 ± 0.77	29.97 ± 2.42	6.82 ± 0.92
20:4 excess	69.32 ± 1.79	45.36 ± 3.01	70.27 ± 0.89

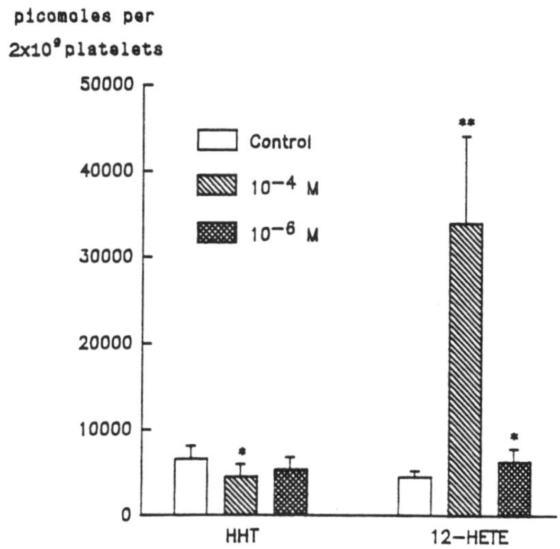

Figure 1. HHT and 12-HETE synthesized by platelets stimulated by 10^{-5} M 20:4 n-6. Results in picomoles per 2 x 10^9 platelets represent the mean ± standard deviation of 8 determinations. Standard paired t test shows statistical differences from the control (* $p < 0.05$ ** $p < 0.001$).

Moreover, when the platelets were preincubated with dicranin a cluster of unknown peaks, not present in the control, was observed. Its retention time indicates that these compounds were more polar than standard OH-18:4. Their uv spectra (results not shown) presented a λ maximum at 234 nm indicating a conjugated diene structure. The clump was resolved and four peaks called A, B, C, D (Fig.2) were analyzed by GC-MS.

Electron impact mass spectra of the hydrogenated form of pentafluorobenzyl ester (PFB)-trimethylsilyl ether (TMS) monohydroxy derivatives of polyunsaturated fatty acids exhibit two main fragments corresponding to the breakage on both sides of the OTMS and including the OTMS (16).

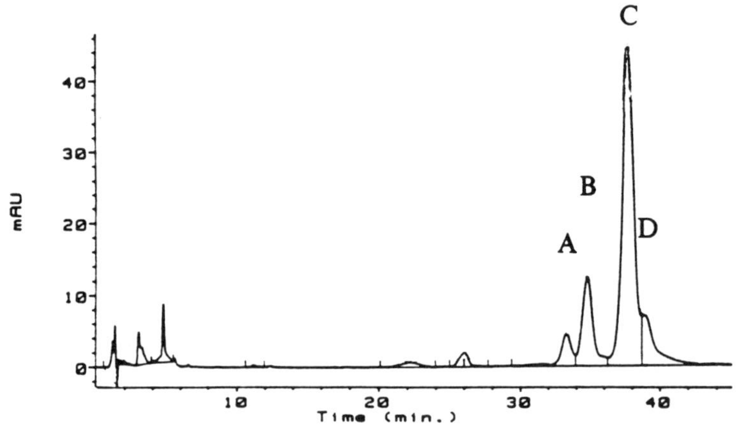

Figure 2: RP-HPLC profile of dicranin metabolites produced by stimulated platelets preincubated with 10^{-4} M of dicranin during 20 min. The eluant was methanol/water pH 3 with acetic acid (62/38 by vol).

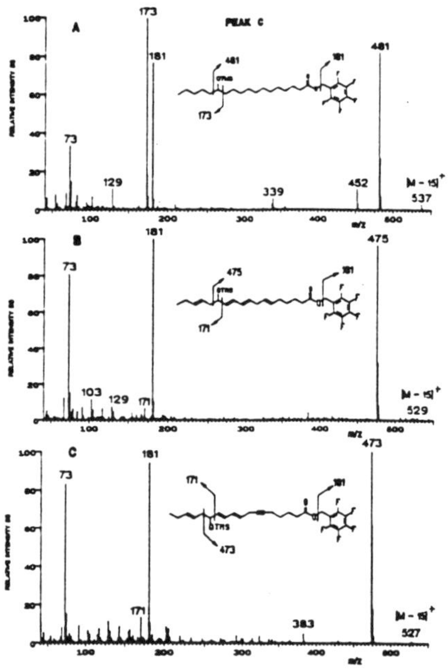

Figure 3: **A**: mass spectrum of compound eluted in the peak C (Fig.2) The molecule were derivatized to PFB-TMS and hydrogenated.

B: mass spectrum of standard 13-OH-18:4 derivatized to PFB-TMS but not hydrogenated.

C: typical mass spectrum of compound eluted in the peak C (Fig.2) derivatized to PFB-TMS and not hydrogenated.

The mass spectrum of the peak A presented two main ions at m/z = 131 and m/z= 523 which indicate the presence of a hydroxy group in position 16 (results not shown).

The mass spectrum of the peak B the ions m/z 187 and 467 revealed a hydroxyl group in position 12 (results not shown).

The mass spectra of the main peak C (figure 3a and 3c) presented two ions at m/z 173 and 481 for the hydrogenated form and m/171 and 473 for the non hydrogenated form, respectively indicating the presence of a 13-hydroxy group.Also their fragmentation indicated clearly that the acetylenic bond between the carbon 6 and 7 remained in these hydroxy derivatives (figure 3c).

The mass spectrum of peak D showed no characteristic ions due to the small amount of material recovered.

Platelet aggregation: (Fig.4). The aggregation of platelets stimulated by 0.1 U/ml of thrombin or by 5x 10^{-6} M of arachidonic acid was not altered by the presence of 10^{-4} M of dicranin unless the platelets had been preincubated.

When platelet were preincubated for 20 min with 10^{-4} M of dicranin aggregation fell from 68 % in the control to 44 %. A 10 min preincubation resulted only in a modification of the velocity of aggregation.

INDUCERS	CONTROL AGGREGATION		10 -4 M Dicranin AGGREGATION		13OH-Dicranin metabolite 10 -6 M AGGREGATION	
	%	VELOCITY	%	VELOCITY	%	VELOCITY
THROMBIN 0.1 U/ml						
without preincubation	65	1.23	70	1.23	58	0.85
10 min preincubation	70	2.11	69	1.52	58	0.85
20 min preincubation	68	1.25	44	0.42		
U46619 1 ug/ml						
without preincubation	66	1.41	0	0	65	1.22
20:4 n-6						
without preincubation	70	3.86	70	3.80		

Figure 4: Effects of 10^{-4} M of dicranin and of 10^{-6} M of 13-OH-dicranin on the platelet aggregation induced by 0.1 U/ml of thrombin or by 5 x 10^{-6} M of 20:4 n-6 or by 1 μg/ml of U-46619. Each value is the mean of two determinations. % represents the percentage of aggregation after 4 min of stimulation and the velocity is the initial slope of the aggregation.

When 1 μg/ml of U-46619 was used as inducer, the platelet aggregation was completely abolished in the presence of 10^{-4} M of dicranin preincubated or not.

The main dicranin metabolite (13-OH-dicranin), isolated was tested at 10^{-6} M with or without prior preincubation. The final aggregation induced by 0.1 U/ml of thrombin was sligthy inhibited and no inhibitory effect was also observed at this concentration when U-46619 was used as inducer.

DISCUSSION

Results show that dicranin preincubated with platelets at 10^{-6} M inhibited weakly the cyclooxygenase activity (HHT) by 18% and that at the same time the lipoxygenase activity (12-HETE) increased by 40 % (Fig 1). This increase was markedly enhanced at 10^{-4} M of dicranin (increase in 12-HETE by 654 %) whereas cyclooxygenase was inhibited only by 31 %. This result indicates that the 12-lipoxygenase activity potentiation was not due to a greater substrate availability resulting from the cyclooxygenase inhibition.

Dicranin was also metabolized by the platelets at 10^{-4} M and at 10^{-6} M . The metabolites were more polar than OH-18:4 (result not shown) and had a maximum UV absorbance at λ max 234 nm indicating the presence of an hydroxy fatty acid with a conjugated diene. The mass spectrum of the hydrogenated main compound (peak C) (figure 3A) showed the same retention time and the same fragmentation as a 13-OH-18:0 standard . The comparison between the mass spectrum of this compound non hydrogenated (figure 3C) and the 13-OH-18:4 standard non hydrogenated (figure 3B) indicated clearly that the acetylenic bond between the carbon 6 and 7 remained intact: m/z 475 for 13-OH-18:4 and 473 for 13-OH-18:3-6-ynoic acids, respectively. Also their fragments $[M-15]^+$ differs of 2 mass units). The ions m/z 171 and 473 for this main compound eluted in the peak C involved a hydroxy group in position 13.

Their origin has not yet been investigated using specific inhibitors but this last major compound has already been found in the moss (10).

Platelet aggregation induced by thrombin was inhibited by dicranin only when platelets were preincubated for 10 or 20 min, suggesting that the inhibitory effect was due to lipoxygenase metabolites. This inhibition can also be explained by the fact that dicranin strongly enhanced the 12-HETE synthesis. It is well established that 12-HETE can hinder platelet aggregation (17-18) by inhibiting the activity of thromboxane synthetase (19-20).

The inhibition of platelet aggregation induced by the U46619, in the presence of dicranin was complete. This suggests that dicranin could interact with the receptor site of the PGH_2. This effect seems to be irreversible because readditions of inducer (U46619) were not able to reverse the inhibition. (result not shown).

Dicranin has an original mecanism compared to the other well known acetylenic fatty acid described in the introduction.

CONCLUSION

Dicranin has a anti-aggregatory properties and potentiates the 12-HETE synthesis. More tests must be done to state the real role of dicranin "in vivo".

ACKNOWLEDGMENTS

The excellent technical assistance of Mrs Tavazzi-Schoenberger is gratefully acknowledged.

REFERENCES

1- Smith, J.B. (1980), in haemostasis and thrombosis Am. J. Pathol. **99**, 742-804.
2- Hamberg, M., Svensson, J. and Samuelsson, B. (1974), Proc. Natl. Acad. Sci. USA **71**, 3824-28.
3- Nugteren, D.H. (1975), Biochim. Biophys. Acta **380**, 299-307.
4- Evans, R.W., Sprecher, H. (1985), Prostaglandins **29**, 431-441.
5- Sun, F.F., McGuire, J.C., Morton, D.R., Pike, J.E., Sprecher, H. and Kunau, W.H. (1981), Prostaglandins, **21**, 333-343.
6- Kuehn, H., Schewe, T. and Rapoport, S.M. (1984), Biomed. Biochim. Acta **43**, 358-61.
7- Wihelm, T.E., Sankarappa, S.K., Van Rollins, M. and Sprecher H. (1981), Prostaglandins **21**, 323-332.
8- Jamieson, G.R. and Reid, E.H. (1976), Chemistry **15**, 1731-1734.
9- Andersson B., Andersson, W.H., Chigault, J.R., Ellison, E.C., Gellerman, J.L., Hawkins, J.H. and Schlenk H. (1974), Lipids, **9**, 506-511.
10-Ichikawa,T., Namikawa, M., Yamada, K., Sakai, K. and Kondo,K. (1983), Tetrahedron Letters, **24**, 3337-3340,
11-Funk, M., Issac, R., and Porter, N. (1976), Lipids **11**, 113-117.
12-Borel, C., Fernadez, I., Welti, D.H., Colmenarez, M. and Guichardant, M. (in preparation).
13-Lagarde, M., Bryon, P.A:, Guichardant, M. and Dechavanne, M. (1980), Thrombos. Res. **17**, 581 - 88.
14-Born, G.V.R. (1962), Nature **194**, 927 - 29.
15-Guichardant, M., Lagarde, M. (1985) Biochim. Biophys. Acta **836**, 210 - 214.
16-Rabinovitch, H. Durand, J. Rigaud,M., Mendy, F. and Breton, J.C. (1981), Lipids, **16**, 518-524.
17-Duthil, C.E., Haddeman, E., Don, J.A.and Ten Hoor, F. (1981), Prostaglandins, **6**, 111-126.
18-Aharony, D., Smith, J.B. and Silver, M.J. (1982), Biochem. Biophys Acta. **718**, 193-200.
19-Hammarstrom, S. and Falardeau, P. (1977),.Proc. Natl. Sci. USA **74**, 3691-3695,.
20-Croset M. and Lagarde M. (1983),. Biochim. Biophys. Res. Commun. **112**, 878-833.

AAS 37
Prostaglandins in the
Cardiovascular System

pH-DEPENDENT BINDING OF THE TXA_2/PGH_2-RECEPTOR OF HUMAN PLATELET MEMBRANES TO VARIOUS LIGANDS

J.G.W. Theis[+] H. Dellweg, E. Perzborn, and R. Groß

Institut für Herz/Kreislauf- und Artheroskleroseforschung, Bayer AG, Wuppertal, Germany; [+]Zentrum für Kinderheilkunde, Philipps-Universität, Marburg, Germany

SUMMARY: [^{3}H]-BAY U 3405 was used to characterize the pH-dependency of the binding of various ligands to the TXA_2/PGH_2-receptor of human platelet membranes.

Maximum binding of [^{3}H]-BAY U 3405 is achieved at pH 5.8. In inhibition studies the ligands Daltroban, CTA_2, and U 46619 also show a higher affinity at pH 5.8 compared to pH 7.4. In contrast, the ligands I-PTA-OH and GR 32191 have a higher affinity at pH 7.4. No difference is seen with SQ 29548.

The ligands I-PTA-OH, GR 32191, and SQ 29548 have a second protonable group in common, which is thought to be the reason for the different pH-dependent binding.

INTRODUCTION

Thromboxane A_2 (TXA_2) is thought to play a pathophysiological role in ischemic cerebro- and cardiovascular diseases, bronchial asthma, and shock. Therefore it is assumed that thromboxane A_2/prostaglandin H_2 (TXA_2/PGH_2)-receptor blocking drugs could have beneficial therapeutic effects in their treatment. (Lefer, 1985; Ogletree, 1987; Lefer and Darius, 1987).

Since many of these diseases are accompanied by significant local or systemic acidosis due to ischemia, blood stasis, or respiratory insufficiency, it is of special interest to investigate the role of pH upon the binding of the TXA2/PGH2-receptor to its natural or pharmacological ligands.

In this study [^{3}H]-BAY U 3405 (Perzborn et al., 1990; Pleiss et al., 1990) was used to characterize the pH-dependency of the binding of the TXA_2/PGH_2-receptor to the ligands depicted in Fig.3.

METHODS

In order to obtain sufficient quantities of platelet membranes, the membranes were prepared from platelets derived from buffy-coat. The buffy-coat resulted from preparation of human blood for transfusions. The blood, not older than 20 h, was centrifuged at 2500 g for 10 min at 10°C and the resulting buffy-coat, usually regarded as waste, was carefully collected. Each preparation of membranes was performed with buffy-coat separated from 40 l of whole human blood using a method modified from Barber and Jamieson (1970).

Binding studies were performed in Tris-NaCl-glucose buffer (50 mM Tris-HCl, 100 mM NaCl, 5 mM glucose, pH 7,4) or MES-NaCl buffer (50 mM MES, 100 mM NaCl, pH 5.8) at 37°C. Different concentrations of [^{3}H]-BAY U 3405 (7.9 Ci/mmol) and 50 µg of membrane protein were incubated for selected times in 250 µl or 1.2 ml (inhibition studies) of assay buffer. Non-specific binding was determined in the presence of a 1000-fold excess of non-labelled BAY U 3405. The binding reaction was terminated by addition of 4 ml of icecold washing buffer (Tris-NaCl-glucose buffer, pH 7.4, or citrat-NaCl buffer, pH 5.8), immediately followed by rapid filtration through Whatman GF/F glass fiber filters and subsequent washing with three times 4 ml of washing buffer. The content of radioactivity was counted in a Liquid Scintillation Counter.

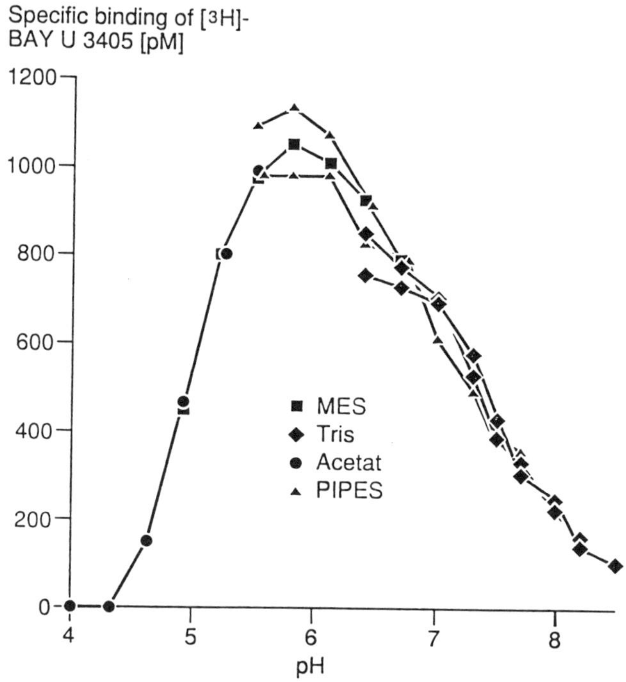

Figure 1: pH-dependency of the binding. 5 nM [^{3}H]-BAY U 3405 and 50 µg membrane protein were incubated for 60 min in 250 µl of the indicated buffer (each line represents one of 6 seperate experiments).

RESULTS

Maximum binding of [^{3}H]-BAY U 3405 to the TXA_2/PGH_2-receptor is achieved at a pH of 5.8 (Fig. 2). Near the physiologic pH-value even small pH-changes have a distinct influence upon receptor-binding.

Scatchard analysis of equilibrium binding studies at pH 7.4 and pH 5.8 (Fig. 3) reveals that the increase of [^{3}H]-BAY U 3405 binding is caused solely by an increase in affinity, the number of binding sites remains constant. At pH 7.4 the affinity constant K_d is 8.7 ± 3.8 nM (B_{max} = 6.6 ± 0.6 pmol/mg protein) compared to 1.2 ± 0.2 nM (B_{max} = 6.1 ± 0.6 pmol/mg protein) at pH 5.8.

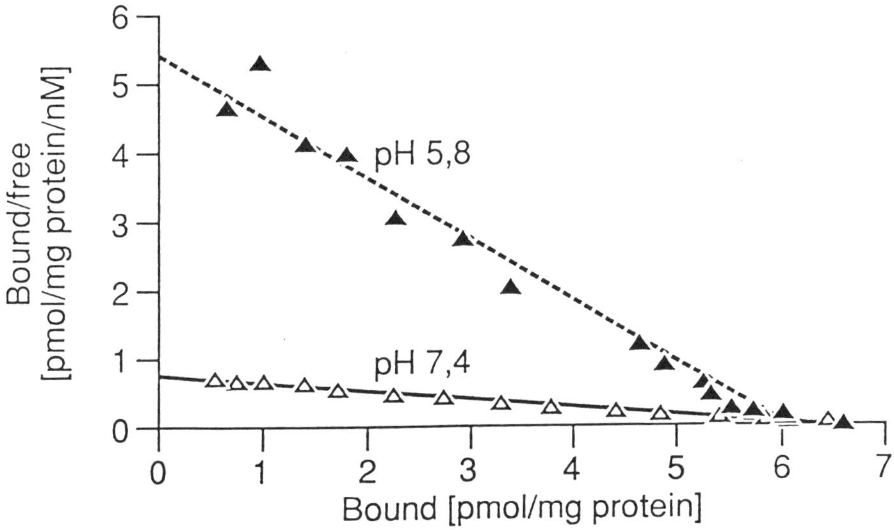

Figure 2: Scatchard plot of the specific binding data. 0.4 - 100 nM [^{3}H]-BAY U 3405 and 50 µg membrane protein were incubated for 60 min at pH 7.4 or for 30 min at pH 5.8.

In inhibition studies the antagonists BAY U 3405 and Daltroban and the agonists CTA_2 and U 46619 show significant higher affinities at pH 5.8 compared to pH 7.4. In contrast, I-PTA-OH and GR 32191 have a higher affinity at pH 7.4. No significant difference is seen with SQ 29548 (Fig. 3).

DISCUSSION

Possible reasons for the increased affinity under acid conditions are changes of the ligand, changes of the receptor, or an increased availability of ligand and/or receptor. The only change of [^{3}H]-BAY U 3405 upon acidification is an increase of the protonation of the α-carbonic acid group from 0.25% at pH 7.4 to 10% at pH 5.8 (pKa = 4.8 ± 0.1). However, studies involving the TXA_2/PGH_2-receptor-ligand [^{3}H]-S-145 and related molecules have shown that modification of the α-carboxyl group

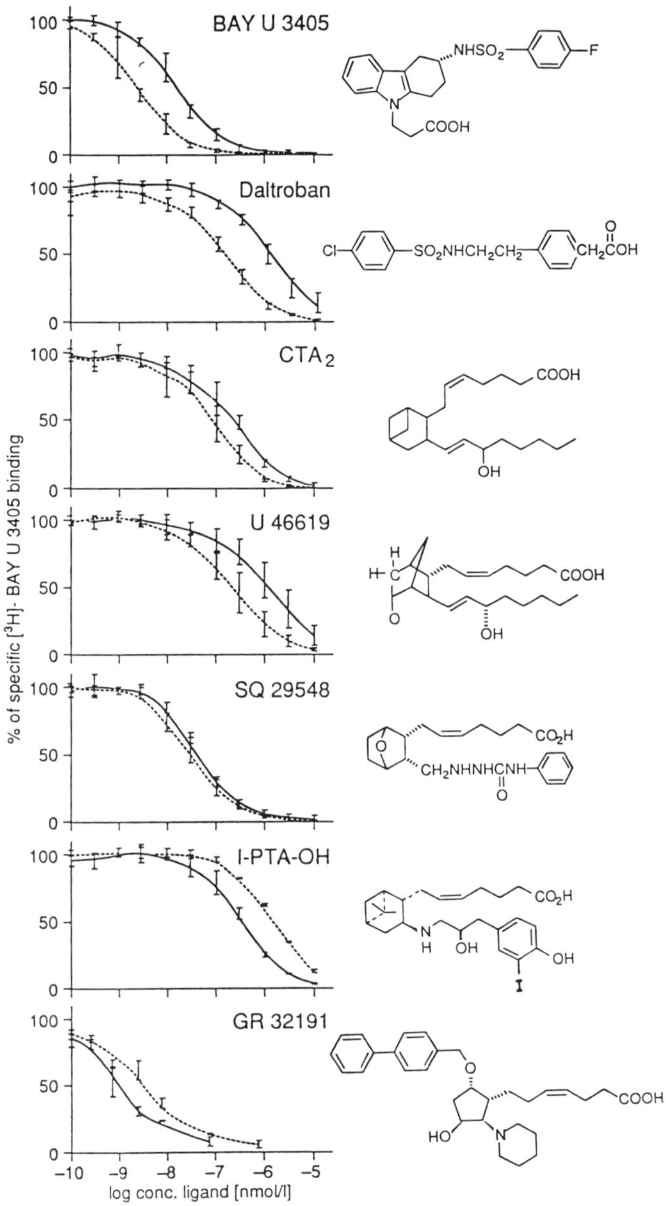

Figure 4: Inhibition curves of the non-labelled ligands. Increasing concentrations of non-labelled TXA_2-antagonists or TXA_2-agonists were incubated with 5 nM (pH 7.4) or 0.8 nM (pH 5.8) [^{3}H]-BAY U 3405 and 50 µg membrane protein under equilibrium conditions (n = 3 - 5).

does not play a major role in binding (Ushikubi et al., 1989). Although an increased availability of ligand and receptor caused by changes in membrane structure cannot be excluded, protonation of amino acid side chains of the receptor upon acidification are thought to be the most likely cause of the observed pH-dependency. These amino acid side chains are most likely histidine residues in the observed pH-range.

Significant differences exist between the pH-influence upon the affinity of the TXA_2/PGH_2-receptor to structurally different ligands. There is only one chemical moiety that is common to all ligands with similar or lower affinity under acid conditions: an alkaline group. Since TXA_2 and PGH_2 do not contain such an alkaline group, they are also thought to have a higher affinity under acid conditions.

These pH-dependent affinity changes may be important for the pathophysiological role of TXA_2 or for the potency of TXA_2-antagonists in local acidosis due to hypoxia or ischemia.

REFERENCES

Barber, A.J. and Jamieson, G.A. (1970). J. Biol. Chem. 245, 6357-6365.

Lefer, A.M. (1985). Federation Proc. 44, 275-280.

Lefer, A.M. and Darius H. (1987). Federation Proc. 46, 144-148

Ogletree, M.L. (1987). Federation Proc. 46, 133-138.

Perzborn, E., Fiedler, V.B., Seuter, F., Stasch, J.P., Weber, H., Sander, E., Böshagen, H., Rosentreter, U. (1990). Stroke 21 (12 Suppl), IV143-145.

Pleiss, U., Radke, M., Schmitt, I. (1990). J. Labelled Comp. Radiopharm. 28, 1081.

Ushikubi, F., Nakajima, M., Yamamoto, M., Ohtsu, K., Kimura, Y., Okuma, M., Uchito, M., Fujiwara, M., Narumija, S. (1989). Eicosanoids 2, 21-27.

AAS 37
Prostaglandins in the
Cardiovascular System

EFFECT OF BN 52256 AND OTHER MEDIATOR ANTAGONISTS ON OUABAIN-INDUCED VENTRICULAR FIBRILLATION IN SENSITIZED GUINEA-PIGS AND ON ISCHEMIA-INDUCED FIBRILLATION IN RATS

H.-J. Mest, T. Rein, A. Riedel, W. Köpernik and C. Brequet*

Department of Pharmacology and Toxicology, Martin Luther University , Halle 4020, Germany. * Institut Henri Beaufour, Le Plessis-Robinson, 92350, France.

SUMMARY: The threshold dose of ouabain necessary to induce ventricular fibrillation is decreased in sensitized guinea-pigs signalizing an enhanced arrhythmogenicity. Esculetine or WEB 2170 antagonists of histamine and PAF, respectively and especially a combination of both can increase the threshold dose of ouabain-induced fibrillation demonstrating an antiarrhythmic effect. BN 52256 a substance with multi-antagonistic properties shows antiarrhythmic effect in this method, too. WEB 2170 and BN 52256 decrease the incidence of ventricular fibrillation after coronary ligation in rats.

INTRODUCTION

In dependence on the pathophysiological situation different mediators are involved in the biochemical regulation of heart rhythm. Besides the importance of sympathetic and parasympathetic transmitters the involvement of eicosanoids in this regulation seems to be relevant (Mest et al., 1987; Parratt & Coker, 1985). In particular pathophysiological conditions further mediators could also be involved in this process. PAF, histamine and 5-HT might be responsible for cardiac arrhythmias during cardiac anaphylaxis (Koltai et al., 1986; Levi et al., 1984; Stewart & Piper, 1988). Antagonists of PAF induced antiarrhythmic effects if the arrhythmogenicity is enhanced by administration of PAF (Riedel et al., 1987; Riedel & Mest, 1987). The arrhythmogenicity of ouabain is enhanced in sensitized guinea-pigs induced by a release of different mediators. The purpose of the present paper was to test antagonists which seems to antagonize mediators released by anaphylaxis and by ischemia.

MATERIAL AND METHOS

Ouabain-induced cardiac arrhythmias in sensitized guinea-pigs: Guinea-pigs were actively sensitized by i.p. injection of 100 µg ovalbumin dispersed in 100 mg $Al(OH)_3$. After a 3-week-period responders and non-responders were separated by an ovalbumin inhalation test using an ultrasonic nebulizer.

The guinea-pigs were anaesthetized with urethane (1.4 g/kg). After 2 min. ovalbumin was administered for challenging and a continuous infusion of ouabain (10 µg/kg/min) was started to determine the threshold dose necessary to induce ventricular fibrillation. The substances used were given intravenously 2 min. before ouabain administration. ECG was recorded continuously until the death of the animals using Einthoven II lead. If it was not possible to induce ventricular fibrillation the threshold dose necessary to induce the death (asystolia) of animals was determined.

Coronary ligation in anaesthetized rats: After anaesthesia with 30 mg/kg pentobarbitone open chest rats were subjected to complete occlusion of left anterior descending coronary artery (LCAO). ECG was continuously recorded. The substances were given before LCAO occlusion. The incidence of ventricular fibrillation and the time until onset of fibrillation were recorded.

Drugs used: WEB 2170 (6-(2-chlorophenyl)-8,9-dihydro-1-methyl-8-(4-morpholinyl-carbonyl)-4H,7H-cyclopenta(4,5) thieno (3,2-f)(1,2,4)-triazolo-(4,3-a)(1,4)diazeoine; Boehringer Ingelheim, FRG), clemastine and ovalbumin (Sigma, St.Louis, USA), cyproheptadine (Serva, Heidelberg, FRG), BN 52256 (4,9-Dihydr-4-(1-methyl-4-piperidinylene)-10H-benzol 4,5 cyclohepta

1,2-b selenophen-10-one; IHB, Les Plessis Robinson, France), esculetine, propranolol and ouabain.
The results are expressed as means and S.E.M. and the incidence of fibrillation was expressed as % compared to animals in which carried out LCAO. Differences between groups are considered as significant when $p < 0.05$. Conservative Approximation of Newman-Keuls-test and Chi^2-test were used.

RESULTS

The threshold dose of ouabain necessary to induce ventricular fibrillation is 140 + 11 µg/kg in non-sensitized guinea-pigs. The threshold dose is decreased to 101 + 4 µg/kg signalizing an enhanced arrhythmogenicity. WEB 2170 (5 mg/kg), clemastine (5 mg/kg) and cyproheptadine (0.5 mg/kg) increase the threshold dose in sensitized guinea-pigs (Fig.1). A combination of WEB 2170 in the inactive dose (2 mg/kg) together with clemastine both in inactive doses (1 mg/kg and 0.1 mg/kg, respectively) induced antiarrhythmic effects (Fig.2). The same effect was received by a combination of WEB 2170 with cyproheptadine. In a further experiment BN 52256 induced an antiarrhythmic effect in a dose range of 20 and 80 µg/kg. In these experiments instead of fibrillation the threshold dose of ouabain for death (asystolia) was determined, because after pretreatment with BN 52256 it was not possible to induce ventricular fibrillation (Fig.3).

The onset of ventricular fibrillation after coronary ligation in rats was only delayed by propranolol. The incidence of ventricular fibrillation was 54 % after coronary ligation in rats. The standard antiarrhythmic propranolol reduced the incidence to 10 %. The PAF-antagonist WEB 2170 and the multi-antagonistic substance BN 52256 could also reduce the incidence of fibrillation in a statistically significant manner (Fig.4).

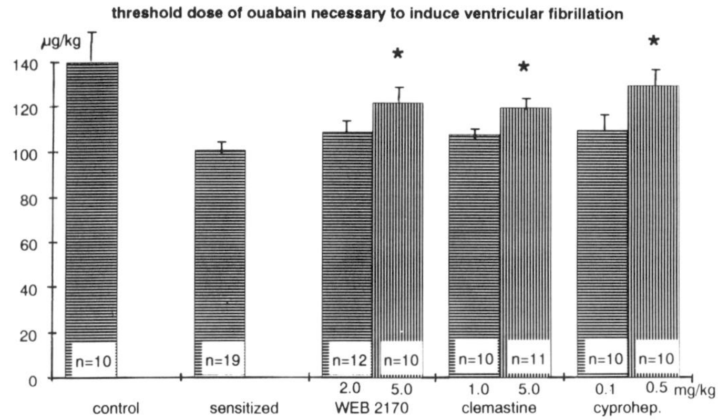

Fig. 1 The threshold dose for fibrillation in non-sensitized (control) and in sensitized guinea-pigs (sensitized) is shown. In the higher dose used WEB 2170, clemastine and cyproheptadine increase the threshold dose compared to the untreated group in sensitized guinea-pigs (* $p < 0.05$).

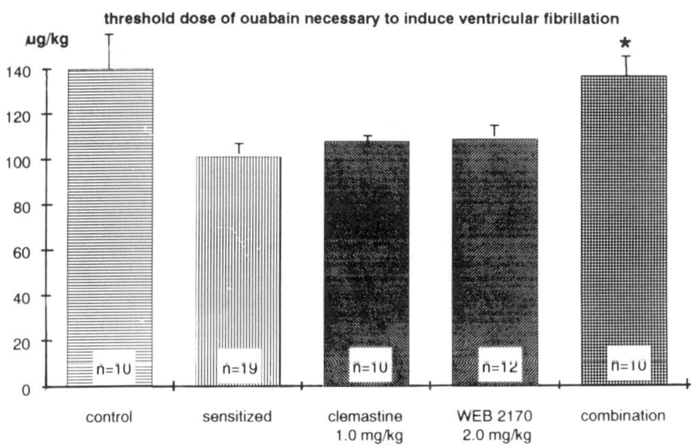

Fig. 2 A combination of WEB 2170 and clemastine both in inactive doses increases the threshold dose for ventricular fibrillation (further explanation see Fig.1).

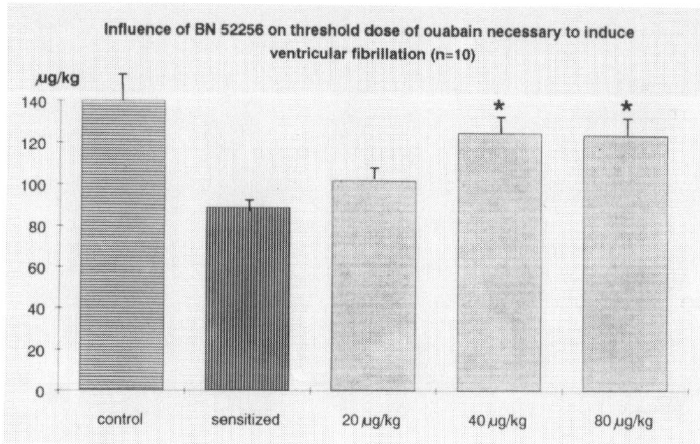

Fig. 3 BN 52256 increases the threshold dose of ouabain necessary to induce ventricular fibrillation in dose of 40 and 80 µg/kg (further explanation see Fig.1).

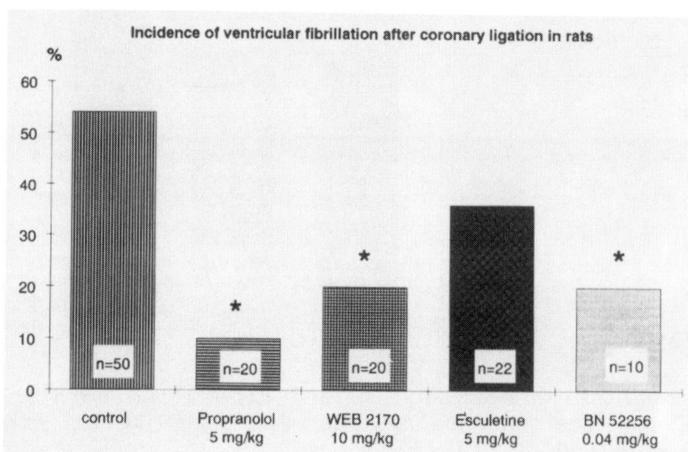

Fig. 4 The incidence of ventricular fibrillation after coronary ligation is reduced by propranolol, WEB 2170 and BN 52256 in a statistically significant manner (* $p < 0.05$).

DISCUSSION

The present results support the assumption that different mediators are involved in anaphylaxis-induced and ischemia-induced ventricular fibrillation. The anaphylactic heart is sensitized against arrhythmogenic stimuli. Different mediators released during anaphylaxis as PAF, histamine, 5-HT, thromboxane and leukotriene could be responsible for rhythm disturbances (Koltai et al., 1986, 1989; Riedel & Mest, 1987; Wainwright et al., 1989). On the other hand, PAF is able to release thromboxane (Ezra et al., 1985) and leukotriene (Voelkel et al., 1982). The involvement (mediators such as histamine and 5-HT are demonstrated in this study. The interaction of mediators seems to be important in dependence on pathophysiological situation. A combination of 2 or 3 different antagonists could be succesful for such kind of cardiac rhythm disturbances. In this study was demonstrated that a PAF-antagonist in combination with a antagonist of histamine induce much more succesful an antiarrhythmic effect in sensitized guinea-pigs as one substance alone. A novel concept is to develop drugs antagonizing various mediators. BN 52256 seems to possess inhibitory activities against H_1, H_2, $alpha_1$, $alpha_2$ and PAF receptors. The lower dose of BN 52256 necessary to induce antifibrillatoric effects has shown potent antiarryhthmic properties in such kind of arryhthmias. In general conclusion it seems necessary to looking for a new way to treat cardiac arrhythmias by influencing different mediators responsible for cardiac rhythm disturbances in specific pathophysiological situations.

REFERENCES

Ezra, D., Feuerstein, G., Ramwell, P. W., Hayes, E., and Goldstein R. E. (1985) Effects of platelet-activating factor on coronary venous plasma levels of TXB_2, 6-keto$PGF_{1}a$ and leukotriene C_4 immunoreacitity in the intact domestic heart. In: Neri, G.G., eds. Adv. Prostaglandin, Thromboxane and Leukotriene Res., New York, Raven Press, 19-21

Koltai, M., Lepran, I., Szekeres L., Viossat, I., Chabrier, E., and Braquet, P. (1986) Effect of BN 52021, as specific PAF- acether antagonist, on cardiac anaphylaxis in Langendorff hearts isolated from passively sensitized guinea-pigs. Eur. J. Pharmacol., 130, 133-136

Koltai, M. Tosaki, A., Hosford, D., and Braquet, P. (1989) Ginkgolide B protects isolated hearts against arrhythmias induced by ischemia but not reperfusion. Eur.J. Pharmacol., 164, 293-302

Levi, R., Burke, J.A., Guo, Z.G., Hattori, Y., Hoppens, C.M., Mc Manus, L.M., Hanahan, D.J.,and Pinckard, R.N. (1984) Acetyl glyceryl phosphorylcholine (AGEPC). A putative mediator of cardiac anaphylaxis in guinea-pig. Circ. Res., 54, 117-124

Mest, H.J., Riedel, A., and Schneider, S. (1987) Relevance of thromboxane/prostacyclin balance for cardiac rhythm disturbances. In: Prostaglandins in Clinical Research. Eds. Sinzinger, H., Schrör, K., Alan R. Liss, Inc., New York, 185-190

Parrat, J.R., Coker, S.J. (1985) Thromboxane, prostacyclin, and the severity of early ischemic and reperfusion arrhythmias - A review of the evidence. In: Prostaglandins and Other Eicosanoids in the Cardiovascular System. Ed. Schrör K.Karger, Basel, 172-182

Riedel, A., Braquet, P., and Mest, H.J., (1987) The effect of the specific PAF antagonist BN 52021 and the calcium blocker diltiazem on PAF-induced arrhythmogenicity. Pharmacol. Res. Comm., 19, 703-712

Riedel, A., Mest, H.J. (1987) The effect of PAF (platelet-activating factor) on experimental cardiac arrhythmias and its inhibition by substances influencing arachidonic acid metabolites. Prostagland. Leuk. Med., 28, 103-109

Steward, A.G., Piper, P.J. (1988) Platelet activating factor and the cardiovascular system involvement in cardiac anaphylaxis. In: Prog. in Biochem., Pharmacol. Ed. Paoletti R., Karger, Basel, 1988, 132-140

Voelkel, N., Worthen, J.T., Henson, P.M., and Murphy, R.C. (1982) Nonimmunologic production of leukotrienes induced by platelet-activating factor. Science, 218, 286-288

Wainwright, C.L., Parrat, J.R., and Bigaud, M. (1989) The effects of PAF antagonists on arrhythmias and platelets during acute myocardial ischaemia and reperfusion. Eur. Heart J., 10, 235-243

AAS 37
Prostaglandins in the
Cardiovascular System

INFLUENCE OF A CHOLESTEROL RICH DIET IN RABBITS ON THE FORMATION OF PGI_2 AND TXA_2

J. Beitz[a], A. Beitz[a], Ch. Giessler[a], P. Mentz[a], A.N. Orekhov[b], E.R. Andreeva[b], H.-J. Mest[a]

[a]Department of Pharmacology and Toxicology, Martin Luther University Halle-Wittenberg, P.O.Box 302, O-4010 Halle, FRG
[b]Cardiology Research Center, Academy of Medical Sciences USSR, Moscow

SUMMARY: In the study was investigated whether the formation of prostanoids is changed in the different regions of aorta or in clotting whole blood in dependence on development of atherosclerosis. For this question New Zealand rabbits were fed for different periods with a cholesterol rich diet (0.5 %). At the end of the different dietary periods the animals were killed and the following parameters estimated: blood: levels of total cholesterol, HDLcholesterol, VLDLcholesterol, cholesterol in the β-migrating lipoprotein fraction, serum lipid peroxides, TXB_2 formation capacity of clotting whole blood; aorta: surface of intima covered with fatty streaks, free and esterified cholesterol, triglycerides, collagen, formation of 6-keto-$PGF_{1\alpha}$ and TXB_2 by abdominal and thoracic aortas.
The lipid parameter demonstrated a relatively strong correlation with the duration of cholesterol rich diet or the macroscopically detectable atherosclerosis, but the prostanoid formation remained unchanged.

The pathogenesis of atherosclerosis is characterized by a multifactorial genesis. Two metabolic changes in early stages are serum dyslipoproteinemia and disturbances in the formation of prostanoids. Many studies of several groups have demonstrated the presence of close connections between both metabolic changes. The formation of PGI_2-like material was diminished (Duhault et al., 1981) and it of TXA_2 was increased at enhanced concentration of cholesterol (Stuart et al., 1982). As the result of it, the aggregability of platelets against ADP or epinephrine was enhanced

(Carvalho et al., 1974). Plasma levels of lipoproteins, influencing the intracellular concentration of cholesterol, are known to modulate the prostanoid formation (Beitz et al., 1986). But in literature are also published data describing a more complex figure, including the hypothesis of increased PGI_2 formation in early stages of atherosclerosis and decreased formation in later stages (Sinzinger et al., 1979) on one side and a normal or diminished formation of TXB_2 or platelet aggregation in hyperlipidemics (Fischer et al., 1984) on the other side. In the present study was investigated whether the formation of prostanoids are changed in different regions of aorta or in clotting blood in dependence on the development of atherosclerosis.

MATERIAL AND METHODS

50 adult New Zealand rabbits were acclimatized for 14 days at standard laboratory conditions (temperature: 21 ± 2 °C, humidity: 50 ± 10 %), a 12-h light/dark cycle, standard pellet diet and were individually cayed in stainless-steel wire bottomed cages. At the end of the acclimatization period the animals were subdivided into 5 groups randomly and kept on an atherogenic diet for different periods (see table I).

Table I: Duration of the treatment with standard pellet diet and atherogenic diet

		standard pellet diet	atherogenic diet
group 1	n=10	12 weeks	0 weeks
group 2	n=10	10 weeks	2 weeks
group 3	n=10	8 weeks	4 weeks
group 4	n=10	4 weeks	8 weeks
group 5	n=10	0 weeks	12 weeks

standard pellet diet: daily 40 g pellets + 0.5 ml olive oil/kg body weight; atherogenic diet: daily 40 g pellets + 0.2 g cholesterol + 0.5 ml olive oil/kg body weight (cholesterol was dispersed in olive oil and this dispersion was mixed with pellets. Water was provided at libitum.

At the end of dietary period animals were anesthetized with pentobarbital. The carotid artery was canulated and blood was taken for estimation of

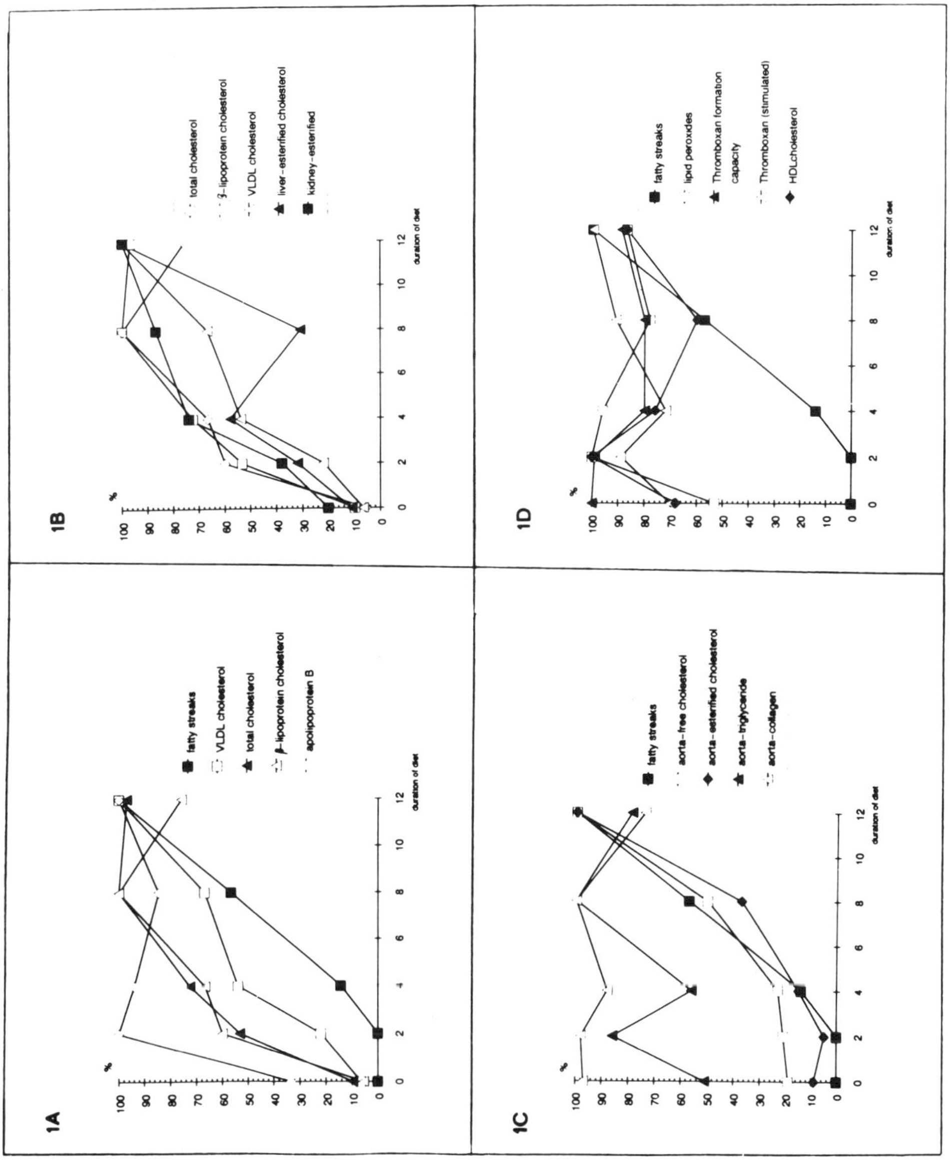

Fig. 1: Relative change (in % of the maximal value of individual parameter) of selected parameters of table II in dependence on duration of atherogenic diet (in weeks)

Table II: Modification of different parameters of blood, serum, liver, kidney and aorta in dependence of cholesterol rich diet in rabbits

	Duration of atherogenic diet				
	0 weeks	2 weeks	4 weeks	8 weeks	12 weeks
serum					
TC	73.6± 14.0	397.7± 96.0**	542.2± 97.0**	748.0± 68.0**	725.3± 44.0**
ß-LP	27.7± 12.0	295.8± 60.0**	329.2± 62.0**	493.2± 69.0**	374.6± 91.0**
VLDL	22.1± 10,0	73.7± 37.0	180.1±115.0*	224.1± 52.0**	334.4± 87.0**
HDL	28.8± 3.0	42.5± 5.0*	32.5± 6.0	25.4± 3.0	36.9± 7.0
apo B	1.5± 0.1	4.5± 0.5**	4.2± 0.2**	3.8± 0.3**	4.5± 0.2**
peroxides	41.0± 5.0	77.0± 8.0**	74.0± 8.0**	60.0± 5.0**	67.0± 6.0**
blood					
TXB_2 (basal)	357.0±161.0	352.0± 41.0	287.0± 64.0	284.0± 49.0	316.0± 37.0
TXB_2 (stimulated)	354.0±111.0	449.0± 92.0	364.0± 49.0	459.0± 47.0	506.0± 77.0
aorta					
fatty streaks	0 ± 0	0 ± 0	10.9± 5.1*	43.0± 7.9**	75.8± 9.0**
FC	7.7± 0.8	8.3± 2.4	8.9± 1.2	19.6± 3.5*	39.3± 6.6**
CE	7.3± 2.4	4.0± 1.6	12.3± 0.4*	31.0± 11.2**	82.7± 19.1**
TG	23.4± 2.4	39.5± 4.6	25.5± 2.6	45.8± 5.6*	36.3± 4.0
collagen	152.8± 2.4	154.1± 13.9	138.8± 10.1	157.0± 12.0	115.4± 9.6
6-keto-PGF_{1a} (a.a.)	453.0± 63.0	734.0±208.0	741.0±329.0	889.0±250.0	1036.0±531.0
6-keto-PGF_{1a} (a.t.)	454.0± 73.0	945.0±222.0	907.0±466.0	552.0±113.0	598.0±188.0
TXB_2 (a.a.)	8.5± 1.0	10.8± 5.3	14.5± 5.2	14.7± 3.7	16.8± 6.8
TXB_2 (a.t.)	4.7± 0.9	6.3± 2.4	4.9± 2.6	5.8± 1.2	4.2± 0.6
liver					
FC	3.1± 0.3	3.0± 0.3	4.3± 0.6	4.3± 0.8	4.1± 0.4*
CE	1.4± 0.3	4.1± 0.4**	7.5± 1.0**	10.1± 1.2**	13.0± 1.6**
kidney					
FC	2.9± 0.3	3.4± 0.1	3.5± 0.1**	3.4± 0.3*	3.8± 0.3*
CE	0.2± 0.1	0.4± 0.1*	0.8± 0.2**	0.9± 0.2**	1.1± 0.2**

thromboxane B_2 formation capacity according to Block et al. (1984); an other aliquot was used for preparation of serum and estimation of different classes of lipoproteins according to earlier published methods (Beitz et al., 1991), of apo B and serum lipid peroxides (Satoh et al., 1978). After collecting blood the animals were killed by an overdosage of anesthetic. The aortas were removed intact from the aortic arch to the iliac bifurcation, stripped of all adventitial delbris and cut lengthwise into two halves. One half of each aorta was used for estimation of per cent of intima covered with fatty streaks (Beetens et al., 1984), the other half was used for estimation of free and esterified cholesterol (FC + CE) according to the earlier described methods (Beitz et al., 1991), collagen and triglycerides (Orekhov et al., 1985). Additionally, segments of thoracic and abdominal aortas were incubated for 3 min at 37 °C in tyrode.

RESULTS AND DISCUSSION

As demonstrated in table II and Fig. 1 the increases in the serum lipoprotein values occur before the macroscopically detectable development of fatty steaks: The fastest increase was observed for the apolipoprotein B value, followed by an increase in total cholesterol (TC) and cholesterol in the β-migrating lipoprotein fraction (β-LP). The increse in the level of VLDLcholesterol (VLDL) reached the level of signifi-

Legend to table II: TC- total cholesterol (in mg/dl); β-LP-cholesterol in the β-migrating lipoprotein fraction (sum of β-VLDL, IDL and LDL) (mg/dl); VLDL- VLDLcholesterol (mg/dl); HDL- HDLcholesterol (mg/dl); apo B-apolipoprotein B (g/l); peroxides- serum lipid peroxides (nmol/ml); TXB_2-thromboxane B_2 formation capacity of clotting blood (ng/ml) with (stimulated) and without (basal) addition of exogenous thrombin (20 U/ml); fatty streaks- area of intima covered with fatty streaks (% of total surface); FC- free cholesterol (mg/g fresh weight); CE- esterified cholesterol (mg/g fresh weight); TG- triglycerides (mg/g fresh weight); collagen- collagen (mg/g fresh weight); a.a.- prostanoid formed by abdominal aorta (pg/mg fresh weight); a.t.- prostanoid formed by thoracic aorta (pg/mg fresh weight).

* $P < 0.05$ in comparison to the value after 0 weeks atherogenic diet

** $P < 0.01$ in comparison to the value after 0 weeks atherogenic diet

cance not before 4 weeks of cholesterol rich diet (Fig. 1A). The increase in the level of serum lipid peroxides was within the first two weeks of cholesterol rich diet, HDLcholesterol was enhanced only after 2 weeks of cholesterol rich diet and the TXB_2 formation capacity remained unchanged during the whole dietary period (Fig. 1B). The changes in serum cholesterol levels in the individual lipoprotein classes correlate with the increases of esterified cholesterol (CE) in different organs: increase in TC or β-LP with CE of kidney; increase in VLDL with it of CE of liver (Fig. 1C); and development of fatty streaks with the increase in the level of CE in the aorta (Fig. 1D). The levels of triglycerides and collagen in the aorta remained unchanged (Tab. 2 or Fig. 1D). The prostanoid formation by the aorta was not statistically significantly changed in dependence on duration of diet, only for the formation of 6-keto-PGF_{1a} and TXB_2 by the abdominal aorta a similar tendency was demonstrated for an increased formation after 12 weeks of cholesterol rich diet compared with it before diet (table II). Beetens et al. (1984) have investigated the same question by feeding rabbits a cholesterol rich diet for different periods. They found an increased PGI_2 formation after 2 weeks of cholesterol rich diet and a diminished PGI_2 formation after longer duration of cholesterol rich diet. The results of our study contradict this result, but support earlier published data (Beitz et al., 1990). As in the study of Beetens et al. (1984) the lipid parameters demonstrated a relatively strong correlation with the duration of diet or the macroscopically detectable atherosclerosis, but the prostanoid formation remained unchanged under our experimental conditions. Neither the TXB_2 formation capacity of clotting whole blood nor the PGI_2 or TXB_2 synthesis by the aorta correlated with the measured lipid parameters of blood, aorta or other organs under our experimental conditions.

ACKNOWLEDGEMENT

We gratefully acknowledge the technical assistance of Mrs. I.Adler and R.Rappold. The study was partially supported by a grant of Deutsche Forschungsgemeinschaft.

REFERENCES

Beetens, J.R., Coene, M.-C., Verheyen, A., Zonnekeyn, L., and Herman, A.G. (1984) Influence of vitamin C on the metabolism of arachidonic acid and the development of aortic lesions during experimental atherosclerosis in rabbits. Biomed. Biochim. Acta 43, S273-S276

Beitz, J., Block, H.-U., Beitz, A., Müller, G., Winkler, L., Dargel, R., Mest, H.-J. (1986) Endogenous lipoproteins modify the thromboxane formation capacity of platelets. Atherosclerosis 60, 95-99

Beitz, J., Kuklinski, B., Beitz, A., Taube, Ch., Oswald, B., Szymanski, Ch., Rath, F.W., Mest, H.-J. (1990) Influence of high density lipoproptein (HDL), prepared from human blood, on prostanoid formation, serum and tissue lipids and development of atherosclerosis in cholesterol fed rabbits. Prostaglandins Leukotrienes and Essential Fatty Acids 40, 211-215

Beitz, J., Beitz, A., Pawelski, K., Szymanski, Ch., Rath, F.W.,and Mest, H.-J. (1991) Influence of the trapidil derivative AR 12463 on serum and tissue lipids and development of aortic lesions during experimental atherosclerosis in rabbits. Biomed. Biochim. Acta 50, 101-107

Block, H.-U., Sziegoleit, W., and Mest, H.-J. (1984) Estimation of thromboxane B_2 in clotting human whole blood by gas chromatography. Biomed. Biochim. Acta 43, S385-S388

Carvalho, A.C.A., Colman, R.W., and Lees, R.S. (1974) Platelet function in hyperlipidemia. N. Engl. J. Med. 290, 434-438

Duhault, J., Lonchampt, M., Anstett, M., Saint-Dizier, D., and Saint-Romas, D. (1981) An inverse correlation between aortic prostacyclin like material and plasma lipids. IRCS Medical Science 9, 423

Fischer, S., Honigmann, G., Hora, C., Schimke, E., Beitz, J., Hanefeld, M., Leonhardt, W., Haller, H., Förster, W., and Schliack, V. (1984) Ergebnisse einer Leinöl- bzw. Olivenöldiät bei hyperlipidämischen Patienten. Dt. Z. Verdau- Stoffwechselkr. 44, 245-251

Orekhov, A.N., Tertov, V.V., Novikov, I.D., Krushinsky, A.V., Andreeva, E.R., Lankin, V.Z., and Smirnov, V.N. (1985) Lipids in cells of athero-sclerotic and uninvolved human aorta. I. Lipid composition of aortic tissue and enzyme isolated and cultured cells. Exp. Mol. Pathol. 42, 117-137

Satoh, K. (1978) Serum lipid peroxide in cerebrovascular disorders determinated by a new colorimetric method. Clin. Chim. Acta 90, 37-43

Sinzinger, H., Clopath, P., Silberbauer, K., and Auerswald, W. (1979) Prostacyclin synthesis in human and experimental atherosclerosis. Atherosclerosis 34, 345-347

Stuart, M.J., Gerrard, J.M., and White, J.G. (1982) Effect of cholesterol on production of thromboxane B_2 by platelets in vivo. N. Engl. J. Med. 302, 6-10

AAS 37
Prostaglandins in the
Cardiovascular System

CONCOMITANT ASPIRIN TREATMENT ABOLISHES THE ANTIATHEROSCLEROTIC EFFECTS OF THE CALCIUM CHANNEL BLOCKER ISRADIPINE MEDIATED BY PGI_2

Ch. Pirich, *Graziana Lupattelli, Irene Virgolini, ***A.Keiler, A. Gerakakis, #P. Angelberger, and H.Sinzinger

Wilhelm-Auerswald Atherosclerosis Research Group (ASF) Vienna, and Atherosclerosis Research Group of the Austrian Academy of Sciences (ATK), Vienna; *2nd Department of Medicine, Policlinic Monteluce, University of Perugia, Italy; ** Department of Surgery , Hospital Ried; and # Chemical Institute, Research Center Seibersdorf, Austria

SUMMARY: 108 male rabbits, aged 6 months, with experimental hypercholesterolemia and experimental abdominal aortic lesioning received different regimen of antiatherosclerotic treatment; 36 of them were treated with isradipine, a dihydropyridine calcium antagonist (0.3 mg/kg/daily), 36 with isradipine in combination with aspirin whereas 36 animals received placebo. The entry of 125I-radiolabelled LDL into the aorta was demonstrated to be significantly diminished in isradipine-treated rabbits as well as positive Sudan-III-staining and aortic cholesterol content were in comparison to placebo. This benefit was almost completely abolished by concomitant aspirin-treatment. The notable increase in vascular prostacyclin (PGI2) is supposed to mediate the strong antiatherosclerotic effect of isradipine resulting in an inhibition of LDL-entry and vascular cholesterol accumulation. Aspirin almost totally blocked the raise in PGI2-synthesis by the inhibition of cyclooxygenase detected in isradipine-treated animals. It can be concluded, that aspirin-treatment may minimize the antiatherosclerotic actions of calcium antagonists which are mediated by the PG-system.

INTRODUCTION

Lipid infiltration, i.e. the entry of cholesterol-rich lipoproteins into the arterial wall is one of the key-events in atherogenesis [12]. Thereby, calcium seems to mediate the pathogenetic effects of cholesterol accumulation, leading to cellular death [2]. Calcium channel blockers have been proven to inhibit this process independently of their antihypertensive effects, acting by the stimulation of PGI2-synthesis; PGI2, like PGE1, is known to decrease LDL-influx into the arterial wall [13]. This study aimed to assess, whether the antiatherogenic efficacy of isradipine, a calcium channel blocker of the dihydropyridine family which stimulates PGI2-synthesis the most [15] is inhibited in hypercholesterolemic rabbits by aspirin.

MATERIAL AND METHODS

Isolation and radiolabelling of LDL: LDL were isolated from fresh human plasma through immunoaffinity chromatography [14]. 10 mg LDL/ml were radiolabelled with iodine 125 using the iodine monochloride technique [9]. Labelling was performed shortly before i.v.-injection to the rabbits. In the meanwhile LDL was stored in dialysis buffer. TCA-precipitation and cellulose acetate paper electrophoresis revealed radiochemical purity.

Prostacyclin formation: Prostacyclin formation was assessed after immediate incubation of tissue samples for 3 min in 300 μl buffer (pH 7.4) at 22°C, using the platelet aggregation bioassay [11]. The inhibition of ADP (1 μM)-induced aggregation in 600 μl platelet-rich plasma (PRP) samples by 100 μl incubation buffer was quantified by means of a synthetic PGI2-standard (The Upjohn Company, Kalamazoo, MI, USA). The tissue wet weight (mg) was estimated thereafter. Values are given in picograms of in vitro synthetized PGI2 per milligram vascular tissue per minute.

Morphological control: The abdominal aorta was removed, segments were fixed in 3.5% phosphate-buffered glutaraldehyde (pH 7.4) and morphologically controlled as to the presence of normal endothelial lining, re- or deendothelialization. In some samples Sudan III-surface staining was performed.

Radioactive counting: Vascular segments punched out were counted in a gamma counter (Packard Instrument Company, Downers Grove, IL,USA)

Experimental studies: In 6-months old male rabbits (n = 108) the abdominal aorta was abraded by a Fogarty catheter [5,10]. A 1% cholesterol-supplemented diet was fed for the following 4 weeks. During this time 36 rabbits were treated with isradipine (0.3 mg/kg/day) alone, another 36 rabbits in combination with aspirin (5mg/kg/day), while 36 rabbits received placebo (isotonic NaCl solution). Drug therapy did not alter food consumption and thus cholesterol intake. After the treatment-period all the animals were injected with 10 μCi 125I-LDL, 1, 3, 6, 12, 24 and 48 hours, respectively after application of radiolabeled LDL 6 animals of each group were killed.

Evaluation of LDL-entry into the abdominal aorta: Morphological examination (including Sudan III-staining) and radioactive counting of the vascular tissue activity per surface area were performed in endo-, de- and reendothelialized segments.

Aortic cholesterol content: Excised vascular specimen were cleaned in ice-cold tris-HCl-buffer. The cholesterol content of the aortic samples was determined after extraction according to Folch [2]. 3H-cholesterol standard was used to control the efficiency of lipid extraction. Cholesterol was estimated with a photometric method (CHOD-PAP reaction, Boehringer Mannheim, Germany); for protein-estimation the Lowry method was used [8].

Statistical analysis: Values are presented as $\bar{x} \pm$ SD. Calculation for significance was performed by Student's t-test for paired data.

RESULTS

Cholesterol feeding induced significant atherosclerotic lesions, even in the non-ballooned thoracic aortic segment (figure 1).

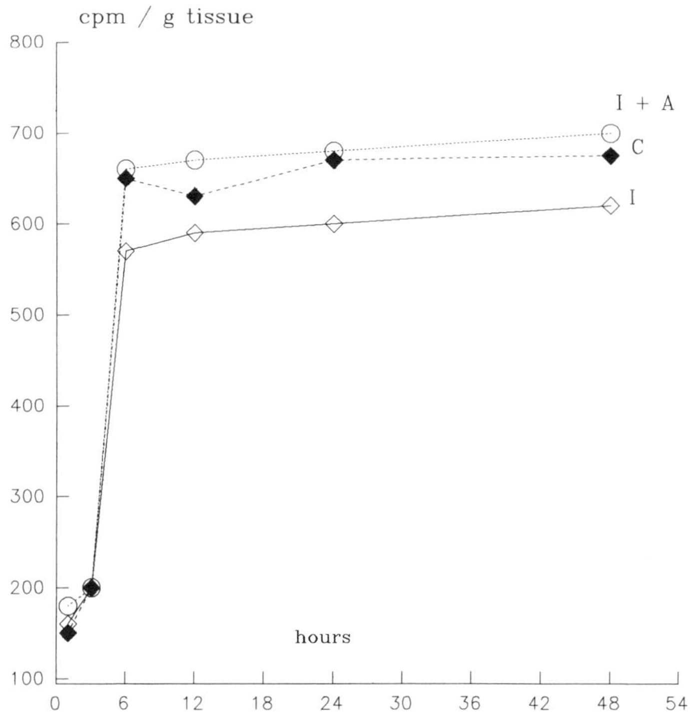

Sudan III-positive surface was significantly smaller in the isradipine treated animals ($p < 0.01$) as compared to controls receiving placebo, but this benefit was almost completely abolished in the group with the combined isradipine-aspirin regimen (table I). Isradipine-treated rabbits showed a significantly lower vascular cholesterol wall content than the placebo group, too . This effect was also reduced by aspirin (table I).

table 1 **Aortic lipid content**

		Sudan III positive areas (% surface)	Cholesterin content (mg/g protein)
TA	I	30 ± 8	27.13 ± 2.80
	I + A	43 ± 6	34.97 ± 4.63
	Co	71 ± 7	44.60 ± 3.27
AA	I	31 ± 6	26.57 ± 3.94
	I + A	40 ± 9	33.02 ± 5.17
	Co	67 ± 8	41.40 ± 4.35

values are given in: $\bar{x}$ ± SD;
I...isradipine; A...asperin; C...controll; TA...thoracic aorta; AA...abdominal aorta

Morphological classification of the endothelial lining was performed. In endothelialized segments the uptake of 125I-LDL by the abdominal aorta was continuously increasing after an initial peak at 6 hours with a maximum at 48 hours after radiotracer injection, the total uptake, however was very low Isradipine-treatment slightly decreased 125I-LDL-uptake, an effect which was completely abolished by aspirin (figure 2).

Deendothelialized segments demonstrated the highest uptake of 125I-LDL into the rabbit aortic wall. They showed a significantly higher ($p < 0.0001$) peak maximum, reached at 12 hours after injection. Isradipine-treatment significantly ($p < 0.001$ to 0.0001) reduced the 125I-LDL-uptake at all the time intervals investigated. This effect was completely abolished by aspirin, too (figure 3).

In reendothelialized segments, the uptake of 125I-LDL was continuously increasing with time, the extent of retention and maximum were significantly ($p < 0.01$ to 0.001) higher. Isradipine-treatment significantly reduced the tracer-uptake, whereas aspirin abolished this effect, with the exception of the 48 hours control interval (figure 4).

Prostacyclin formation, cholesterol content: The vascular PGI2-production in vitro was most pronounced for segments with intact endothelial lining and lowest in deendothelialized areas (table 2). In the isradipine treated group, the PGI2-synthesis in vitro generally was higher than in controls. Aspirin almost totally suppressed PGI2-synthesis. The reduction in cholesterol-content of the abdominal aorta which could be detected after isradipine-treatment was reversed again by aspirin (see table 1).

table 2 Aortic PGI2-generation in vitro (pg PGI2/mg/min)

		I	I + A	Co
TA	E	19.83 ± 2.80	<1*	17.21 ± 4.06
	D	14.61 ± 2.35	<1*	13.02 ± 2.24
	R	19.17 ± 3.60*	<1*	15.36 ± 2.57
AA	E	22.87 ± 4.01*	<1*	18.34 ± 3.21
	D	15.88 ± 3.57	<1*	14.57 ± 3.17
	R	20.85 ± 3.41*	<1*	16.19 ± 3.07

*...p < 0.01 (vs. control)

E...endothelialized;D...deendothelialized;R...reendothelialized

figure 2) Kinetic curve of LDL-entry into rabbit aorta. Isradipine-treated segments show a lower LDL-entry in endothelialized segments.

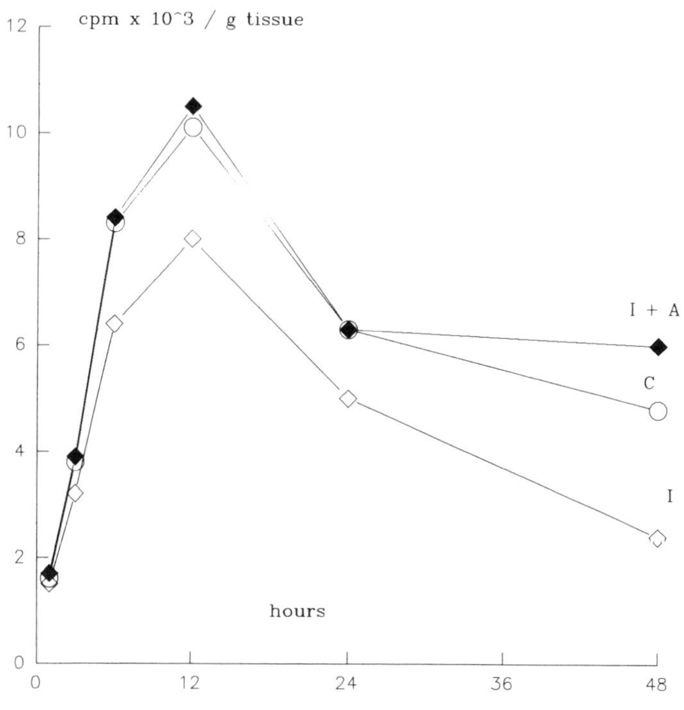

figure 3) The vascular LDL-entry kinetics demonstrate a higher peak maximum in deendothelialized segments than endo- or reendothelialized segments do. Concomitant aspirin treatment abolishes significantly ($p < 0.01 - 0.0001$) the effect induced by isradipine alone.

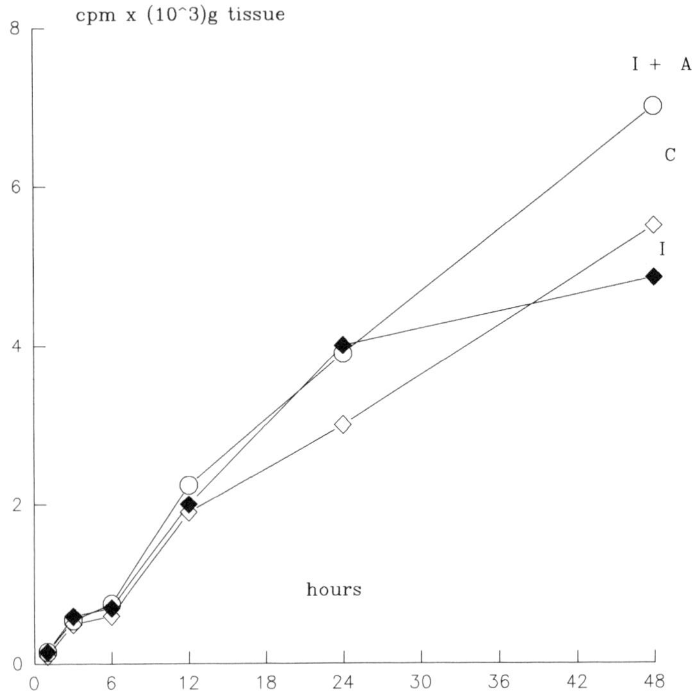

figure 4) Reendothelialized segments show a continous time-dependent increasing uptake. Aspirin together with isradipine significantly ($p < 0.01-0.0001$) abolishs the benificial effect of isradipine alone.

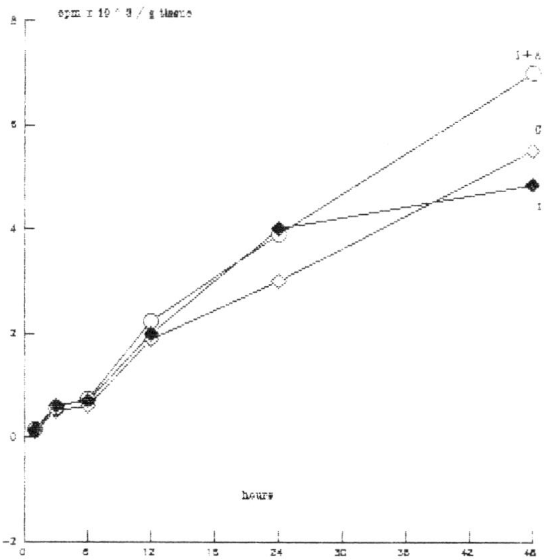

DISCUSSION

These results clearly demonstrate the beneficial effect of the calcium channel blocker isradipine in experimental endothelial injury in rabbit abdominal aortic wall by reducing LDL-entry as well as cholesterol accumulation. Isradipine, one of the most potent PGI2-stimulators among the calcium antagonists [15] strongly enhances vascular PGI2-formation which might be the mediator of the antiatherosclerotic properties reported for this substance class [4,5,7]. Thereby, the local release of PGI2 may change proliferative activity e.g. depression of platelet-derived growth factor (PDGF) liberation, decrease cholesterol esterification and accelerate its mobilization from the arterial wall. Calcium channel blockers may inhibit the deleterious necrosis of foam cells, too. They prevent the cell membrane from lipid-overloading by the blockade of transmembrane calcium movements [6]. The beneficial effect of isradipine concerning LDL-entry as well as cholesterol content is almost completely abolished by a concurrent aspirin therapy, inhibiting the synthesis of the suggested key substance PGI2 by the blockade of cyclooxygenase. There is need for validation of these experimental findings by appropriate clinical studies in humans.

LITERATURE

1 Blumlein SL, Sievers R, Kidd P, Parmley WW (1984). Mechanism of protection from atherosclerosis by verapamil in the cholesterol-fed rabbit. Am J Cardiol 54: 884-889

2 Folch J, Lees M, Stanley HS (1957) A simple method for the isolation and purification of total lipids from animal tissues. J Biol Chemistry 226: 497-509

3 Gleason MM, Medow MS, Tulenko TN (1989). Excess cholesterol alters calcium flux and membrane fluidity in cultured arterial smooth muscle cells. Circulation 80: 63

4 Habib JB, Bosaller C, Wells D, Williams C, Morisett JD, Henry PD (1986) Preservation of endothelium-dependent vascular relaxation in cholesterol-fed rabbits by treatment with the calcium channel blocker PN 200-110. Circ Res 58: 305-309

5 Handley DA, Van Volen RG, Melden MK, Saunders RN (1986) Suppression of rat carotid lesion development by the calcium channel blocker PN 200-110. Amer J Pathol 124: 88-93

6 Henry D, Bentley KI (1981) Suppression of atherogenesis in cholesterol-fed rabbit treated with nifedipine. J Clin Invest 68: 1366-1369

7 Jackson CL, Bush RC, Bowyer DE (1989) Mechanism of antiatherogenic action of calcium antagonists. Atherosclerosis 80: 17-26

8 Lowry OH, Rosenbrough NJ, Farr AL, Randall RJ (1951) Protein measurement with the Folin phenol reagent. J Biol Chem 193: 265-275

9 McFarlane AS (1958) Efficient trace labelling of proteins with iodine. Nature 182: 53-57

10 Nait M, Kuzuya F, Asai K, Shibata K, Yoshimina N (1984) Ineffectiveness of Ca-antagonists nicardipine and diltiazem on experimental atherosclerosis in cholesterol-fed rabbits. Atherosclerosis 51: 343-350

11 Sinzinger H, Firbas W, Cromwell M (1982) Alterations in rabbit aortic prostacyclin formation. Prostaglandins 24: 323-329

12 Anitschkow N (1933) Experimental arteriosclerosis in animals. In: Cowdry EC (ed) Arteriosclerosis. McMillan, New York, pp 271-322

13 Smith DL, Willis AL, Mahmud I (1984) Eicosanoid effects on cell proliferation in vitro-relevance to atherosclerosis. Prostgl Leukotr Med 16:10-16

14 Virgolini I, Angelberger P, Lupattelli G, Li SR, Banyai M, Pidlich J, Sinzinger H (1991) Comparison of different methods for LDL-isolation and radioiodine labelling in liver receptor binding. J Nucl Med Biol (in pr.)

15 Weiss K, Fitscha P, O'Grady J, Sinzinger H (1989) Isradipine: a potent calcium blocker with beneficial effects on platelet function and vascular prostacyclin production. Thromb Res 54: 311-317

AAS 37
Prostaglandins in the
Cardiovascular System

EFFECT OF PROSTACYCLIN ANALOGUE ILOPROST ON HAEMODYNAMIC PARAMETERS DURING FEMORO-CRURAL RECONSTRUCTION.

FCT Smith, CP Shearman.

University Department of Vascular Surgery
Queen Elizabeth Hospital, Birmingham B15 2TH, UK.

SUMMARY:A randomised placebo-controlled trial was conducted to investigate the effects of iloprost, a stable prostacyclin analogue, on peripheral resistance, graft blood flow and mean systemic arterial blood pressure (MABP) during femoro-crural arterial bypass. 3000ng of iloprost, infused into the graft, produced an immediate drop in peripheral resistance by a mean (range) of 40% (4-80%)(P<0.01, Wilcoxon). Decreased peripheral resistance persisted to 20 minutes. Graft flow during the same period increased by 52% (-7 to 294%) (P<0.01). A transient maximal drop in mean MABP of 22% from 83-65 mmHg occurred 5 minutes post iloprost infusion but caused no detrimental effects and recovered to baseline values by 10 mins.

Iloprost produces an immediate decrease in peripheral resistance associated with a prolonged increase in graft blood flow. This may reduce graft failure in the early postoperative period.

INTRODUCTION

Arterial bypass to distal calf vessels may be necessary for lower limb salvage in critical ischaemia. However, 20-40% of distal grafts still occlude unexpectedly in the early postoperative period (Reichle et al 1980, Bandyk et al 1987). Factors predisposing to graft failure include high peripheral resistance, low blood flow and graft thrombogenicity.

Following distal vascular reconstruction, leucocyte activation, endothelial cell swelling and vasospasm contribute to high peripheral resistances, predisposing to graft failure

(Beard et al,1989). Pharmacological manipulation to reduce or attenuate these changes may have a beneficial effect on early graft patencies.

Iloprost, a stable prostacyclin analogue, is an effective vasodilator, has antithrombotic, leucocyte- and endothelium-stabilising properties (De Gaetano et al,1990), and reduces reperfusion injury after prolonged ischaemia (Simpson et al,1987). Topical application of the drug increases the patency of microvascular anastomoses (Kort et al, 1987).

This study was undertaken to investigate the effect, on haemodynamic parameters, of a single bolus infusion of 3000ng iloprost, administered into the graft during femoro-crural reconstruction.

MATERIALS AND METHODS

Ethical committee permission and informed consent of patients were obtained. All patients underwent vascular reconstruction for critical lower limb ischaemia, using autologous in-situ long saphenous vein with distal anastomosis to a single crural vessel.

On completion of the graft, the calf vessel proximal to the distal anastomosis was temporarily occluded to prevent retrograde flow. Steady state baseline blood flow and mean graft pressure were established using an operative Doppler flowmeter, (OpDop 130, SciMed, UK.), and a pressure transducer, (Baxter Healthcare Corporation, Netherlands), connected to a silastic cannula introduced into the graft through an unligated sidebranch. Peripheral resistance, was expressed in peripheral resistance units (PRU) where 1 PRU = 1mmHg $ml^{-1}min^{-1}$.

Patients then received either 3000ng of Iloprost or placebo, according to randomisation. This was infused into the graft, in 15ml of normal saline, over 2 mins, via the pressure cannula. Graft blood flow and peripheral resistance measurements were recorded at 5, 10, 15, and 20 mins post-infusion until skin closure. Systemic blood pressure measurements were recorded simultaneously via radial artery cannula.

Postoperatively, graft blood flow was measured by duplex Doppler ultrasonography (Diasonics DRF 300) at 60 minutes post infusion and daily for 7 days. Graft patency and ankle-brachial pressure index (ABPI) were assessed at 1 week.

RESULTS

Eighteen patients received iloprost (mean age 72(62-86); 9M,9F), and 15, placebo,(mean age 75(59-82); 8M,7F).

Mean baseline peripheral resistance on graft completion was similar for both groups of patients,(iloprost 1.14 PRU ± 0.1 SEM; controls 1.13 PRU ± 0.14 SEM). Iloprost produced an immediate decrease in peripheral resistance in all patients by a mean of 40% (range 4% to 80%), compared to controls in whom there was a mean 5.3% increase in resistance, (range -8% to +36%, $P<0.01$ Wilcoxon; Fig.1). Decreased peripheral resistance in iloprost-treated patients persisted to 20 minutes ($P<0.01$). Largest decreases in peripheral resistance tended to occur in those patients with high initial resistances ($r=.56$, $P<0.02$).

During the same period, there was a mean increase in graft blood flow of 52% (range -7% to 294%) in the iloprost-treated group, compared to controls in whom there was a mean increase of 6%, (range -17% to 26%, $P<0.01$, Wilcoxon; Fig.2).

No difference in response to iloprost was seen between those patients who underwent epidural anaesthesia and those who did not, or between diabetics and non diabetics.

A transient maximal decrease in mean MABP, from 83 to 65 mmHg,

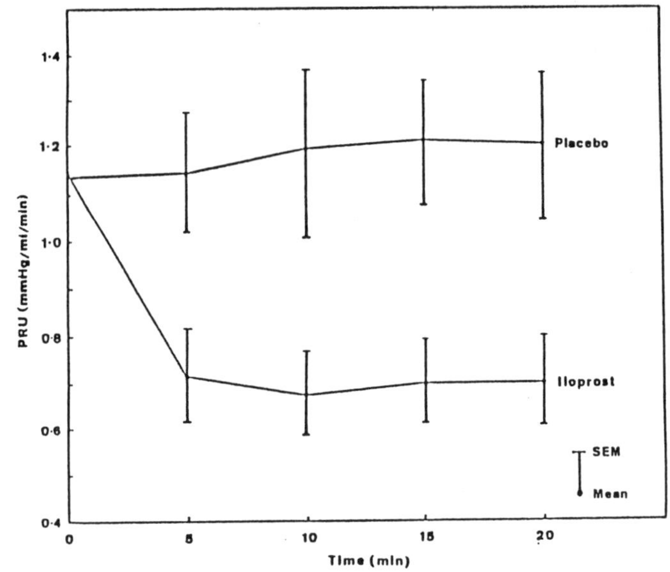

Figure 1 Decrease in peripheral resistance after iloprost infusion.

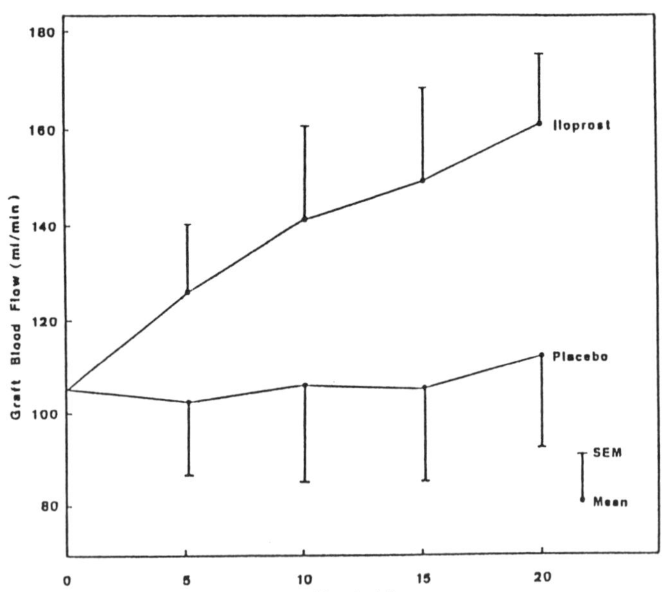

Figure 2 Increase in graft blood flow after iloprost infusion.

was recorded at 5 minutes post-infusion, in patients who received iloprost. This caused no detrimental effects and returned to baseline values within 10 minutes. No other side-effects were noted.

In patients with patent grafts, there was no significant difference in ABPI at one week, between the iloprost-treated group (mean 1.02, range 0.88-1.3) and controls (mean 0.96, range 0.8-1.03).

DISCUSSION

Iloprost produced an immediate decrease in peripheral resistance which persisted until skin closure. This was reflected by graft blood flow which was still increasing 20 minutes after infusion. Decreased peripheral resistance and increased graft blood flow are unlikely to be due solely to vasodilation since systemic blood pressure, which decreased following iloprost infusion, presumably because of a generalised vasodilatory effect, returned to baseline levels after 10 minutes. Moreover, iloprost has a short half life of less than 30 minutes (Krause and Krais,1986). This suggests that beneficial effects on peripheral resistance initiated by iloprost, are subsequently sustained through other mechanisms.

Iloprost reduces neutrophil aggregation (Belch et al,1987), and adherence to damaged endothelium (Müller et al 1988). It increases the density of perfused capillaries and antagonises effects of leukotrienes (Müller et al 1987). Iloprost protects ischaemic muscle against reperfusion injury (Belkin et al,1990) and preservation of microvascular patency may contribute to the reduced peripheral resistances which occurred in iloprost-treated patients in this study.

In conclusion, infusion of a single 3000ng dose of iloprost, into the graft during femoro-distal bypass, causes an immediate decrease in peripheral resistance, persisting until skin closure. This is associated with increased graft blood flow which remains elevated during the early postoperative period. The use of iloprost as an adjunct to distal bypass is particularly appropriate in those patients with low graft blood flows due to high peripheral resistances on graft completion. Iloprost may reduce the risk of graft failure during this vulnerable early postoperative period.

Acknowledgements
Iloprost for this study was kindly supplied by Schering Health Care, Burgess Hill, West Sussex, UK

REFERENCES

Bandyk DF, Kasbnick HW, Stewart GW, Towne JB. Durability of the in-situ saphenous vein bypass. (1987) A comparison of primary and secondary patency. J Vasc Surg 5:256-8.

Beard JD, Scott DJA, Skidmore R, Baird RN, Horrocks M. (1989) Operative assessment of femorodistal bypass grafts using a new Doppler flowmeter. Br J Surg 76:925-928.

Belch JJF, Saniabadi A, Dickson R. Sturrock RD, Forbes CD.(1987) Effect of iloprost (ZK 36374) on white cell behaviour. In Gryglewski RJ, Stock G eds. Prostacyclin and its stable analogue Iloprost. Berlin Springer-Verlag 97-102.

Belkin M, Wright G, Hobson RW. (1990) Iloprost infusion decreases skeletal muscle ischaemia-reperfusion injury. J Vasc Surg 11:77-83.

De Gaetano G, Bertelé V, Cerletti C. (1990) Mechanism of action and clinical use of prostanoids. In Dormandy J and Stock G eds. Critical leg ischaemia - its pathophysiology and management. Berlin Springer-Verlag 117-143.

Kort WJ, De Kam J, Westbroek DL. (1987) Peroperative topical administration of ZK 36374 (iloprost) acts favourably on patency of small arterial anastomoses in rats. Microsurgery 8;17-21.

Krause W, Krais Th. Pharmacokinetics and pharmacodynamics of the prostacyclin analogue Iloprost in man. (1986) Eur J Clin Pharmacol 30:61-68.

Müller B, Schmidtke M, Witt W. (1988) Adherence of leucocytes to electrically damaged venules in vivo. Effects of iloprost, PGE_1, indomethacin, forskolin, BW 755 C, sulotroban, hirudin, and thrombocytopenia. Eicosanoids 1:13-17.

Müller B, Schmidtke M, Witt W. Action of the stable prostacyclin analogue iloprost on microvascular tone and permeability in the hamster cheek pouch. (1987) Prostagl Leukotr Med 29:187-198.

Reichle FA, Martinson MW, Rankin KP. Infrapopliteal reconstruction in the severely ischemic lower extremity. (1980) Ann Surg 191:59-65.

Simpson PJ, Mickelson J, Fantone JC, Gallagher KP, Lucchesi BR. (1987) Iloprost inhibits neutrophil function in vitro and in vivo and limits experimental infarct size in canine heart. Circ Res 60:666-673.

AAS 37
Prostaglandins in the
Cardiovascular System

FIBRINOLYTIC ENHANCEMENT WITH A PROSTAGLANDIN ANALOGUE ILOPROST

D C Berridge, R Lonsdale, S Jallihal, J C Westby, B R Hopkinson, G S Makin.

University Hospital, Queen's Medical Centre, Nottingham, NG7 2UH.

SUMMARY:

Earlier workers have suggested a possible fibrinolytic effect using prostaglandin or prostaglandin analogues. Despite using maximum tolerated doses of the prostaglandin analogue Iloprost, we have been unable to demonstrate any significant effect on fibrinolysis in patients with stage IV peripheral vascular disease (Fontaine classification).

INTRODUCTION:

There have been several studies which have suggested an important role for endogenous fibrinolysis in maintaining the patency of aorto-coronary (Arnesen, 1983), and saphenous vein bypass grafts (Hamer et al, 1973: Wu, 1981). A reduced fibrinolytic potential is associated with a significantly higher risk of early graft failure (Earnshaw et al, 1987), an effect which is compatible with the fibrinolytic shutdown which is known to occur after major surgery (Griffiths, 1979).

Prostacyclins can enhance fibrinolytic activity (Utsunomiya et al, 1980; Szczeklik et al, 1983), which may be due to an induction of vascular t-PA release (Crutchley et al, 1982). Iloprost (Schering Health Care Limited, Burgess Hill) is a chemically stable carbacyclin analogue of prostacyclin and shows a similar pharmacological profile. In vitro, iloprost has been shown to reduce the euglobulin lysis time (Korbut et al, 1983), and in rats produces thrombolysis of pre-formed clots. The effect of short duration intermittent infusions (6 hours per day) of iloprost appear to enhance fibrinolysis by reducing the release of alpha-2-antiplasmin from platelets (Beitele et al, 1988). Impaired fibrinolytic potential in patients with atherosclerotic disease has also been corrected with intermittent infusions of iloprost (Beitele et al, 1988). The effects of longer term therapy with this agent have not been studied, and has therefore formed the basis of a pilot study.

PATIENTS AND METHODS:

Ten patients with ischaemic rest pain and distal skin necrosis were entered into the study. They received a maximum tolerated infusion of iloprost for six hours a day for 21 days. A comprehensive fibrinolytic screen was performed throughout the treatment period to define the onset, depth and persistence of any fibrinolytic effect detected. Venous blood samples were taken prior to the infusion, on day 4, day 7, day 14 and day 21. Post-infusion samples were also taken on days 22 and 28 (1 and 7 days post-therapy respectively). Samples were taken for thrombin clotting time (TCT), activated partial thromboplastin time (APTT), international normalised ration (INR), euglobulin lysis time, fibrinogen, plasminogen, alpha-2-antiplasmin, fibrin/fibrinogen degradation products, cross-linked fibrin degradation products and tissue plasminogen activator. In addition, a further sample was taken for euglobulin lysis time following a 10 minute period of venous occlusion as described above. In addition to the fibrinolytic and haematological tests, a standard biochemical screen (urea and electrolytes, liver function tests) was performed at each assessment period. Exclusion criteria are listed in Table 1.

All results are expressed as median values with interquartile ranges unless otherwise stated. Statistics were performed using the Mann-Whitney U test.

TABLE 1 - EXCLUSION CRITERIA FOR THE ILOPROST STUDY

1. Under the age of eighteen years.
2. Pregnant women and women of childbearing potential.
3. Patients in whom reconstructive surgery of angioplasty is indicated at the time of entry into the study.
4. Patients who have suffered a myocardial infarction or cerebrovascular accident within the preceding four months.

5. Patients with unstable angina pectoris, cardiac failure, or hypertension despite treatment (systolic consistently above 160mmHg and/or diastolic consistently greater than 95mmHg).
6. Patients with bleeding diatheses or platelet counts less than 80 x 10^6/ml or greater than 500 x 10^6ml.
7. Patients with Raynaud's disease as a primary diagnosis.
8. Patients requiring dialysis.
9. Patients with serious concurrent illnesses (eg gastrointestinal bleeding) whose peripheral vascular disease is not of primary importance.
10. Patients unable to give informed consent.

RESULTS

Ten patients received intra-venous infusions of iloprost for six hours per day for 21 days at the maximum tolerated dose for each patient. The mean dose administered was 1.9+/-0.3 nanograms/Kg/minute. There was no consistent effect of iloprost on any of the coagulation or fibrinolytic parameters measured. For each parameter, subsequent venous samples were compared with their respective initial value using the Mann-Whitney U test. There were no significant changes in any of the parameters at any time during the study (Tables 2, 3).

DISCUSSION:

Patients with arteriosclerosis of the lower limbs are known to have an impaired fibrinoiytic capacity which is dependent on the severity of the ischaemia (Browse et al 1977). In comparison to the upper limbs, fibrinolytic activity in the lower limbs is reduced, and is exacerbated by ischaemia. This difference is ascribed to chronic hydrostatic pressure depleting the local vasculature of plasminogen activator. Karaca and Nilsson (1970) found that hemiplegic patients confined to bed for a long time, had almost the same fibrinolytic activity in the legs as in the arms. Furthermore in patients who were partly mobilised, the fibrinolytic activity in the legs decreased relative to that in the arms. This phenomenon may help to explain the benefit derived from bed rest on ulcers of ischaemic or

TABLE 2 COAGULATION AND FIBRINOLYTIC PARAMETERS DURING ILOPROST THERAPY

	PRE	DAY 4	DAY 7	DAY 14	DAY 21	DAY 22	DAY 28
TCT (seconds)	13 (13-14.1)	13.8 (13.5-14)	13.8 (13.1-14.8)	14 (13.5-15)	13.8 (13.4-15.4)	13.8 (12.9-15.8)	13.3 (12.5-13.9)
APTT (seconds)	38 (30-42)	34 (32-39)	34 (33-41)	34 (32-38)	35 (33-43)	37 (34-43)	36 (35-38)
INR	1 (0.9-1.4)	0.9 (0.9-0.9)	0.9 (0.9-1.0)	0.9 (0.9-0.9)	0.9 (0.9-1.3)	0.95 (0.9-1.45)	0.9 (0.88-1.03)
ELT pre	225 (135-345)	180 (150-278)	248 (150-300)	180 (135-315)	225 (158-394)	285 (221-360)	255 (240-285)
post (minutes)	83 (49-233)	150 (75-275)	105 (60-150)	90 (30-285)	135 (83-248)	165 (38-251)	150 (135-345)
Fibrinogen (g/l)	3.93 (3.51-5.87)	3.54 (2.99-4.47)	3.86 (3.06-4.48)	3.7 (3.02-4.94)	3.81 (3.20-4.94)	3.92 (3.00-4.91)	3.37 (2.96-4.11)
PAI	3.0 (0.0-5.5)	1.5 (0.0-8.0)	2.0 (0.0-7.3)	2.5 (0.3-8.8)	5.0 (0.0-16.3)	7.0 (2.3-13.3)	9.0 (2.0-22.0)

TABLE 3 COAGULATION AND FIBRINOLYTIC PARAMETERS DURING ILOPROST THERAPY

	PRE	DAY 4	DAY 7	DAY 14	DAY 21	DAY 22	DAY 28
Plasminogen (%)	113 (102-133)	110 (86-126)	102 (94-125)	112 (89-130)	106 (94-129)	107 (100-130)	112 (95-150)
Alpha-2-AP (%)	86 (80-99)	84 (76-104)	82 80-94)	84 (80-101)	91 (82-96)	92 (84-99)	80 (78-92)
FDP'S (mg/ml)	Undetectable i.e less than 8 mg/ml for all samples						
XDP'S (ng/ml)	185 (154-596)	175 (138-248)	260 (130-770)	215 (169-300)	125 (110-250)	190 (118-263)	210 (151-490)
TPA (units)	0.13 (0.05-1.70)	0.30 (0.09-1.54)	0.25 (0.08-0.65)	0.63 (0.09-1.38)	0.25 (0.05-0.65)	0.65 (0.24-1.19)	0.20 (0.05-1.20)

venous origin. It may also explain why thrombosis is much less common in the arms than in the legs.

Although earlier work has suggested that prostacyclins can exert an independent fibrinolytic effect, these studies have tended to use higher doses in in-vitro or animal models than can be used in humans (Korbut et al, 1983; Vaughan et al, 1989). This latter study showed a 42+/-14% lysis in a rabbit jugular vein model. However, a dose of 1.2 micrograms/Kg/hour was used which is approximately ten times the maximum tolerated dose in our patients (2 nanograms/Kg/minute). Belch et al (1984) infused iloprost at up to 2 nanograms/Kg/minute in ten male healthy volunteers. No effect on plasma fibrinogen, plasminogen or plasminogen activator was detected.

More recently prostacyclins have been shown to enhance the thrombolytic effect of recombinant tissue plasminogen activator (rt-PA) (Vaughan et al, 1989). Bolus graft administration of iloprost has also been shown to double graft flow (Shearman et al, 1990).

In summary, despite using maximum tolerated doses, we have been unable to demostrate any significant effect on fibrinolysis in patients with stage IV peripheral vascular disease (Fontaine classification). Its benefits in this group of patients must therefore be ascribed to its other important effects - namely anti-aggregatory/disaggregatory effects on both platelets and leucocytes, vasodilation and also its cytoprotective properties for ischaemic tissue (Vane, 1985).

REFERENCES:

Arnesen H, Semb G, Hol R et al. Scand J Haematol. 1983; 30; supp 39: 43-6.

Beitele V, Mussoni L, Del Rossee G et al. Thromb Haemostas. 1988; 60; 2: 141-4.

Belch JJF, Greer I, McLaren M et al. Prostaglandins 1984; 28; 1: 67-77.

Browse NL, Gray L, Jarrett PEM, Morland M. Br J Med. 1977; 1: 478-81.

Crutchley DJ, Cananan LB, Maynard JR. J Pharmacol Exp Therap. 1982; 222: 544-9.

Earnshaw JJ, Westby JC, Makin GS, Hopkinson BR. Br J Surg. 1987; 74: 932-5.

Griffiths NJ. Ann Roy Coll Eng. 1979; 61: 12-6.

Hamer JD, Ashton F, Meynell MJ. Br J Surg. 1973; 60; 5: 386-89.
Karaca M, Nilsson IM. Acta Mec Scand. 1971; 189: 325-9.
Korbut R, Byrska-Danek A, Gryglewski RJ. Thromb Res. 1983; 29: 655-60.
Shearman CP, Hickey NC, Simms MH. Eur J Vasc Surg. 1990; 4: 455-7.
Szczeklik A, Kopec M, Sladek K et al. Thromb Res. 1983; 29: 655-60.
Utsunomiya T, Krausz MM, Valei CR, Shepo HB, Hechtman HB. Surgery 1980; 88: 25-30.
Vane JR. IN Shroer K ed. Prostaglandins and Eicosanoids in the Cardiovascular System. Proceedings 2nd International Symposium Basel; Karger 1985; 7-28.
Vaughan DE, Plavin SR, Schafer AI, Loscalzo J. Blood 1989; 73; 5: 1213-17.
Wu AVO, Wolfe JHN, Mannick JA, Br J Surg. 1981; 68: 367.

AAS 37
Prostaglandins in the
Cardiovascular System

CARDIOPROTECTION BY MOLSIDOMINE AND ILOPROST IN MYOCARDIAL ISCHAEMIA IN ANAESTHETIZED CATS

R. J. Gryglewski and J. Święs

Department of Pharmacology, Copernicus Academy of Medicine, Grzegórzecka 16, 31-531 Cracow, Poland

SUMMARY: In ten anaesthetized open chest cats the ligation of left descending coronary artery (LLDCA) resulted in 80 percent of mortality with survival time of 40.9 ± 8.6 min. The death of animals was preceded by premature ventricular contractions which occurred with frequency 7.3 ± 0.6/min after 2.1 ± 0.3 min following LLDCA. Molsidomine at a dose of 20 µg/kg given i.v. to 10 cats 15 min before LLDCA affected none of the above characteristics of acute myocardial ischaemia. The pretreatment with iloprost(2 µg/kg given i.v. to 10 cats) diminished frequency of premature ventricular contractions and elongated a period of time required for their occurrence after LLDCA, however, iloprost was also unable to diminish mortality of LLDCA cats. Only a combined administration of molsidomine and iloprost significantly diminished mortality among LLDCA cats down to 20 percent and doubled their survival time as compared to the controls. It is concluded that NO-donors (molsidomine) exert permissive effect towards the cardioprotective action of prostacyclin analogues (iloprost) in cats with myocardial ischaemia. LLDCA cats pretreated with molsidomine + iloprost enjoyed a more complete cardioprotection than those pretreated with a high dose (3000 units/kg i.v.) of superoxide dismutase.

Molsidomine, N-ethoxycarbonyl-3-morpholino-sydnonimine is metabolized to 3-morpholinosydnonimine (SIN-1) that after ring opening gives rise to a direct nitric oxide (NO) donor, N-morpholino-N-nitrosaminoacetonitrile (SIN-1A)(Bohn & Schönafinger, 1989). Molsidomine not only competes with organic nitrates as a therapeutic agent for the treatment of ischaemic heart disease but also it prevents experimental occlusive coronary thrombosis (Just & Martorana, 1989). Both actions of molsidomine are likely to be associated with the stimulation of soluble guanylate cyclase by NO similar or identical with that of endogenous EDRF (Vanhoutte, 1989).

Iloprost is a stable carbacyclin analogue of endogenous prostacyclin. Prostacyclin and iloprost are stimulators of membrane-bound adenylate cyclase. In experimental myocardial ischaemia the cardioprotective action of prostacyclin and iloprost seems to be associated with accumulation of c-AMP (Müller et al., 1991).

Nitric oxide and EDRF share with prostacyclin its vasodilator, platelet-suppressant, cytoprotective and fibrinolytic properties. In vitro iloprost or prostacyclin were reported to synergize with NO-donors as platelet suppressants (Radomski et al., 1987; Bult et al., 1989; Gryglewski et al., 1989; Lidbury et al., 1989) and as leukocyte cytoprotectors (Gryglewski et al., 1989; Korbut et al., 1989) but not as vasodilators (Gryglewski et al., 1989).

We put forward a conception that NO-induced rise in c-GMP has a permissive effect on prostacyclin-induced responses which are mediated by a rise in c-AMP in platelets or leukocytes. In line with that conception, we are presently looking for an interaction between molsidomine and iloprost in ischaemic myocardium in vivo.

MATERIALS AND METHODS

53 mongrel cats, body weight of 2 -3 kg were anaesthetized with sodium pentobarbitone (30 mg/kg i.p.). The chest was open along the sternum. Breathing was supported with a respiratory pump (20

strokes per minute, 20 ml/kg volume each, acc. to Schrör et al., 1988). A silk thread was introduced under the left descending coronary artery at the site of its branching from the left coronary artery. In 3 sham-operated cats the thread was left loose for 2 hours of the observation period. The remaining 50 cats were left for 15 min to recover from surgical procedure and then they were injected into femoral vein either with saline (1 ml) or molsidomine (20 µg/kg) or iloprost (2 µg/kg) or molsidomine (20 µg/kg) and iloprost (2 µg/kg) or superoxide dismutase (3000 units/kg). Fifteen minutes after the treatment the left descending coronary artery was completely occluded by a ligature (LLDCA). Mean arterial blood pressure (BP) was measured in right carotid artery. ECG, the first lead, was recorded in a typical tripolar system. Also measured were: a period of time (T_o) that relapsed from LLDCA to occurrence of premature ventricular contractions (PVC), frequency of PVC/min during 90 minutes of the observation period or during survival time (T_s), finally T_s in minutes and mortality rate (M) within each group of 10 cats.

Statistics: Except for M, all other measurements were presented as mean ± S.E. and statistical significance of a difference between control and treated animals was calculated using unpaired Student's t test at levels of p 0.05 and 0.01. A difference from M within the groups was calculated by χ^2 test.

Drugs: Molsidomine (Corvaton) Casella-Riedel. Iloprost (Schering). Superoxide dismutase (peroxinorm) Grünenthal.

RESULTS

In three sham operated cats neither PVC nor a fall in BP occurred within 2 hours of the observation period. In fifty cats with LLDCA none type of pretreatment could prevent an acute fall in BP that occurred immediately following the ligation of coronary artery (Fig.1, Fig.2). In ten cats pretreated with saline severe PVC appeared 2 min following LLDCA and these PVC increased their severity and eventually led to the death of 80 percent of animals within 40 min or so(Table 1). This mortality (M) in the control group was statistically diminished by none of pharmacological treatments except for one - a concomitant administration of molsidomine and iloprost. In this group of cats M dropped to 20 percent and the survival time (T_s) was doubled as compared with control. The pretreatment with molsidomine alone affected none of the parameters studied whereas the pretreatment with iloprost diminished the frequency of PVC, elongated T_o and marginally elongated T_s. The pretreatment with superoxide dismutase affected only this last sign of myocardial ischaemia (Table 1).

Table 1.

The effect of saline or pharmacological treatment on premature ventricular contraction (PVC), onset of PVC (T_o), survival time (T_o) and mortality (M) in anaesthetized open chest cats after occlusion by ligation of their left descending coronary artery (LLDCA). Except for the ratio M all other values are presented as mean ± S.E. Levels of statistical significance are $^{*}p < 0.05$ and $^{**}p < 0.01$; & - for statistical purposes 90 min was taken as maximum T_s in survivals.

Treatment	Dose(i.v.)	PVC/min	T_o(min)	T_s(min)$^{\&}$	M
0.9% Saline	1 ml/kg	7.3 ± 0.6	2.1 ± 0.3	40.9 ± 8.6	8/10
Molsidomine	20 µg/kg	7.3 ± 0.9	3.0 ± 0.4	55.2 ± 7.8	7/10
Iloprost	2 µg/kg	3.6 ± 0.4**	9.1 ± 1.9**	66.6 ± 7.6*	6/10
Molsidomine + Iloprost	2 µg/kg + 20 µg/kg	4.2 ± 0.4**	6.6 ± 0.9**	81.6 ± 5.6**	2/10
SOD	3000 u/kg	6.1 ± 0.7	2.3 ± 0.4	64.5 ± 7.2*	6/10

Figure 1.

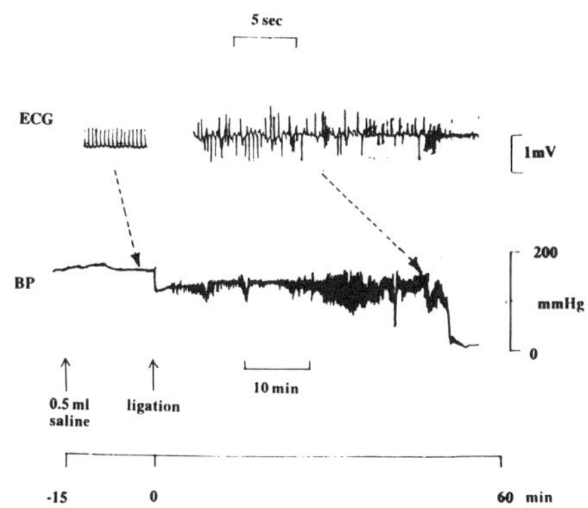

A typical tracing of mean arterial blood pressure (BP) and ECG in an anaesthetized control cat before and after LLDCA (ligation).

Figure 2.

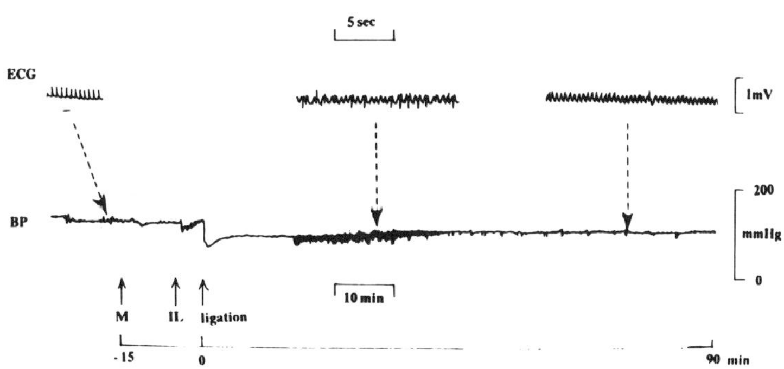

A typical tracing of BP and ECG in an anaesthetized cat which was pretreated with molsidomine (m, 20 µg/kg i.v.) and iloprost (2 µg/kg i.v.) before and after LLDCA (ligation)

DISCUSSION

In experimental animals iloprost was reported to reduce the size of myocardial infarction, to enhance anatomical and functional recovery of ischaemic heart, to suppress postischaemic arrhythmias and to prevent coronary thrombosis (Müller et al., 1991). In contrast with the experimental efficacy of iloprost, prostacyclin has no therapeutical use for treatment of patients with angina pectoris or myocardial infarction (Gryglewski et al., 1991).

Recently, we have proposed that prostacyclin requires for its thrombolytic action the permissive effect of nitric oxide. In vitro in full blood, nitric oxide has little of thrombolytic effect of its own (Gryglewski et al., 1989). A synergism between NO-donors and prostacyclin in their platelet-suppressant action (Radomski et al.,1987; Bult et al.,1989; Lidbury et al.,1989), in their cytoprotective action on leukocytes (Gryglewski et al.,1989) and in their fibrinolytic action (our unpublished observation) may contribute to the permissive effect of NO-induced rise in cyclic GMP on thrombolysis by prostacyclin.

Lack of beneficial therapeutical effects of prostacyclin and its analogues for the treatment of patients with myocardial ischaemia (Gryglewski et al.,1991) might be due to the impairement of the generation of EDRF(NO) by their coronary arteries (Ganz et al., 1991), and thus, deficiency in cyclic GMP. Could it be that a "permissive effect" of this last is indispensable also for cardioprotective action of prostacyclin? Indeed, we have presently demonstrated that molsidomine, an NO-donor,at a dose that has no cardioprotective effect of its own,allows iloprost to develop its full-scale cardioprotective action in cats whose hearts were made ischaemic by ligation of left descending coronary artery, without subsequent reperfusion. Cardioprotective effect of a combined administration of molsidomine and iloprost not only surpasses the protection offered by iloprost alone but also it is stronger than cardioprotection by a megadose of superoxide dismutase. Therefore, we conclude that there exists an experimental rationale for undertaking clinical trials of a combined therapy with NO-donors and prostacyclin analogues in patients with myocardial ischaemia.

REFERENCES

Bohn, H., and Schönafinger, K. (1989) Oxygen and oxidation promote the release of nitric oxide from sydnonimines. J. Cardiovasc. Pharmacol. 14, S6-S12.

Bult, H., Fret, H.R.L., and Herman, A.G. (1989) Interaction between SIN-1 and prostacyclin in inhibiting platelet aggregation. J. Cardiovasc. Pharmacol. 14, S120-S123.

Ganz, P., Vekshtein, V.I., Yeung, A.C., Treasure, C.B., Weidinger, F.F., Vita, J.A., Ryan,Jr., T.J., McLenachan, J.M., and Selwyn, A.P. (1991) Impaired endothelial vasodilator function in human coronary arteries. In: Cardiovascular Significance of Endothelium-Derived Vasoactive Factors (G.M. Rubanyi, Ed), Futura Pub.Co Mount Kisco, New York, pp.113-124.

Gryglewski, R.J., Korbut, R., Trąbka-Janik, E., Zembowicz, A., and Trybulec, M. (1989) Interaction between NO-donors and iloprost in human vascular smooth muscle, platelets and leukocytes. J. Cardiovasc. Pharmacol. 14, S124-S128.

Gryglewski, R.J., Botting, R.M., and Vane, J.R. (1991) Prostacyclin: from discovery to clinical application. In: Cardiovascular Significance of Endothelium-Derived Vasoactive Factors ((G.M. Rubanyi, Ed), Futura Pub.Co, Mount Kisco, New York,pp.3-38.

Just, M., and Martorana, P.A. (1989) Effect of molsidomine on thrombus formation in stenosed coronary arteries of dogs and pigs. J. Cardiovasc. Pharmacol. 14, S129-S136.

Korbut, R., Trąbka-Janik, E., and Gryglewski, R.J. (1989) Cytoprotection of human polymorphonuclear leukocytes by stimulators of adenylate and guanylate cyclases. Eur. J. Pharmacol. 165, 171-172.

Lidbury, P.S., Antunes, E., de Nucci, G., and Vane, J.R. (1989) Interactions of iloprost and sodium nitroprusside on vascular smooth muscle and platelet aggregation. Br. J. Pharmacol. 98, 1275-1280.

Müller, B., Witt, W., and McDonald, F.M. (1991) Iloprost: stable prostacyclin analogue. In: Cardiovascular Significance of Endothelium-Derived Vasoactive Factors (G.M. Rubanyi, Ed), Futura Pub.Co, Mount Kisco, New York, pp.309-333.

Radomski, M.W., Palmer, R.M.J., and Moncada, S. (1987) The antiaggregating properties of vascular endothelium: interaction between prostacyclin and nitric oxide. Br. J. Pharmacol.92, 639-646.

Schrör, K., Smith III, E.F., and Lefer, A.M. (1988) The cat as an in vivo model for myocardial ischaemia and infarction. In: Progress in Pharmacology. Vol.6/4. Gustav Fischer Verlag, Stuttgart New York, pp.31-91.

Vanhoutte, P.M. (1989) Molsidomine is a donor of EDRF. J. Cardiovasc. Pharmacol. 14, S139-S140.

AAS 37
Prostaglandins in the
Cardiovascular System

EICOSANOIDS, OTHER FATTY ACID METABOLITES AND THE CARDIOVASCULAR SYSTEM: ARE THE PRESENT ANTITHROMBOTIC APPROACHES RATIONAL?

M.R. Buchanan[1,2] S.J. Brister[2] and M.C. Bertomeu[1]
McMaster University, Dept Pathology[1] and Surgery[2]
McMaster Clinic, Hamilton General Hospital
237 Barton Street East, Hamilton, L8L 2X2, CANADA

SUMMARY

Antiplatelet ± anticoagulant drugs are currently used as the standard treatment to prevent and treat thrombosis. While this approach is beneficial, it is not optimal. Recent evidence suggests that constituents of the vascular endothelium play an important role in regulating vessel wall thrombogenecity, thereby inhibiting thrombogenesis. These include constituents such as PGI_2, tissue plasminogen activator, thrombomodulin and the lipoxygenase fatty acid metabolite derived from linoleic acid, 13-hydroxyoctadecadienoic acid (13-HODE).

Consequently, new strategies have been developed to maximize the use of these agents for antithrombotic therapy. We will review these different approaches, discuss their rationale, and based upon recent experimental data, introduce an alternative approach for antithrombotic therapy which may circumvent a number of limitations and side-effect of the currently used drugs.

1. INTRODUCTION

"Antiplatelet" drugs are used to prevent and treat thrombosis, based upon the concept that activated platelets secrete constituents which facilitate thrombogenesis. Normally, platelets circulate as discoid-shaped, inert cell bodies which do not interact either with other blood cells or with the vessel wall (1,2). However, when the vessel wall is injured, it becomes thrombogenic, and platelets are activated, adhere to the damaged vessel wall, and secrete a number of constituents which facilitate haemostasis and vessel wall repair (3-12). However, if these platelet-associated responses are not regulated, further vessel wall damage and thrombus formation occur.

Consequently, the concept of treating patients with agents which inhibit the synthesis and/or release of these factors, or interfere with their effects, has evolved as a rationale approach to prevent and treat thrombosis. For example, both aspirin and sulphinpyrazone inhibit platelet cyclooxygenase (13,14), thereby preventing the metabolism of platelet arachidonic acid into thromboxane A_2 (TxA_2). As a result, platelet function is impaired. Alternatively, agents which compete with the platelet TxA_2 receptor are also thought to be useful (15). Persantine[R] (dipyridamole) has also been shown to render platelets hyporesponsive. The mechanism by which persantine inhibits platelet function is not clear. Its effect has been attributed to changes in the platelet metabolic pool and adenosine metabolism, and to an increase on PGI_2 synthesis (16-18). However, none of these drugs have been shown to be consistently effective clinically, and many patients receiving these drugs still suffered thromboembolic complications. There are a number of possible explanations for this. First, inhibition of platelet function by any of these drugs may not render the platelet sufficiently hyporesponsive to the initiating thrombogenic stimuli *in vivo*. These "antiplatelet" drugs may also inhibit the function of other cells, such as the endothelium, thereby masking the beneficial effect associated with decreased platelet function. Or these drugs may enhance thrombosis in some situations by mechanisms previously not considered.

2. LIMITATIONS OF ANTIPLATELET THERAPY

There is an abundance of evidence to support all three possibilities. It is well-documented that inhibition of platelet function by any "antiplatelet" agent, renders the platelets "haemostatically defective", thereby increasing the risk for bleeding side-effects. What is not so obvious, but which may be equally important to consider, is that the inhibitory effect on platelets can be overcome, simply by increasing the stimulus which activates the platelets, as is well documented in vitro or ex vivo (4,17,24).

This suggests that the inhibitory effect of "antiplatelet" agents in vivo can be easily overcome, as the severity of the "thrombotic" disease increases, despite any apparent inhibition of platelet function, as assessed either in vitro or ex vivo. If so, it is expected that "antiplatelet" drugs will be relatively weak in preventing thrombogenesis in patients with severe vascular disease or vessel wall injury; such, in fact, is the case with peripheral vascular disease.

The third aspect of "antithrombotic" therapy which receives little or no attention, concerns the role of lipoxygenase metabolites of arachidonic acid and platelet function, and the effects of "antiplatelet" drugs. When platelets are stimulated, arachidonic acid which is liberated from the phospholipid stores, is metabolized not only by the cyclooxygenase enzyme into TxA_2, but also by the lipoxygenase enzyme into the monohydroxide fatty acid, 12-hydroxyeicosatetraenoic acid (12-HETE) (Figure 1). The amount of 12-HETE produced is at least 10-fold greater than the amount of TxA_2 produced by the platelets (25-26). Little attention is given to the importance of this metabolite when developing "antiplatelet" drugs for antithrombotic therapy.

A number of in vitro studies suggest that 12-HETE and/or its precursor, 12-HPETE facilitate or are necessary for platelet function (25, 26-31). Platelets obtained from patients with myeloproliferative disease, have a lipoxygenase deficiency; the greater the deficiency, the greater the tendency for bleeding, i.e. the less the ability of the platelets to synthesize 12-HETE, the less haemostatically effective the platelets (28,31). The precursor of 12-HETE, 12-HPETE, increases arachidonic acid-induced platelet aggregation (35). It was suggested that 12-H(P)ETE alters platelet membrane permeability, thereby making more arachidonic acid available for metabolism. Studies by us and others suggest that irreversible platelet aggregation is dependant in part, upon the generation of 12-HETE (25,32). We have also demonstrated that by selectively inhibiting the 12-lipoxygenase pathway in platelets, platelet adhesion is impaired, independent of any effect on platelet aggregation (25,32). More importantly, inhibition of 12-HETE synthesis and subsequent platelet adhesion are associated with increased TxA_2 synthesis and increased collagen-induced platelet aggregation. In contrast, when platelets are exposed to low dose aspirin and their ability to aggregate to a collagen stimulus is impaired, they had an **increased ability to adhere** to a collagen-coated surface (25). The latter effect is associated with enhanced 12-HETE synthesis. These results suggest that low dose aspirin will enhance thrombogenesis in some clinical settings in which platelet adhesion per se, dominates as the platelet response to injury. This, in fact, has been confirmed experimentally. Low dose aspirin which enhances platelet adhesivity in vitro, also increases thrombus formation in vivo (33).

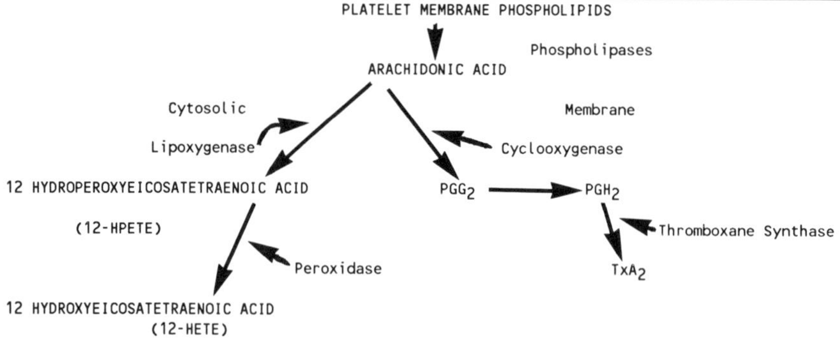

Figure 1. Metabolism of arachidonic acid by cyclo- and lipoxygenase.

Thus, a number of clinical and experimental data obtained from in vitro, ex vivo and in vivo studies, provide evidence that 12-HETE facilitates platelet adhesion, independent of aggregation. If 12-HETE plays an important role in thrombogenesis in man, it suggests that other drugs which are designed to block platelet aggregation per se, may inadvertantly increase the capacity of the platelets to adhere, for example, to an injured vessel wall. Thus, while aspirin may be useful in preventing TxA_2 synthesis, thereby impairing platelet aggregation, such as in patients suffering transient ischemic attacks (19,22,23), the possibility that low dose aspirin facilitates thrombogenic events eg. myocardial infarction, in other patients receiving the same treatment, cannot be excluded, without first demonstrating that platelet adhesion and platelet 12-HETE synthesis are not increased in these patients.

3. ALTERNATIVE APPROACHES TO ANTIPLATELET THERAPY

The rationale for giving a patient drugs to inhibit the interaction of platelets (and other blood cells as well) with the vessel wall does not include using agents which might alter the thrombogenic properties of the vessel wall itself. Instead, we have exploited the concept that constituents released from the vessel wall, which may contribute to the antithrombotic properties of the vascular endothelium, may also alter platelet/vessel wall interactions during thrombogenesis. For example, endothelial cells metabolize arachidonic acid into the prostanoid, PGI_2 which in turn, is thought to act synergistically with endothelial cell-derived relaxant factor and endothelin to inhibit platelet function (34-36). Endothelial cells also synthesize and secrete tissue plasminogen activator (tPA) and its inhibitor (PAI), thereby regulating thrombolysis (37,38). The potent antithrombotic effects of these constituents are thought to optimize antithrombotic therapy during or following thrombosis, such as the rapid lysis of a coronary thrombus following myocardial infarction with tPA (39,40). It is important to note however, that despite a rapid dissolution of the coronary thrombus by tPA, acute vessel wall reocclusion will occur unless the patient is also given heparin and/or antiplatelet drugs (for review, see 41). Furthermore, maintenance of vessel wall patency can only be achieved with chronic anticoagulant and/or antiplatelet therapy. Such long term therapy, while partially reducing recurrent myocardial infarction and general mortality, is however, fraught with an increased risk of bleeding side-effects, particularly haemorrhagic stroke (42).

4. VESSEL WALL THROMBOGENECITY

One possible explanation for this limited "antithrombotic" benefit of these agents is, that none of these agents alters the thrombogenic properties of the stimulus, namely, the thrombogenecity of the damaged vessel wall. It is likely therefore, that thrombogenesis will continue unchecked unless the vessel wall thrombogenecity is also decreased. This also suggests however, that an alternative approach to achieve an antithrombotic effect is, to reduce vessel wall thrombogenecity.

It has also been suggested that many of the "antithrombotic" constituents derived from the vessel wall, in particular, from the endothelium, not only inhibit thrombogenesis following vessel wall injury, but also contribute to the biocompatibility of the uninjured vessel wall. We would argue against that concept, since synthesis and/or secretion of tPA, PGI_2, and endothelin requires **endothelial cell stimulation** (34-38). There is little evidence that healthy uninjured vessel wall cells synthesize any of these components. What then, is (are) the component(s) of the healthy, intact endothelium which render(s) the healthy vessel wall non-thrombogenic?

5. LINOLEIC ACID AND THE LIPOXYGENASE PATHWAY

Endothelial cells are metabolically active under basal conditions. Denning et al (43) and others have demonstrated that triglycerides are continuously turned over in unstimulated endothelial cells (44). Linoleic acid released from this cytosolic triglyceride pool is metabolised intracellularly by the endothelial cell enzyme, 15-lipoxygenase, into the monohydroxide, 13-hydroxyoctadecadienoic acid or 13-HODE, (44-46). 13-HODE is retained in vesicles inside endothelial cells and is not released from the endothelial cells into the ambient surroundings. When endothelial cells are stimulated, however, 13-HODE synthesis rapidly decreases, such as in response to thrombin, endotoxin, Interleukin 1, or other cytokines (44-47). In contrast, the level of intracellular 13-HODE increases when the intracellular levels of cAMP are elevated, both in vitro and in vivo (44,47). The increased synthesis of 13-HODE associated with increased cAMP levels, appears to be a result of increased availability of free linoleic acid released from the triglyceride pool (44). The amount of 13-HODE synthesized by the resting endothelial cell is inversely correlated with the thrombogenecity of the endothelial cell surface. When 13-HODE synthesis is increased, the endothelial cell surface becomes less reactive to platelets, tumour cells and other circulating blood cells (44-47). When 13-HODE synthesis is decreased, the endothelial cell surface becomes more reactive to the circulating blood cells. These observations suggested to us that 13-HODE contributes to the regulation of vessel wall adhesivity.

In further studies, we found that stimulated endothelial cells express the vitronectin receptor on the endothelial cell surface (48). [The vitronectin receptor is a two chain glycoprotein belonging to the adhesion molecule or "integrin" family (49)]. In addition, we found that the vitronectin receptor also appears to be contained in vesicles lying immediately below the plasma membrane of unstimulated endothelial cells (50). Therefore, we determined the physiochemical relationship between the vitronectin receptor in endothelial cells, 13-HODE synthesis and platelet/endothelial cell adhesion. We found that 13-HODE and the vitronectin receptor are co-localized within the same vesicles of non-adhesive endothelial cells (50-51). When the endothelial cells are stimulated, the vitronectin receptor and 13-HODE dissociate, and the vitronectin receptor relocates on the apical surface of the cells, i.e. at a time when the endothelial cells become more adhesive to platelets (51).

We postulate that 13-HODE interacts with the lipophilic site of the alpha chain of the vitronectin receptor, down-regulating its adhesivity and/or its expression on the endothelial cell surface. Consistent with this possibility, namely, that fatty acid metabolites can alter the ability of integrins to recognize their specific ligands, and hence alter their adhesivity, Conforti et al (52) demonstrated that the ability of the vitronectin receptor to recognize its specific ligands was altered by varying the fatty acid with which it associated. Other investigators have found similar relationships between the linoleic and arachidonic acid-derived lipoxygenase metabolites, and glycoprotein IIb/IIIa dependent adhesion of tumour cells, platelets and endothelial cells (47,53,54). Thus, a battery of evidence supports the concept that adhesion molecule expression necessary for cell adhesion, be it to endothelial cells, platelets or to other circulating blood cells, can be manipulated by altering the fatty acid milieu, in particular, by altering the relative amounts of lipoxygenase products derived from linoleic and arachidonic acids. The linoleic acid metabolite, 13-HODE, appears to down-regulate the expression of adhesion molecules while the arachidonic acid metabolites (12-HETE in platelets, 15-HETE in tumour cells), appear to up-regulate the expression of these adhesion molecules.

We also found that when the vessel wall is de-endothelialized by selectively removing the endothelium, the exposed subendothelium is not initially thrombogenic, but rather, as thromboresistant as the healthy intact vessel wall (55,56). These results seemed, at first glance, to contradict the many studies which demonstrate that the injured vessel wall is highly thrombogenic (1,2,7,8). To resolve this apparent inconsistency, experiments were performed to determine whether the amount of 13-HODE present in the basement membrane altered basement membrane thrombogenecity. We found that basement membrane thrombogenecity varied inversely with the amount of 13-HODE associated with it (57-59). These observations have been confirmed in vivo and ex vivo, using both animal and human tissue (58-61).

6. ALTERNATIVE ANTITHROMBOTIC STRATEGIES: Altering Vessel Wall Thrombogenecity

The concept of achieving an antithrombotic effect by impairing or blocking adhesion molecule expression is not new. It has been suggested that an antithrombotic effect can be achieved by blocking adhesion molecules on platelets, such as with glycoprotein IIb/IIIa antibodies (62,63). Not surprisingly however, this approach has been fraught with bleeding side-effects similar to those seen with other antiplatelet agents (64). The recognition that adhesion molecules expressed on the vessel wall may also contribute to thrombogenesis, however, suggests an alternative approach to achieve an antithrombotic effect, namely, to alter vessel wall thrombogenecity, and ideally, without impairing platelet function. A number of recent studies performed both in animals and humans, suggest that this approach is feasible. Our first approach exploited our earlier _in vitro_ observations that by increasing cAMP, we could increase endothelial cell triglyceride turnover and 13-HODE synthesis. If relevant to the _in vivo_ situation, we hypothesized that by increasing vessel wall cAMP and subsequent triglyceride turnover, we would increase the amount of linoleic acid available for 13-HODE synthesis. As a result, we would decrease the adhesivity of both the intact and the injured vessel wall. If so, fewer platelets should adhere to the vessel wall surface, and following injury, thrombogenesis should be ameliorated. We also argued that if 13-HODE synthesis was impaired, thrombogenesis would increase.

Rabbits were pretreated with salicylate or dipyridamole. Salicylate was used to inhibit the peroxidation of the unstable precursor, 13-HPODE to 13-HODE (45,46,65). Dipyridamole was used to inhibit phosphodiesterase, thereby increasing vessel wall cAMP, (18,44,47,56). After one week of oral treatment with either drug, or an appropriate control, both carotid arteries of each animal were isolated and the endothelium was selectively removed using an air-injury technique (55). Three hours later, the animals were injected with ^{3}H-platelets, and the number of ^{3}H-platelets adherent to the injured vessel wall one hour later, was determined as a measure of vessel wall thrombogenecity. Other vessel wall segments (either proximal or distal to the injury site) were also removed, and analyzed for 13-HODE and cAMP levels.

Platelet adhesion to the injured carotid arteries increased two-fold in the salicylate-treated animals, as compared to platelet adhesion to injured carotid arteries in untreated rabbits. This increase in platelet adhesion was associated with a 67 % decrease in vessel wall 13-HODE (58). In contrast, platelet adhesion to the injured carotid arteries in the dipyridamole-treated animals decreased by 50%. This decrease was associated with an increase in 13-HODE synthesis, which correlated significantly with both the dipyridamole plasma level and vessel wall cAMP level. Neither the dipyridamole nor the salicylate treatment altered platelet function significantly, as assessed _ex vivo_ (58). Thus, this study provided direct _in vivo_ evidence that the amount of 13-HODE associated with the vessel wall, correlated with vessel wall thromboresistance, and supported the possibility that manipulating vessel wall thromboresistance per se, is as effective a treatment to inhibit platelet/vessel wall interactions _in vivo_ following vessel wall injury as that obtained using "antiplatelet" agents.

Our second approach was to alter vessel wall thrombogenecity by diet. The rationale was based in part upon i) our _in vitro_ observations that increasing the availability of linoleic acid results in increased 13-HODE synthesis (44,58), and ii) epidemiological studies which suggest that the incidence of cardiovascular disease is significantly lower in populations who ingest diets rich in linoleic acid (66,67). We fed rabbits semi-purified synthetic diets rich either in linoleic acid, linoleic acid and δ-linolenic acid, or eicosapentaenoic acid (EPA) for 4 weeks. Then, injured carotid artery thrombogenecity was measured in the rabbits as described above.

There was an increased synthesis of 13-HODE and a decrease in platelet/vessel wall adhesion in those animals fed a diet rich in linoleic acid ± δ-linolenic acid. Again, platelet adhesion and platelet aggregation were not significantly impaired. Interestingly, EPA had less effect on platelet/vessel wall adhesion, but significantly impaired platelet adhesion, providing further evidence that impairing platelet function does not necessitate an "antithrombotic" effect. Interestingly, the EPA effect on platelets was associated with an inhibition of platelet 12-HETE production. The selectivity of the different diet effects on platelet and vessel wall adhesivity were due to the selective uptake of these fatty acids by the different cells. EPA was selectively incorporated into the platelet, decreasing platelet 12-HETE synthesis and impairing platelet adhesivity as measured ex vivo. In contrast, linoleic acid was selectively incorporated into the blood vessel wall, facilitating increased 13-HODE synthesis (58).

In summary, vessel wall thrombogenecity can be selectively altered in vivo either by drugs or diet, and this effect can be achieved without impairing platelet function. Whether achieving such an acute antithrombotic effect decreases long term thrombogenesis is, at present, not known, but some recent clinical data are suggestive of this possibility. Harker et al (68) found [aspirin + persantine] was not effective in preventing hyperplasia in patients following carotid endartectomies. In that study, persantine was given 2 hours pre-operative, and [aspirin + persantine] was given for 12 months post-operative. In another study, Chesebro (69) found that [aspirin + persantine] was effective in preventing hyperplasia in patients undergoing elective coronary artery bypass grafting. In this study, the patients were given persantine for 48 hours before the surgery, and [aspirin + persantine] for 12 months post-operative. While the two clinical situations are considerably different, the end-point measured in each, was similar, i.e. vessel wall hyperplasia. Is it possible that in the Chesebro study, the two day pre-treatment with persantine was sufficient to increase vessel wall cAMP levels, thereby increasing 13-HODE synthesis and decreasing vessel wall thrombogenecity? If so, the decreased platelet/vessel wall interaction immediately post-surgery, may have been reduced enough to minimize platelet PF4 and PDGF secretion, thereby reducing chronic vessel wall hyperplasia. This is consistent with our in vivo studies, in which we had to pretreated the rabbits for at least one week to ensure consistent and sustained effects of dipyridamole (persantine) on vessel wall cAMP and 13-HODE, and our in vitro studies in which endothelial cells had to be incubated with dipyridamole for at least 24-48 hours to achieve similar effects (44,58).

More recently, we demonstrated that human blood vessels also synthesize 13-HODE, and that the level of 13-HODE in both veins and arteries correlates with vessel wall thrombogenecity (61). Segments of internal mammary arteries and saphenous veins obtained from patients undergoing elective coronary artery bypass surgery, both produce 13-HODE. The arteries produce 6-fold more 13-HODE than the veins, but more interestingly, 13-HODE synthesis in both the arteries and the veins decreases with age. Furthermore, this decrease in 13-HODE synthesis is parallelled by an increase in vessel wall thrombogenecity (61). Studies presently ongoing in our laboratory in a similar patient population, will determine whether increasing 13-HODE synthesis pre-operatively is associated with a corresponding decrease in vessel wall thrombogenecity at the time of surgery.

7. CONCLUSIONS AND IMPLICATIONS

The concept of altering vessel wall thrombogenecity rather than impairing platelet function as a strategy to decrease thrombogenesis, has at present, been limited to cardiologic and surgical intervention, such as angioplasty and coronary artery bypass grafting, with concomitant antiplatelet and anticoagulant treatment (68,69,71). Other approaches suggested to render the vessel wall less thrombogenic after injury, are to target specific thrombin inhibitors at thrombin bound to fibrin or the injured vessel wall (72-75), or to seed genetically altered endothelial cells onto artificial grafts or damaged vessel walls (76). The results of the experimental data discussed above however, suggest an alternative strategy, namely, to change the inherent thrombogenic properties of the vessel wall, thereby reducing the "stimulus" to thrombose. This strategy may involve the manipulation of 13-HODE synthesis in an attempt to regulate adhesion molecule reactivity, not only on the apical surface of the intact endothelium, but also on the surface of the subendothelial which is exposed following injury.

ACKNOWLEDGEMENTS

The studies performed by us and referred to in this chapter were supported, in part, by the Ontario Heart and Stroke Foundation of Canada and the Medical Research Council of Canada.

REFERENCES

1. Ross, R. (1986). The pathogenesis of atherosclerosis - an update. N. Engl. J. Med. 314:488-500.
2. Packham, M.A., Mustard, J.F. (1986). The role of platelets in the development and complications of atherosclerosis. Semin. Hematol. 23:8-26.
3. Moore, S., Pepper, D.S., Cash, J.D. (1975). The isolation and characterisation of platelet factor 4 release from thrombin-aggregated washed human platelets and its dissociation into subunits and the isolation of membrane-bound antiheparin activity. Biochim. Biophys. Acta. 379:370-384.
4. Mustard, J.F., Perry, D.W., Kinlough-Rathbone, R.L., Packham, M.A. (1975). Factors responsible for ADP-induced release reaction of human platelets. Am. J. Physiol. 228(6):1757-1768.
5. Hamberg, M., Svensson, J., Samuelsson, B. (1974). Prostaglandin endoperoxides. A new concept concerning the mode of action and release of prostaglandins. Proc. Natl. Acad. Sci. USA 71:3824-3828.
6. Ross, R. (1987). Platelet derived growth factor. Ann. Rev. Med. 38:71-79.
7. Stemerman, M.B., Spaet, T.H. (1972). The subendothelium and thrombogenesis. Bull. N.Y. Acad. Med. 48:289-301.
8. Mustard, J.F., Packham, M.A., Kinlough-Rathbone, R. (1978). Platelets, thrombosis and atherosclerosis. Adv. Exp. Med. Biol. 104:127-144.
9. Keenan, J.P., Solum, N.O. (1972). Quantitative studies on the release of platelet fibrinogen by thrombin. Br. J. Haematol. 23:461-466.
10. Lajmanovich, A., Hudry-Clergeon, G., Freyssinet, J.M., Marguerie, G. (1981). Human factor VIII procoagulant activity and phospholipid interaction. Biochim. Biophys. Acta. 678:132-136.
11. Lipscomb, M.S., Walsh, P.N. Human platelet factor XI. (1979). Localization in platelet membranes of factor XI-like activity and its function distinction from plasma factor XI. J. Clin. Invest. 63:1006-1014.
12. Tuszynski, G.P., Bevacona, S.J., Schmaier, A.H., Colman, R.W., Walsh, P.N. (1982). Factor XI antigen and activity in platelets. Blood 59:1148-
13. Al-Mondhiry, H., Marcus, A.J., Spaet, T.H. (1970). On the mechanism of platelet function inhibition by acetylsalicylic acid. Proc. Soc. Exp. Dial. Med. 133:632-636.
14. Ali, M., McDonald, J.W.D. (1977). Effects of sulfinpyrazone on platelet prostaglandin synthesis and platelet release of serotonin. J. Lab. Clin. Med. 89:868-875.
15. Willerson, J.T., Golino, P., McNatt, J. Eidt, J., Yao, S-K., Buja, L.M. (1991). Role of new antiplatelet agents as adjunctive therapies in thrombolysis. Am. J. Cardiol. 67:12A-18A.
16. German, D.C., Kredich, N.M., Bjornsson, T.D. (1989). Oral dipyridamole increases plasma adenosine levels in human beings. Clin. Pharmacol. Ther. 45:80-84.
17. Smith, J.B., Mills, D.C.B. (1970). Inhibition of adenosine 3':5'-cyclic monophosphate phosphodiesterase. Biochem. J. 120: 20P.
18. Moncada, S., Korburt, R. (1978). Dipyridamole and other phosphodiesterase inhibitors act as antithrombotic agents by potentiating endogenous prostacyclin. Lancet 1:1286- 1289.
19. Hennekens, C.H., Buring, J.E., Sandercock, P., Collins, R., Peto, R. (1989). Aspirin and other antiplatelet agents in the secondary and primary prevention of cardiovascular disease. Circ. 80:749-756.
20. Harker, L.A., Slichter, S.J. (1972). Platelet and fibrinogen consumption in man. N. Engl. J. Med. 287:999-1005.
21. The Anturane Reinfarction Trial Research Group. (1980). Sulfinpyrazone in the prevention of sudden death after myocardial infarction. N. Engl. J. Med. 302:250-256.
22. Canadian Cooperative Study Group. (1978). A randomized trial of aspirin and sulfinpyrazone in threatened stroke. N. Engl. J. Med. 299:53-59.
23. Cairns, J., Turpie, A.G.G., ISIS-2. (1988). Randomized trial of intravenous streptokinase, oral aspirin, both, or neither among 17, 187 cases of suspected acute myocardial infarction: ISIS-2. Lancet 350-360.
24. Marcus, A.J. (1978). The role of lipids in platelet function with particular reference to the arachidonic acid pathway. J. Lipid Res. 19:793-826.
25. Buchanan, M.R., Butt, R.W., Hirsh, J., Markham, B.A., Nazir, D.J. (1986). Role of lipoxygenase metabolism in platelet function: effect of aspirin and salicylate. Prost. Leuk. Med. 21:157-168.
26. Broekman, M.J., Eiroa, A.M., Marcus, A.J. (1989). Albumin redirects platelet eicosanoid metabolism toward 12(S)-hydroxyeicosatetraenoic acid. J. Lipid Res. 30:1925-1932.
27. Dutilh, C.E., Haddeman, E., Don, J.A., Hoor, F.T. (1981). The role of arachidonate lipoxygenase and fatty acids during irreversible blood platelet aggregation in vitro. Prost. Med. 6:111-126.
28. Gibson, B.E.S., Buchanan, M.R., Barr, R.D., White J.G. (1987). Primary thrombocythaemia in childhood: Symptomatic episodes and their relationship to thromboxane A2, 6-keto-PGE1 and 12-hydroxyeicosatetraenoic acid production. A case report. Prost. Leuko. Med. 26:221-231.

29. Morita, I., Murota S.I. (1987). Role of 12-lipoxygenase products of arachidonic acid on platelet aggregation. Adv. Prost. Thromb. Leuko. Res. 17:219-223.
30. Herrman, K.S. (1985). Lipoxygenase Products: Leukotrienes C4, D4, A4s breakdown products and 12-HPETE influence platelet aggregation in vivo. Prostaglandins 29, No 3:459-465.
31. Okuma, M., Uchino, H. (1979). Altered arachidonate metabolism by platelets in patients with myeloproliferative disorders. Blood 13:1258-1271.
32. Van Ryn-McKenna, J., Buchanan, M.R. (1989). Relative effects of flurbiprofen on platelet 12-hydroxyeicosatetraenoic acid and thromboxane A2 production: Influence on collagen induced platelet aggregation and adhesion. Prost. Leuko. and Med. 36:171-174.
33. Buchanan, M.R., Dejana, E., Gent, M. (1981). Enhanced platelet accumulation onto injured carotid arteries in rabbits after aspirin treatment. J. Clin. Invest. 67:503-508.
34. Moncada, S., Gryglewski, R., Bunting, S., Vane, J.R. (1976). An enzyme isolated form arteries transforms prostaglandin endoperoxides to an unstable substance that inhibits platelets aggregation. Nature 263:663-665.
35. Doni, M.G., Whittle, B.J.R., Palmer, R.M.J., Moncada, S. (1988). Actions of nitric oxide on the release of prostacyclin from bovine endothelial cells in culture. Eur. J. Pharm. 151:19-25.
36. Lopez, J.A., Armstrong, M.L. Piegors, D.J., Heistad, D.D. (1990). Vascular responses to endothelin-1 in atherosclerotic primates. Arteriosclerosis 10:1113-1118.
37. Levin, E.G., Marzec, U., Anderson, J., Harker, L.A. (1984). Thrombin stimulates tissue plasminogen activator release from cultured human endothelial cells. J. Clin. Invest. 74:1988-1995.
38. Hekman, C.M., Loskutoff, D.J. (1985). Endothelial cells produce a latent inhibitor of plasminogen activators that can be activated by denaturants. J. Bio. Chem. 260, No 21:11581-11587.
39. Hsia, J., Hamilton, W.P., Kleiman, N., Roberts, R., Ghaitman, B.R., Ross, A.M. (1990). A comparison between heparin and low-dose aspirin as adjunctive therapy with tissue plasminogen activator for acute myocardial infarction. N. Engl. J. Med. 323:1433-1437.
40. Collen, D., Topol, E.J., Tiefenbrunn, A.J. et al. (1984). Coronary thrombolysis with recombinant human tissue-type plasminogen activator: a prospective, randomized-placebo controlled trial. Circ. 70:1012-1017.
41. Prins, M.H., Hirsh J. (1991). Heparin as an adjunctive treatment after thrombolytic therapy for acute myocardial infarction. Am. J. Cardiol. 67:3A-11A.
42. Lotto, A., Colombo, A., Talarico, G., Fratianne, G., Lettino, M. (1990). Heparin and secondary prevention of acute myocardial infarction. Haemostasis 20:132-141.
43. Denning, G.M., Figard, P.H., Kaduce, T.L., Spector, A. (1983). Role of triglycerides in endothelial cell arachidonic acid metabolism. J. Lipid Res. 24:993-1011.
44. Haas, T.A., Bertomeu, M.C., Bastida, E., Buchanan, M.R. Cyclic AMP regulation of endotheial cell triglyceride turnover, 13-hydroxyoctadecadienoic acid (13-HODE) synthesis and endothelial cell thrombogenecity. Biochim. Biophys. Acta. 1031:174-178.
45. Buchanan, M.R., Butt, R.W., Magas, Z., Van Ryn, J., Hirsh, J., Nazir, D.J. (1985). Endothelial cells produce a lipoxygenase derived chemorepellant with influences platelet/endothelial cell interactions: effect of aspirin and salicylate. Thromb. Haemost. 53:306-311.
46. Buchanan, M.R., Haas, T.A, Lagarde, M., Guichardant, M. (1985). 13-hydroxyoctadecadienoic acid is the vessel wall chemorepellant factor, LOX. J. Biol. Chem. 260:16056-16059.
47. Lauri, D., Bertomeu, M.C., Orr, F.W., Bastida, E., Sauder, D., Buchanan, M.R. (1990). Interleukin-1 increases tumor cell adhesion to endothelial cells through an RGD dependant mechanism: in vitro and in vivo studies. Clin. Expl. Metastasis 8:27-32.
48. Lafrenie, R.M., Podor, T.J., Buchanan, M.R., Orr, F.W. (1990). Interleukin 1α induced vitronectin receptor expression and tumor cell endothelial cell adhesion. FASEB 4:A1134.
49. Hynes, R.O. (1987). Integrins: a family of cell surface receptors. Cell 48:549-554.
50. Buchanan, M.R., Bertomeu, M.C., Haas, T.A., Gallo, S., Eltringham-Smith, L. (1991). Endothelial cell 13-HODE synthesis and tumor cell endothelial cell adhesion. Adv. Prost.Thromb.Leuko.Res. 20:909-912.
51. Aznar-Salatti, J., Bastida, E., Buchanan, M.R., Castillo, R., Ordinas, A., Escolar, G. (1990). Differential localization of von Willebrand factor, fibronectin and 13-HODE in human endothelial cell cultures. Histochemistry 93:507-514.
52. Conforti, G., Zanetti, A., Pasquali-Ronchetti, I., Quaglino, D. Jr., Neyroz, P., Dejana, E. (1990). Modulation of vitronectin receptor binding by membrane lipid composition. J. Biol. Chem. 265:4011-4019.
53. Bastida, E., Bertomeu, M.C., Haas, T.A., Almirall, L., Lauri, D., Orr, F.W., Buchanan, M.R. (1990). Regulation of tumor cell adhesion by intracellular 13-HODE:15-HETE ratio. J. Lipid Med. 2:281-293.
54. Grossi, I.M., Fitzgerald, L.A., Umbarger, L.A., Nelson, K.K., Diglio, C.A., Taylor, J.D., Honn, K.V. (1989). Bidirectional control of membrane expression and/or activation of tumor cell IRGpIIb/IIIa receptor and tumor cell adhesion by lipoxygenase products of arachidonic acid and linoleic acid. Canc. Res. 49:1029-1037.
55. Buchanan, M.R., Richardson, M., Haas, T., Hirsh, J., Madri, J. (1987). The basement membrane underlying the vascular endothelium is not thrombogenic. Thromb. Haemost. 58:698-704.
56. Buchanan, M.R., Bastida, E. (1988). Endothelium and underlying membrane reactivity with platelets,

leukocytes and tumor cells: regulation by the lipoxygenase-derived fatty acid metabolites, 13-HODE and HETE's. Med. Hypothesis, 27:317-325.

57. Aznar-Salatti, J., Bastida, E., Haas, T.A., Escolar, G., Ordinas, A., de Groot, P.H.G., Buchanan, M.R. (1991). The reactivity of the extracellular matrix with platelets is dependant upon the method of its preparation. Arterosclerosis, 11:In Press.

58. Weber, E., Haas, T.A., Mueller, T.H., Eisert, W.G., Hirsh, J. Richardson, M., Buchanan, M.R. (1990). Relationship between vessel wall 13-HODE synthesis and vessel wall thrombogenecity following injury. Influence of salicylate and dipyridamole treatment. Thromb. Res. 57:383-392.

59. Bertomeu,M.C.,Crozier,G.L.,Haas,T.A.,Fleith,M.,Buchanan, M.R.(1990). Selective effects of dietary fats on vascular 13-HODE synthesis and platelet/vessel wall interactions. Thromb. Res. 59:819-830.

60. Simon, T.C., Makheja, A.N., Bailey, J.M. (1989). The induced lipoxygenase in atherosclerotic aorta converts linoleic acid to the platelet chemorepellant factor 13-HODE. Thromb. Res. 55:171-178.

61. Brister, S.J., Haas, T.A., Bertomeu, M.C., Austin, J., Buchanan, M.R. (1990). 13-HODE synthesis in internal mammary arteries and saphenous veins: Implications in cardiovascular surgery. In: Adv. Prost. Thromb. Leuko. Res. 21:667-670.

62. Roth, G.J. (1991). Developing relationships: arterial platelet adhesion, glycoprotein 1b, and leucine-rich glycoproteins. Blood 77:5-19.

63. Coller, B.S., Folts, J.D., Smith, S.R., Scudder, L.E., Jordan, R. (1989). Abolition of in vivo platelet thrombus formation in primates with monoclonal antibodies to the platelet GPIIb/IIIa receptor:correlation with bleeding time, platelet aggregation, and blockade of GPIIb/IIIa receptors. Circ. 80:1766-1774.

64. FitzGerald, D.J. (1989). Platelet inhibition with an antibody to glycoprotein IIb/IIIa. Circ. 80:1918-1919.

65. Siegel, M.I., McConnell, R.T., Cuatrecasas, P. (1979). Aspirin-like drugs interfere with arachidonate metabolism by inhibition of the 12-hydroperoxy-5,8,10,14-eicosatetraenoic acid peroxidase activity of the lipoxygenase pathway. Biochemistry 76:3774-3778.

66. Wood, D.A., Riemeisma, R.A., Butler, S., Thomson, M., MacIntyre, C., Elton, R.D., Oliver, M.F. (1987). Linoleic and eicosatetraenoic acids in adipose tissue and platelets and risk of coronary heart disease. Lancet 1:177-183.

67. Oliver, M.F., Riemeisma, R.A., Thomson, M., Fulton, M., Abraham, R.A., Wood, D.A. (1989). Linoleic acid and coronary heart disease. Br. J. Hosp. Med. 42:298-300.

68. Harker, L., Bernstein, E., Scala, T. (1990). Effect of aspirin/dipyridamole on restenosis after carotid endarterectomy: randomized placebo controlled clinical trial. Circulation 80:III-5.(Abstr.)

69. Chesebro, J.H. (1990). Effect of dipyridamole and aspirin on vein graft patency after coronary bypass operations. Thromb. Res. XII:5-10.

70. Dehmer, G.J., Popma, J.J., Van Den Berg, M.D., Eichhorn, E.J., Prewitt, J.B., Campbell, W.B., Jennings, L., Willerson, J.T., Schmitz, J.M. (1988). Reduction in the rate of early restenosis after coronary angioplasty by a diet supplemented with n-3 fatty acids. N. Engl. J. Med. 319:733-740.

71. GISSI-2. (1990). A factorial randomised trial of alteplase versus streptokinase and heparin versus no heparin among 12,490 patients with acute myocardial infarction. Lancet 336:65-71.

72. Jang, I-K., Gold, H.K., Ziskind, A.A., Leinbach, R.C., Fallon, J.T., Collen, D. (1990). Prevention of platelet-rich arterial thrombosis by selective thrombin inhibition. Circ. 81:219-225.

73. Eisenberg, P.R. (1991). Role of new anticoagulants as adjunctive therapy during thrombolysis. Am. J. Cardiol. 67:19A-24A.

74. Marzec, U.M., Kelly, A.B., Hanson, S.R., Lasslo, A., Harker, L.A. (1990). Inhibition of thrombus formation in vivo by novel antiplatelet agent. Arteriosclerosis 10:367-371.

75. Okwusidi, J., Falcone, M., Van Ryn-McKenna, J., Hirsh, J., Ofosu, F.A., Buchanan, M.R. (1990). In vivo catalysis of thrombin inhibition by antithrombin III and heparin co-factor II and antithrombotic effect: Differential effects of dermatan sulfate and unfractioned heparin. Thromb. & Haemorrh. Dis. 1/2:77-80.

76. Dichek, D.D., Neville, R.F., Zwiebel, J.A., Freeman, S.M., Leon, M.B., Anderson, W.F. (1989). Seeding of intravascular stents with genetically engineered endothelial cells. Circ. 80:1347-1353.

AAS 37
Prostaglandins in the
Cardiovascular System

ANTIATHEROSCLEROTIC PROPERTIES OF ORAL CICAPROST IN HYPERCHOLESTEROLEMIC RABBITS

M. Braun, M. Sarbia*, P. Kienbaum, Th. Hohlfeld, A. Weber, and K. Schrör

Institut für Pharmakologie and *Institut für Pathologie, Heinrich-Heine-Universität Düsseldorf, Moorenstr. 5, D-4000 Düsseldorf 1, FRG

SUMMARY: The effects of the orally active prostacyclin mimetic cicaprost on morphologic and functional alterations of rabbit aorta was investigated in experimental hypercholesterolemia. Oral cicaprost resulted in a significantly reduced aortic atheromatous plaque formation and partially prevented hypercholesterolemia-induced impairment of endothelium-dependent relaxations. It is concluded that long-term substitution with PGI_2 may beneficially influence the progression of atherosclerosis.

INTRODUCTION

Prostacyclin has a number of properties which might retard or even prevent the progression of atherosclerotic lesions. This includes the inhibition of mitogen release from platelets, endothelial cells and macrophages as well as effects on cholesterol metabolism in macrophages and the vessel wall (Willis, 1989). Defibrotide, which stimulates endogenous prostacyclin formation has been shown to protect the vessel wall from development of atheromatous plaques in hypercholesterolemia (Löbel and Schrör, 1989). This study investigates whether exogenous prostacyclin substitution can also exhibit beneficial effects in cholesterol-fed rabbits.

MATERIALS AND METHODS

Model: New Zealand White Rabbits (6-9 per group) were fed either a standard diet (CON) or a cholesterol (1%) - enriched diet (CHOL) for 12 weeks. Olive oil (3%) has been used as binding agent. Cicaprost (5 µg/kg x day) was given orally (drinking water) during the whole feeding period. The substance was withdrawn 72 h before the acute experiments in order to exclude any direct actions.

Measurements:

Serum lipids: Total cholesterol, triglycerides, LDL- and HDL-cholesterol were measured in the serum using standard laboratory assays provided by Boehringer Mannheim, FRG.

Morphology: Atheromatous plaque formation was evaluated by two different methods, planimetrically in percent of total aortic surface or by an empiric atherosclerosis grading score [0 - 5] (Löbel and Schrör, 1989). Additionally, aortic intimal proliferation was investigated by light microscopy.

Functional studies were performed on isolated segments of thoracic aorta in 10 ml organ bathes containing oxygenated Krebs-Henseleit solution (5% CO_2 in O_2; pH 7.4; 37°C) supplemented with indomethacin (3 µmol/l). Vascular tension was measured isometrically (Statham transducer U2) and continuously registered. The vessels were equilibrated for 60-90 min at a resting tone of 25 mN. Standard contractions were evoked by potassium chloride (KCl,

40 mmol/l) and $PGF_{2\alpha}$ (10 µmol/l). Standard maximum relaxations were elicited by linsidomine (SIN-1; 100 µmol/l), the active metabolite of molsidomine, that spontaneously releases nitric oxide (NO) during hydrolysis. Substance P (30 nmol/l) and acetylcholine (ACh; 1 nmol/l - 10 µmol/l) both acting by an endothelium-dependent release of NO.

Substances and solutions: Acetylcholine hydrochloride (Dispersa, Germering, FRG), cicaprost (Schering, Berlin, FRG), indomethacin (Luitpold Pharma, München, FRG), $PGF_{2\alpha}$ (Serva, Heidelberg, FRG), linsidomine (Cassella-Riedel, Frankfurt, FRG), substance P (Sigma, Deisenhofen, FRG). Cicaprost, indomethacin and linsidomine were kindly provided by the respective manufacturers.

Calculations: Relaxations were expressed in % of precontraction. Data are given in mean ± s.e.m. of n observations. P values < 0.05 were considered significant.

RESULTS

Serum lipids: Cholesterol feeding resulted in a 16-fold increase of total cholesterol and a 66-fold increase of LDL-cholesterol, whereas serum triglycerides and HDL-cholesterol remained unchanged. Cicaprost had no direct effects on serum cholesterol and lipoprotein profile (not shown).

Morphology: Cholesterol feeding resulted in a severe, almost homogenous atheromatous plaque formation at the aortic surface. Cicaprost treatment significantly reduced aortic plaque formation, by approximately 20 % (n=9; p<0.05) (Table I).

Histologic examination of aorta demonstrated significant and generalized intimal proliferation in CHOL-rabbits which was considerably reduced in cicaprost-treated animals. The intimal extension ranged from 0.4 - 4.4 mm^2 in the CHOL group compared to 0.2 - 2.2 mm^2 in the cicaprost treated hypercholesterolemic rabbits. Endothelium and smooth muscle cells showed light microscopically normal features.

Table I: Atheromatous plaque formation expressed as percent of total aortic surface or using the atherosclerosis score (AS-Score)

Group	Plaques [% surface]	AS-Score [0-5]
CON	2 ± 0.3	0.4 ± 0.2
CON + CICA	1 ± 0.3	0.1 ± 0.1
CHOL	84 ± 4^{+}	4.6 ± 0.2^{+}
CHOL + CICA	63 ± 5*	3.6 ± 0.2*

n=9; +) $p<0.05$ vs CON; *) $p<0.05$ vs CHOL

Vascular function: Contractile effects of KCl and $PGF_{2\alpha}$ did not differ between the groups. The relaxing effect of SIN-1 was also similar in all groups whereas the endothelium-dependent relaxations differed considerably. Cholesterol feeding resulted in a massive impairment of ACh and substance P-induced relaxations. Endothelium-dependent relaxations were significantly improved in the cicaprost-treated hypercholesterolemic rabbits (CHOL + CICA) as compared to untreated cholesterol-fed animals (Table II).

Table II: Relaxation [% precontraction] of thoracic aorta by SIN-1 (100 µmol/l), ACh (1 µmol/l) and substance P (30 nmol/l).

Group	SIN-1	ACh	Substance P
CON	92 ± 3	80 ± 5	45 ± 4
CON + CICA	91 ± 4	78 ± 4	45 ± 4
CHOL	84 ± 3^{+}	17 ± 7^{+}	12 ± 2^{+}
CHOL + CICA	87 ± 6*	45 ± 8*	27 ± 6*

n=6-9; +) $p<0.05$ vs CON; *) $p<0.05$ vs. CHOL

DISCUSSION

The present study demonstrates beneficial effects of oral cicaprost in experimental hypercholesterolemia of rabbits. Atheromatous plaque formation was significantly reduced by the prostacyclin mimetic. Histological studies demonstrated considerably less intimal proliferation in cicaprost-treated animals.

These findings are in accordance to previous studies from our laboratory demonstrating antiatherosclerotic properties of an enhanced endogenous prostacyclin formation in hypercholesterolemic rabbits (Löbel and Schrör, 1989). Similar beneficial results have been reported for the stable prostacyclin mimetic iloprost in lipofundin-induced atherosclerosis in rats (Jellinek et al., 1985).

Several studies demonstrated an impairment of endothelium-dependent relaxation by different stimuli in experimental hypercholesterolemia (Verbeuren et al., 1986; Habib et al.,1986) as well as in atherosclerotic human coronary arteries (Bossaller et al., 1987; Ludmer et al., 1986; Zeiher et al., 1991). Our data confirm a marked loss of endothelium-dependent relaxation by ACh and substance P in hypercholesterolemic rabbits. In contrast, response to maximum concentration of exogenous NO was unaffected. Similar observations were made by others using sodium nitroprusside and nitroglycerin (Bossaller et al., 1987; Guerra et al., 1989; Dusting et al., 1990) as NO-Donors or nitric oxide solution. However, a rightward shift of the concentration response curve for nitroglycerin and a diminished response to NO in atherosclerotic rabbit aorta have also been reported (Verbeuren et al., 1990). Most investigators agree that a diminished release of NO from atheromatous vessels may account for the impaired endothelium-dependent relaxations. Accordingly, L-arginine substitution has been shown to improve the altered endothelium-dependent relaxation of resistance vessels in the perfused hind-limb of hypercholesterolemic rabbits (Girerd et al., 1990). In contrast, a recent report demonstrated an increased release of nitrogen oxide from hypercholesterolemic rabbit aorta which however was less effective on detector vessels (Minor et al., 1990). Similar results were obtained in the coronary circulation of hypercholesterolemic rabbits (Woditsch et al., 1991). Improved vessel relaxation after SOD suggested an increased inactivation of NO by oxygen radicals in hypercholesterolemic rabbit aorta (Tagawa et al., 1991).

This study demonstrates that oral cicaprost partially prevents hypercholesterolemia-induced impairment of endothelium-dependent relaxation. There was a significant correlation between the reduction of atheromatous plaque formation and improved endothelium-dependent relaxation to ACh. These data suggest beneficial effects of long-term oral prostacyclin substitution for endothelial function in hypercholesterolemia.

REFERENCES

Bossaller, C., Habib, G.B., Yamamoto, H., Williams C., Wells, S., and Henry, P.D. (1987) Impaired muscarinic endothelium-ependent relaxation and cyclic guanosine 5'-monophosphate formation in atherosclerotic human coronary artery and rabbit aorta. J. Clin. Invest. 79, 170-174.

Dusting, G.J., Cucio, A., Harris, P.J., Lima, B., Zambetis, M., and Martin, J.F. (1990) Supersensitivity to vasoconstrictor action of serotonin precedes the development of atheroma-like lesions in the rabbit. J. Cardiovasc. Pharmacol. 16, 667-674.

Girerd, X.J., Hirsch, A.T., Cooke, J.P., Dzau, V.J., and Creager, M.A. (1990) L-arginine augments endothelium-dependent vasodilation in cholesterol-fed rabbits. Circ. Res. 67, 1301-1308.

Guerra, R., Brotherton, A.F.A., Goodwin, P.J., and Clark, C.R. (1989) Mechanisms of abnormal endothelium-dependent vascular relaxation in atherosclerosis: Implications for altered autocrine and paracrine functions of EDRF. Blood Vessels 26, 300-314.

Habib, J.B., Bossaller, C., Wells, S., Williams, C., Morrisett, J.D. and Henry, P.D. (1986) Preservation of endothelium-dependent vascular relaxation in cholesterol-fed rabbit by treatment with the calcium blocker PN 200110. Circ. Res. 58, 305-309.

Jellinek, H., Stock, G., and Takács, E. (1985) Lipofundin arteriosclerosis and iloprost treatment. In: Prostacyclin and its stable analogue iloprost (R.J. Gryglewski and G. Stock, Eds.) Springer Verlag, Berlin, Heidelberg, pp. 269-278

Löbel, P., and Schrör, K. (1989) Stimulation of vascular prostacyclin and inhibition of platelet function by oral defibrotide in cholesterol-fed rabbits. Atherosclerosis 80, 69-79.

Ludmer, P.L., Selwyn, A.P., Shook, T.L., Wayne, R.R.,Mudge, G.H., Alexander, W., Ganz,P. (1986) Paradoxical vasoconstriction induced by acetylcholine in atherosclerotic arteries. New Engl. J. Med. 315, 1046-1051.

Minor, R.L., Myers, P.R., Guerra, R., Bates, J.N., and Harrison, D.G. (1990) Diet-induced atherosclerosis increases the release of nitrogen oxides from rabbit aorta. J. Clin. Invest. 86, 2109-2116.

Tagawa, H., Tomoike, H., and Nakamura, M. (1991) Putative mechanisms of the impairment of endothelium-dependent relaxation of the aorta with atheromatous plaque in heritable hyperlipidemic rabbits. Circ. Res. 68, 330-337.

Verbeuren, T.J., Jordaens, F.H., Zonnekeyn, L.L., Van Hove, C.E., Coene, M.-C., and Herman, A.G. (1986) Effect of hypercholesterolemia on vascular reactivity in the rabbit. Circ. Res. 58, 552-564.

Verbeuren, T.J., Jordaens, F.H., Van Hove, C.E., Van Hoydonck, A.-E., and Herman, A.G. (1990) Release and vascular activity of endothelium-derived relaxing factor in atherosclerotic rabbit aorta. Eur. J. Pharmacol. 191, 173-184.

Willis, A.L., Smith, D.L. (1989) Therapeutic impact of eicosanoids in atherosclerotic disease. Eicosanoids 2, 69-99.

Woditsch, I., Hohlfeld, Th., Strobach, H., Schrör, K. (1991) Oral cicaprost protects from hypercholesterolemia-induced impairment of coronary vasodilation. Eicosanoids 4 (Suppl), S 52

Zeiher, A.M., Drexler, H., Wollschläger, H., and Just, H. (1991) Modulation of coronary vasomotor tone in humans. Circulation 83, 391-401.

AAS 37
Prostaglandins in the
Cardiovascular System

ORAL CICAPROST REDUCES PLATELET AND NEUTROPHIL ACTIVATION IN EXPERIMENTAL HYPERCHOLESTEROLEMIA

Th. Hohlfeld, A. Weber, and K. Schrör

Institut für Pharmakologie, Heinrich-Heine-Universität Düsseldorf, Moorenstr.5, D-4000 Düsseldorf, Germany

SUMMARY: Oral treatment of cholesterol-fed rabbits with the PGI_2 mimetic cicaprost largely reduces hypercholesterolemia-induced platelet and neutrophil hyperreactivity. In addition, cicaprost prevents atherosclerosis-induced platelet desensitization for PGI_2. These effects persist after cicaprost treatment is withdrawn. Since platelets and leukocytes are supposed to contribute to atherogenesis, this suggests a favourable effect of long-term oral PGI_2 substitution in hypercholesterolemia.

INTRODUCTION

Platelet and leukocyte activation appear to be involved in the pathogenesis of vascular lesions induced by endothelial injury (Kristensen et al., 1990) or hypercholesterolemia (Fagiotto et al., 1984). Anti-platelet agents have been reported to reduce the severity of atherosclerotic lesions in experimental endothelial injury (Harker et al., 1983). However, little is known how platelet and leukocyte function are affected by long-term treatment with anti-platelet agents in hypercholesterolemia.

The carbacyclin derivative cicaprost is a stable PGI_2 mimetic that is orally active (Stürzebecher et al., 1986). This study investigates the effect of long-term PGI_2 substitution by oral cicaprost on platelet function in hypercholesterolemic rabbits. In addition, the effect of cicaprost on atherosclerosis-induced neutrophil granulocyte activation has been investigated, an index for the inflammatory response in atherosclerosis.

MATERIALS AND METHODS

Male New Zealand White rabbits (1800-2000 g, n=8-9 per group) were fed either a standard diet or a cholesterol-enriched diet, consisting of 150 g/day rabbit pellets (Deuka, Bramsche, FRG) supplemented with 1% cholesterol and 3% olive oil. The animals were fed these diets for 3 months. Blood was drawn from the central ear artery and was used for measurement of serum cholesterol and platelet and neutrophil activity at the end of the cholesterol feeding period. Cicaprost (5 µg/kg·day, Schering AG, Berlin-Bergkamen, FRG) was given orally with the drinking water. Three days before blood was obtained, Cicaprost treatment was withdrawn to exclude a direct effect on blood cell function.

Platelet activity was measured by collagen (0.3-10 µg/ml)-induced aggregation ex vivo (Labor aggregometer, Hamburg, FRG) of citrated platelet rich plasma (Biostabil^R, Biotest, Frankfurt, FRG, 7:1, v/v). Platelet sensitivity to PGI_2 was studied ex vivo by inhibition of ADP (6 µM)-induced platelet ATP secretion by iloprost (1-300 nM, Schering AG, Berlin-Bergkamen, FRG). ATP was measured by luciferase-generated luminescence (CLS reagent, Boehringer, Mannheim, FRG). Neutrophil activity was measured by zymosan (20 µg/ml)-induced formation of reactive oxygen metabolites, detected by luminol (100 µg/ml)-enhanced chemiluminescence in citrated whole blood.

All data are mean ± SEM of n experiments. Statistical significance was analysed by the two-tailed t-test. P values of ≤ 0.05 were considered significant.

RESULTS

Cicaprost did not change serum cholesterol in any group of animals. However, it significantly attenuated platelet aggregation in both rabbits fed standard and cholesterol diet at 2 months (Fig. 1).

Hypercholesterolemia markedly increased collagen-induced platelet aggregation. This hyperreactivity was significantly reduced in rabbits receiving cicaprost at collagen concentrations lower than 5 µg/ml (Fig. 2), although treatment had been stopped 3 days before measurement. In contrast, in rabbits fed standard diet, platelet inhibition by cicaprost disappeared and turned into a moderate increase of aggregation at high collagen concentrations.

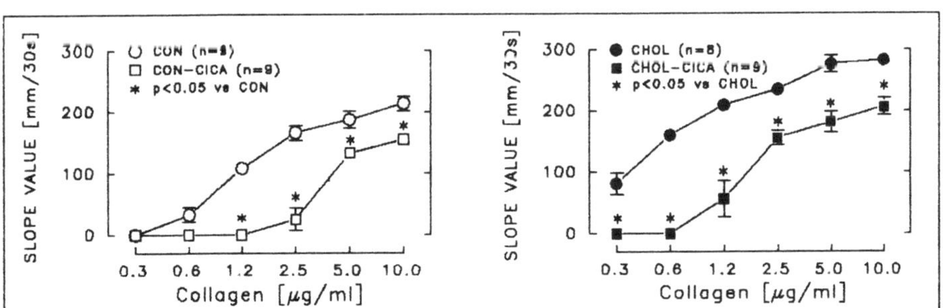

Figure 1: Collagen-induced platelet aggregation ex vivo after 2 months of standard (CON) or cholesterol-enriched diet (CHOL) during oral treatment with cicaprost (CICA). Cicaprost inhibited platelet aggregation regardless of the diet fed.

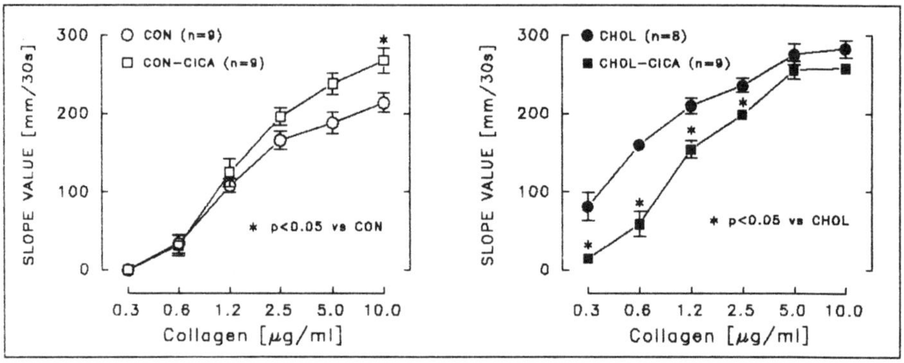

Figure 2: Collagen-induced platelet aggregation ex vivo after 3 months of standard (CON) or cholesterol-enriched diet (CHOL). Although cicaprost treatment (CICA) had been stopped for 3 days before measurements, platelet hyperreactivity in hypercholesterolemia was reduced in this group.

Platelets of hypercholesterolemic rabbits showed a considerable loss of sensitivity to iloprost in vitro, as indicated by a 3-fold increase of the IC_{50} for iloprost to inhibit ADP-induced platelet ATP secretion (Fig. 3). Cicaprost completely prevented platelet desensitization in cholesterol-fed rabbits, but did not induce major changes of platelet sensitivity to iloprost in rabbits fed the standard diet.

Cholesterol feeding stimulated neutrophil activity ex vivo. This was shown by an increase of zymosan-induced chemiluminescence from 1.5 ± 0.2 cpm/10^3 cells (standard diet) to 7.0 ± 0.7 cpm/10^3 cells (cholesterol diet), ($p < 0.05$). Cicaprost treatment reduced neutrophil hyperreactivity in cholesterol fed animals to 4.7 ± 0.9 cpm/10^3 cells ($p < 0.05$ vs cholesterol-enriched diet). Cicaprost did not change neutrophil-dependent chemiluminescence in rabbits fed standard diet (1.6 ± 0.3 cpm/10^3 cells), ($p > 0.05$ vs standard diet without treatment).

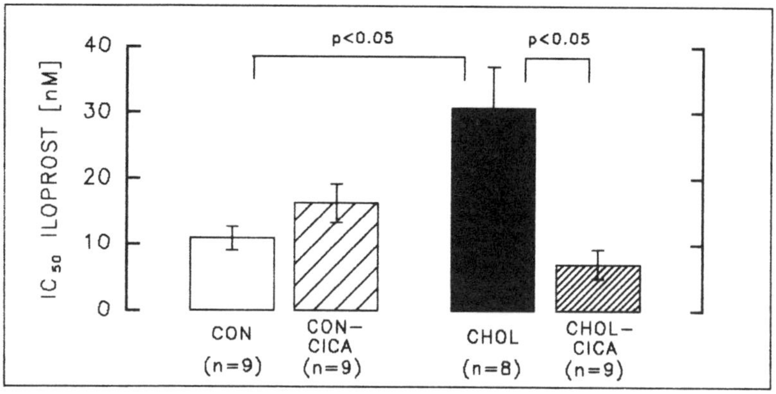

Figure 3: IC_{50} values for inhibition of ADP-induced platelet ATP-secretion by iloprost. Rabbits were fed either a standard (CON) or a cholesterol-enriched diet (CHOL) for 3 months. Cicaprost treatment (CICA) prevented platelet desensitization towards iloprost in vitro hypercholesterolemic animals animals but id not alter platelet sensitivity to iloprost in animals fed the standard diet.

DISCUSSION

Cholesterol-induced platelet hyperreactivity, as reported previously by others (Carvalho et al., 1974, Wörner & Patscheke, 1980) and ourselves (Löbel & Schrör, 1989), is related to changes in membrane lipid composition, in particular an increased arachidonic acid content (Dalal et al., 1990). This may increase thromboxane formation and feedback amplification of aggregation in atherosclerotic animals (Weber et al., 1991).

In this study, cicaprost markedly inhibited ex vivo platelet aggregation during the feeding period in rabbits fed standard or cholesterol-enriched diet. This indicates that plasma levels of cicaprost were sufficient to directly inhibit platelets.

However, the reduction of platelet hyperreactivity by cicaprost cannot be totally explained by a direct inhibitory effect, since it persisted for at least 3 days after cicaprost was withdrawn. At this time, direct platelet inhibition by cicaprost had disappeared and turned to a certain degree of rebound increase of platelet activity in rabbits fed the standard diet. Eventually, in cicaprost-treated hypercholesterolemic rabbits less reactive platelets due to a lower membrane cholesterol content were formed.

PGI_2 has been shown to stimulate cholesterol ester hydrolysis (Pomerantz & Hajjar, 1990), an effect which may also be shared by cicaprost.

An atherosclerosis-related decrease of platelet sensitivity for PGI_2 and PGI_2 mimetics, as observed in the present study, has also been reported for hypercholesterolemic patients (Strano et al., 1982, Schrör et al., 1989). In cholesterol-fed rabbits, cicaprost treatment preserved a completely normal response of platelets for iloprost. Similar results have previously been described for hypercholesterolemic rabbits treated with defibrotide, a stimulator of endogenous PGI_2 generation (Löbel & Schrör, 1989). Ligand binding studies with platelet membranes prepared from these animals, which will be published elsewhere, did not support the contention that this effect of cicaprost may be due to an increased PGI_2 receptor affinity or density in hypercholesterolemia. A different site of action, eventually related to post-receptor signal transduction pathways, appears to be more probable, but requires further studies.

In addition to platelets, neutrophils were also hyperreactive in hypercholesterolemia. Elevated neutrophil activity has also been found in hypercholesterolemic men (Croft et al., 1990). It is currently unknown to which extent neutrophils contribute to atherogenesis and whether they do it by release of oxygen radicals, proteolytic enzymes or factors chemotactic for other classes of leukocytes. However, neutrophil activity may be considered as an index of the inflammatory response in athero-sclerosis and may be representative for the activity of monocytes and macrophages which are known to promote atherosclerotic lesions (Cotran & Munro, 1988). PGI_2 mimetics and probably cicaprost do not directly inhibit neutrophil-dependent oxygen radical formation (Schrör & Hecker, 1986). However, since platelet-leukocyte interactions are relevant in atherosclerosis (Curtiss et al., 1987), it may be assumed that the reduction of neutrophil activity by cicaprost is indirect in nature and potentially results from inhibition of platelet hyperreactivity.

CONCLUSION

Long-term PGI_2 substitution by oral cicaprost in hypercholesterolemic rabbits reduces platelet hyperreactivity and prevents platelet desensitization for PGI_2. This, together with a decrease of leukocyte hyperreactivity, may reduce the severity of vascular lesions in atherosclerosis.

REFERENCES

Carvalho, A.C.A., Colman, R.W., and Lees R.S. (1974) Platelet function in hyperlipoproteinemia. New Engl. J. Med. 290, 434-438.

Munro, R.S., and Cotran, J.M. (1988) The pathogenesis of atherosclerosis: Atherogenesis and inflammation. Lab. Invest. 58, 249-261.

Croft, K.D., Beilin, L.J., Vandongen, R., Rouse, I., and Masarei, J. (1990) Leukocyte and platelet function and eicosanoid production in subjects with hypercholesterolemia. Atherosclerosis 83, 101-109.

Curtiss, L.K., Black, A.S., Takagi, Y., and Plow, E.F. (1987) New mechanism of foam cell formation in atherosclerotic lesions. J. Clin. Invest. 80, 367-373.

Dalal, K.B., Ebbe, S., Mazoyer, E., Carpenter, D., and Yee, T. (1990) Biochemical and functional abnormalities in hypercholesterolemic rabbit platelets. Lipids 25, 86-92.

Fagiotto, A., Ross, R., and Harker, L. (1984) Studies of hypercholesterolemia in the nonhuman primate. I. changes that lead to fatty streak formation. Arteriosclerosis 4, 323-340.

Harker, L.A., Harlan, J.M., and Ross, R. (1983) Effect of sulfinpyrazone on homocysteine-induced endothelial injury and atherogenesis in baboons. Circ. Res. 53, 731-739.

Kristensen, S.D., Roberts, K.M., Kishk, Y.T., and Martin, J.F. (1990) Accelerated atherogenesis occurs following platelet destruction and increases in megakaryocyte size and DNA content. Eur. J. Clin. Invest. 20, 239-247.

Löbel, P., and Schrör, K. (1989) Stimulation of vascular prostacyclin and inhibition of platelet function by oral defibrotide in cholesterol-fed rabbits. Atherosclerosis 80, 69-79.

Pomerantz, K.B., and Hajjar, D.P. (1990) High-density-lipoprotein-induced cholesterol-efflux from arterial smooth muscle cell-derived foam cells: functional relationship of the cholesteryl ester cycle and eicosanoid biosynthesis. Biochemistry 29, 1892-1899.

Schrör, K., and Hecker, G. (1987) Potent inhibition of superoxide anion generation by PGE_1 and the PGE_1 analog OP 1206 in human PMN's - unrelated to its antiplatelet, PGI_2-like activity. VASA, Suppl. 17, 11-16.

Schrör, K., Löbel, P., and Steinhagen-Thiessen, E. (1989) Simvastatin reduces platelet thromboxane formation and restores normal platelet sensitivity against prostacyclin in type IIa hypercholesterolemia. Eicosanoids 2, 39-45.

Strano, A., Davi, G., Averna, M., Rini, G.B., Novo, S., DiFede, G., Mattina, A., and Notarbartolo, A. (1982) Platelet sensitivity to prostacyclin and thromboxane production in hyperlipidemic patients. Thromb. Haemostasis 48, 18-20.

Stürzebecher, S., Haberey, M., Müller, B., Schillinger, E., Schröder, G., Skuballa, W., Stock, G., Vorbrüggen, H., and Witt, W. (1986) Pharmacological profile of a novel carbacyclin derivative with high metabolic stability and oral activity in the rat. Prostaglandins 31, 95-109.

Weber, A., Hohlfeld, Th., and Schrör, K. (1991) ADP-induced second-wave aggregation in platelet rich plasma from hypercholesterolemic rabbits. Thromb. Res., in press

Wörner, P., and Patscheke, H. (1980) Hyperreactivity by an enhancement of the arachidonate pathway of platelets treated with cholesterol-rich phospholipid dispersions. Thromb. Res. 18, 439-451.

AAS 37
Prostaglandins in the
Cardiovascular System

ORAL CICAPROST PROTECTS FROM HYPERCHOLESTEROLAEMIA-INDUCED IMPAIRMENT OF CORONARY VASODILATION

I. Woditsch, Th. Hohlfeld, H. Strobach, and K. Schrör

Institut für Pharmakologie der Heinrich-Heine-Universität Düsseldorf, Moorenstraße 5, D-W-4000 Düsseldorf 1, FRG

SUMMARY: Isolated Langendorff-hearts prepared from cholesterol fed rabbits (1 % cholesterol for 3 months) showed a significant impairment in endothelium-dependent relaxation after short-term infusion of bradykinin (0.05 µmol/l) and carbamoylcholine (0.1 µmol/l). Generation of the endothelial mediators nitric oxide and prostacyclin by bradykinin was enhanced in hypercholesterolemia. Cicaprost treatment (5 µg/kg x d) largely prevented the hypercholesterolemia-related impairment of coronary vasodilation and nitric oxide release. It is concluded that (i) impairment of endothelium-dependent relaxation in the coronary microcirculation of hypercholesterolemic rabbits is not due to diminished endothelium-dependent mediator release but rather to accelerated inactivation or reduced activity of the released mediators and that (ii) oral cicaprost beneficially influences these alterations.

INTRODUCTION

It is well established that hypercholesterolemia results in diminished endothelium-dependent relaxation of aorta and coronary arteries. These observations have been frequently made in bioassay experiments by measuring relaxation of detector vessels (e.g. Verbeuren et al. 1986, Sellke et al. 1990, Tagawa et al. 1991). Whether this impairment is due to diminished release of the mediator(s), decreased action of the mediator(s) on the target tissue or a more rapid inactivation of the mediator(s) remains to be determined. Only few attempts have been made for direct quantification of the mediator nitric oxide under the conditions of hypercholesterolemia (Minor et al 1990).

Hypercholesterolemia-related alterations in the generation of prostacyclin (PGI_2), another mediator of endothelium-dependent vasodilation, is also subject of controversy. Several authors have described a diminshed PGI_2 formation in atherosclerotic vessels (Dembinska-Kiec et al. 1977), while others found a transient increase, followed by a decrease depending on the stage of hypercholesterolaemia (Beetens et al. 1986).

This study was designed to (i) investigate the action of endothelium-dependent vasodilators on the coronary microcirculation of hypercholesterolemic rabbits in correlation to nitric oxide (NO) and PGI_2 release, and (ii) to study whether oral administration of the PGI_2 analog cicaprost (Stürzebecher et al. 1986) does modify any hypercholesterolemia related alterations in mediator generation or function.

MATERIALS AND METHODS

White New Zealand rabbits (n=9) were fed for 3 months standard rabbit pellets (Deuka, Bramsche, FRG) supplemented by 1 % cholesterol and 3 % olive oil. Another group of animals (n=9) received cicaprost (5 µg/kg x d) together with the cholesterol-rich diet (CHOL+CICA). Animals of two control groups were either given the standard diet alone (CON) or standard diet supplemented with cicaprost (CICA) for the same period of time. Cicaprost was administered with the drinking water and was withdrawn 72 h before the acute experiments to avoid any direct effects.

Langendorff-hearts were prepared at the end of the feeding period according to standard laboratory procedures (Schrör et al. 1982). The hearts were perfused at a constant rate of 40 ml/min with oxygenated Krebs-Henseleit-buffer (pH 7.4, 37°C). Endothelial function was stimulated by short-term (3 min) infusion of carbamoylcholine (0.1 µmol/l), bradykinin (0.05 µmol/l) and substance P (0.05 µmol/l). These concentrations were previously found to be equieffective with respect to release of NO and coronary vasodilation (Woditsch et al. 1990). As endothelium independent control, an equieffective, submaximal concentration of glyceroltrinitrate (20 µmol/l) was used. Coronary perfusion pressure (CPP) was measured continuously. NO was determined in the coronary effluent by the oxyhemoglobin technique (Schrör et al. 1991). Oxyhemoglobin (3 µmol/l) was added to the perfusion buffer immediately after carbamoycholine and was present during the stimulation with bradykinin and substance P. PGI_2 was determined in the coronary effluent in terms of 6-oxo-$PGF_{1\alpha}$ by radioimmunoassay.

Bovine hemoglobin, sephadex G-25-150, bradykinin, substance P were obtained from Sigma (Deisenhofen, FRG), glyceroltrinitrate from Schwarz-Pharma (Monheim, FRG), cicaprost and iloprost from Schering AG (Berlin, FRG). All other chemicals were purchased from Merck, Darmstadt (FRG).

The data are mean ± SEM of n determinations. Statistical analysis was performed by the two-tailed t-test. p levels of ≤ 0.05 were considered significant.

RESULTS

There was a comparable level of resting coronary perfusion pressure in all groups of animals studied, the means ranging between 31 and 33 mmHg. In hypercholesterolemic animals, vasodilation by carbamoylcholine and bradykinin was significantly reduced as compared to controls ($p < 0.05$). These changes were independent of the presence of HbO_2. The impaired vasodilation was largely prevented by oral cicaprost treatment during cholesterol feeding ($p < 0.05$) (Fig. 1, Table I), while cicaprost treatment did not alter endothelium-dependent relaxation in the control group fed the standard diet. Endothelium-independent vasodilation by glyceroltrinitrate amounted to 8.0 ± 0.6 mmHg in control animals and was not different between the groups.

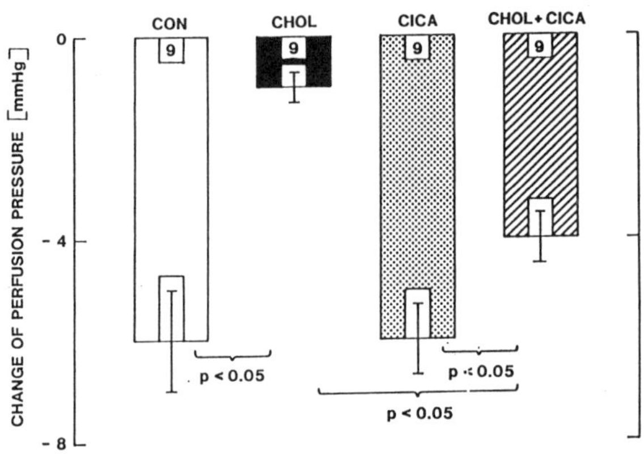

Fig. 1: Decrease of coronary perfusion pressure in Langendorff-perfused rabbit hearts by carbamoylcholine (0.1 µmol/l) (CON) and its alteration by cholesterol (CHOL) feeding and/or cicaprost treatment (CICA). The bars are mean ± SEM of the number of experiments indicated at the bars.

Basal release of NO was also similar in all groups. For example, hearts of control rabbits released 30.4 ± 2.5 nmol/l NO (n=6). Bradykinin stimulated NO release (Table I). This endothelium-dependent NO release was significantly enhanced in hearts of hypercholesterolemic rabbits. Cicaprost treatment during cholesterol feeding largely prevented these cholesterol-related alterations in NO release. In contrast, cicaprost treatment alone, did not modify bradykinin-induced NO release.

Table I : Bradykinin-(0.05 µmol/l) induced decrease of CPP in Langendorff perfused rabbit hearts and release of NO and 6-oxo-PGF$_{1\alpha}$ into the coronary effluent (area under the curve) in control animals (CON) compared to alterations by cicaprost (CICA) and/or cholesterol enriched diet (CHOL)

	CON	CICA	CHOL	CHOL+CICA
CPP [mmHg]	5.4 ± 0.6	4.4 ± 0.5	1.1 ± 0.5*	3.8 ± 1.0+
NO [nmol]	1.5 ± 0.2	1.6 ± 0.3	2.3 ± 0.3*	1.5 ± 0.3+
6-oxo-PGF$_{1\alpha}$ [nmol]	0.09 ± 0.02	0.21 ± 0.04*	0.24 ± 0.04*	0.17 ± 0.03

The data are mean ± SEM of 9 experiments in each group. *)p < 0.05 vs. CON, +)p<0.05 vs. CHOL

Basal release of 6-oxo-PGF$_{1\alpha}$ was not different between the several groups of rabbits, amounting to 0.30 ± 0.04 in the control and 0.36 ± 0.05 nmol/l in the cholesterol-fed animals, respectively ($p > 0.05$, $n = 9$). Bradykinin stimulated 6-oxo-PGF$_{1\alpha}$ formation above basal levels in control hearts. This effect was enhanced in hypercholesterolemic animals (Table I). Cicaprost treatment also caused enhanced 6-oxo-PGF$_{1\alpha}$ formation in response to bradykinin in control hearts. However, there was no further stimulation in cholesterol-fed animals treated with cicaprost. Similar findings on endothelium-dependent relaxation and mediator release were obtained after short-term infusion of substance P (data not shown).

DISCUSSION

These data demonstrate an impaired relaxation of the coronary microcirculation in hypercholesterolemia. This is in line with previous findings by others (Sellke et al. 1990, Osborne et al. 1989). Importantly, impairment of endothelium-dependent relaxation is here obtained in early stages of atherosclerosis where overt plaque formation has not yet developed.

Our data show that this reduced coronary relaxation in response to vasodilating stimuli, such as bradykinin, cannot be explained by reduced generation of endothelium-derived mediators. In contrast, formation of NO and PGI_2 is rather enhanced in the coronary microcirculation of cholesterol fed rabbits. Eventually, there might be differences in mediator release between large arteries and small resistance vessels, dependent on the degree of tissue injury. Thus, Beetens et al. (1986) described an initially enhanced 6-oxo-$PGF_{1\alpha}$ production by aortic segments in hypercholesterolemia which was followed by a severly diminished production after a longer time of cholesterol feeding. It is possible that similar considerations are also true for the enhanced NO formation found in this study and also in a previous investigation of Minor et al (1990).

Alternatively, the discrepancy between enhanced mediator generation and reduced vasomotor response may be due to enhanced inactivation of the liberated mediator. Several mechanisms for such inactivation processes have been postulated including radical-associated reactions (Tagawa et al. 1991, Minor et al. 1990). Finally, a reduced sensitivity of the vasculature to NO or PGI_2 may be involved. However, the unchanged relaxation to endothelium-independent NO donors, such as glyceroltrinitrate, would not support this concept.

Oral cicaprost largely prevented this hypercholesterolemia related impairment of coronary relaxation as well as the alterations in NO release. Orekhov et al (1983) have previously shown antiproliferative actions of PGI_2 in cultured human vascular smooth muscle cells. Eventually, similar effects, as well as prevention of platelet and white cell-derived growth factor and cytokine release are involved in these long-term effects of the prostacyclin analog.

In summary, there is an impaired endothelium-dependent vasodilation in the coronary microcirculation of hypercholesterolemic rabbits. This is probably not due to diminished mediator formation, but rather to an enhanced degradation and/or reduced sensitivity of the coronary vasculature against NO and PGI_2, respectively. Oral treatment with the prostacyclin mimetic cicaprost prevents this impairment of endothelium-dependent relaxation in the coronary microcirculation at unchanged plasma cholesterol levels. It is concluded that hypercholesterolemia is associated with enhanced PGI_2 formation to maintain endothelial control of vessel tone. This can be mimicked by continuous exogenous substitution of PGI_2.

REFERENCES

Beetens, J.R., Coene, M.-C., Verheyen A., Zonnekeyn, L., and Herman A.G. (1986) Biphasic response of intimal prostacyclin production during the development of atherosclerosis, Prostaglandins, 32, 3, 319-334.

Dembinska-Kiec, A., Gryglewska, T., Zmuda, A., and Gryglewski, R.J. (1977) The generation of prostacyclin by arteries and by the coronary vascular bed is reduced in experimental atherosclerosis, Prostaglandins 14, 1025-1034.

Minor, R.L., Myers, P.M., Guerra, R., Bates, J.N., and Harrison, D.G. (1990) Diet-induced atherosclerosis increases the release of nitrogen oxides from rabbit aortas, J. Clin. Invest. 86, 2109-2116.

Orekhov, A.N., Tertov V.V., and Smirnov V.N. (1983) Prostacyclin analogues as antiatherosclerotic drugs, Lancet, 27, 521.

Osborne, J.A., Siegman, M.J., Sedar A.W., Mooers S.U., and Lefer, A.M. (1989) Lack of endothelium-dependent relaxation in coronary arteries of cholesterol-fed rabbits, Am. J. Physiol. 256, C591-C597.

Schrör, K., Darius, H., Addicks, K., Köster R., and Smith III, E.F. (1982) PGI_2 prevents ischemia-induced alterations in cardiac catecholamines without influencing nerve-stimulation induced catecholamine release in nonischemic conditions, J. Cardiovasc. Pharmacol. 4, 741-748.

Schrör, K., Förster, S., and Woditsch, I. (1991) On-line measurement of nitric oxide release from organic nitrates in the intact coronary circulation, Naunyn-Schmiedeberg's Arch. Pharmacol. 344, 240-246.

Sellke, F.W., Armstrong, M.L. and Harrison, D.G. (1990) Endothelium-dependent vascualr relaxation is abnormal in the coronary microcirculation of atherosclerosis primates, Circulation 81, 1586-1593.

Stürzebecher, S., Haberey, M., Müller, B., Schillinger, E., Schröder, G.S., Kuballa, W., Stock, G., Vorbrüggen H. and Witt W. (1986), Pharmacological profile of a novel carbacyclin derivative with high metabolic stabilitiy and oral activity in the rat, Prostaglandins 31, 95-109

Tagawa, H., Tomoike, H., and Nakamura, M. (1991) Putative mechanisms of the impairment of endothelium-dependent relaxation of the aorta with atheromatous plaque in Watanabe heritable hyperlipidemic rabbits, Circ. Res. 68, 330-337.

Verbeuren, T.J., Jordaens, F.H., Zonnekeyn, L.L., Van Hove, C.E., Coene, M.-C., and Herman, A.G. (1986) Effect of hypercholesterolemia on vascular reactivity in the rabbit, Circ. Res. 58, 552-564.

Woditsch, I., Strobach, H. and Schrör, K. (1990) Endothelium-dependent vasodilation in the reperfused ischemic rabbit heart, Circulation, 82, 4, Suppl. III - 378.

AAS 37
Prostaglandins in the
Cardiovascular System

EFFECTS OF CIPROSTENE ON RESTENOSIS RATE DURING THERAPEUTIC TRANSLUMINAL CORONARY ANGIOPLASTY

Harald Darius, Uwe Nixdorff, Johannes Zander,

Hans-Jürgen Rupprecht, Raimund Erbel and Jürgen Meyer

Department of Medicine II, Johannes Gutenberg - University,
Langenbeckstrasse 1, 6500 Mainz 1, Germany

SUMMARY

Ciprostene, a chemically stable prostacyclin analog was studied for its effects on restenosis in patients with coronary artery disease undergoing therapeutic percutaneous transluminal coronary angioplasty (PTCA). In a double-blind, randomized trial 32 patients were randomized to receive either ciprostene or the respective placebo. The infusion started intracoronarily at a rate of 40 ng/kg/min 20 min before introduction of the balloon catheter into the coronary artery. Thereafter infusion was continued intravenously for 36 hours at a rate of 120 ng/kg/min and a tapering off period until 48 hours. The quantitive analyses of the degree of coronary artery stenoses on the angiographic films before PTCA, after PTCA and after 6 month of follow-up was performed in 24 patients available.

In patients receiving placebo (n=12) coronary artery stenoses was 81 ± 3 % before PTCA and was reduced to 34 ± 3 % by angioplasty. At the 6 month follow up angiography stenoses diameter was measured as 63 ± 8 %, being not significantly different from the % stenoses before PTCA. In contrast, coronary artery stenoses in patients receiving ciprostene (n=12) measured 83 ± 3 % before PTCA, 31 ± 4 % after PTCA and 55 ± 9 % at 6 month, being still significantly different from pre-PTCA value ($P<0.05$). When patients were characterized according to their clinical status, these differences were accounted for by patients with unstable angina receiving ciprostene.

Ciprostene seems to reduce restenosis 6 month after coronary angioplasty in patients with unstable angina. The infusion rate of 40 ng/kg/min i.c. followed by 120 ng/kg/min i.v. was tolerated well, although the incidence of catheter associated bleedings was increased.

INTRODUCTION

Since introduction of percutaneous transluminal coronary angioplasty (PTCA) into clinical medicine this is the method of choice for the treatment of patients with coronary artery disease and high degree stenoses of proximal segments in one or two major arteries. One of the main clinical problems is the rate of restenoses during the 6 month period following the angioplasty. The studies performed to reduce the incidence of restenosis suggest, that treatment with platelet inhibitor drugs may reduce the risk of acute thrombotic complications during or early after the angioplasty procedure, however no effective medication for the prevention of restenosis after PTCA was reported (Corcos etal, 1985; Schwartz etal, 1988).

The mechanism of restenosis seems to involve initial platelet adherence at the site of balloon dilatation and in a second phase growth of fibroblasts and vascular smooth muscle cells. Platelets are able to release vasoconstrictor and proaggregatory mediators like TXA_2 or serotonin resulting in vasoconstriction, spasm, and acute thrombotic occlusions. Additionally, platelets release chemotactic mediators like 12-HETE stimulating smooth muscle cell movement and mitogens like PDGF (platelet derived growth factor) inducing smooth muscle cell proliferation. Therefore, effective inhibitors of platelet activation like PGI_2 may be able to prevent early vessel occlusion and late restenosis following PTCA.

This study was designed as a double-blind, randomized and placebo controlled trial to evaluate the effects of the chemically stable PGI_2 analog ciprostene (Linet etal, 1986) on restenosis rate in 32 patients undergoing therapeutic PTCA.

STUDY DESIGN AND METHODS

Study design and patient recruitment

The study was designed to compare the effects of ciprostene to placebo in patients undergoing single vessel PTCA. The design was randomized and double-blind. Main endpoint was the percent stenoses of the coronary artery dilated at the 6 month follow-up coronary angiography.

All 32 patients recruited for this study (25 males, 7 females; mean age 52.8 $\pm$ 8,6 yrs, range 31-68 yrs) were referred to our center for a balloon angioplasty of a coronary artery stenoses and gave their written informed consent. Patients with recent myocardial infarction, recent cerebrovascular accidents, known bleeding disorders, poorly controlled diabetes or arterial hypertension as well as premenopausal women were not included in this trial.

Patients were classified as suffering from unstable angina when anginal attacks occurred spontaneously and ECG changes typical of ischemia like ST-segment alteration or T-wave inversion had been documented during the anginal attacks.

Coronary angiography, balloon dilatation and drug administration

Coronary angiography was performed according to the Judkins technique using a 9F guiding catheter. The catheter was introduced into the coronary artery to be dilated and the infusion of ciprostene or placebo was started intracoronarily at a dose of 40 ng/kg/min for 20 min. Immediately after termination of the intraarterial infusion an intravenous infusion at a rate of 40 ng/kg/min was started. Infusion rate increased by 20 ng/kg/min every 30 min, until a final infusion rate of 120 ng/kg/ min was administered, which was maintained for 36 hrs. In order to avoid the development of a rebound phenomenon, the infusion rate was tapered off by 20 ng/kg/min every two hrs until cessation of infusion 48 hrs after the angioplasty procedure.

Balloon angioplasty was performed immediately after termination of the intracoronary infusion using balloons of 2.0 to 3.5 mm in diameter. The coronary artery to be dilated was visualized by injection of contrast medium in two orthogonal views, which were chosen identical before and after PTCA and at the 6 month follow up angiography. For measurement of luminal diameters cine films were analyzed from a twentyfold magnified projection. Vessel contours were outlined manually using an ultrasonic pen and analyzed by a computer system (Cardiograph 200, Kontron Instruments). The degree of obstruction was calculated as the mean of the narrowest segments of all projections, in which the stenotic segment was clearly visible (Meyer etal, 1982).

Concomitant medication

All patients received aspirin (100 mg/d) and nifedipine (3 x 20 mg/d) as a local routine medical therapy until the follow up angiography at 6 month. During the PTCA procedure patients received organic nitrates, calcium antagonists, and heparin (10000 IU i.v. and 3000 IU i.c.). Patients with unstable angina were treated with aspirin and continuous infusion of heparin (15 IU/kg) additionally.

Miscellaneous

The study protocol was reviewed and approved by the institutional ethical committee (Ethikkommission bei der Ärztekammer Rheinland- Pfalz). The study was supported by The Upjohn Company, Kalamazoo, Michigan, USA.

All data presented are mean $\pm$ SEM of n observations. Longitudinal statistical analyses was performed by analysis of variance (ANOVA), means were compared by Student's t-Test for paired data using a commercially available computer program (Primer of Biostatistics, McGraw-Hill, New York, 1988).

RESULTS

Thirty two patients were recruited for the study and received ciprostene (n=17) or placebo (n=15). Final assessment including analyses of the three coronary angiography films before, after PTCA and at 6 month follow up was performed in 24 patients with successful PTCA (12 ciprostene, 12 placebo). In 4 patients with unstable angina (3 ciprostene, 1 placebo) plasma CK levels rose to more than twice the normal level indicating myocardial ischemia and a non successful dilatation, three patients rejected 6 month follow up coronary angiography, and one patient (placebo) underwent bypass surgery within 48 hrs after PTCA because of a large intimal dissection but without any signs of acute ischemia.

With respect to medical history and cardiovascular risk factor profile both groups of patients were comparable and did not show any significant differences.

Coronary angiography at 6 month

The alterations in the degree of coronary artery stenoses after PTCA and during the 6 month follow up in all patients are depicted in Figure 1. In patients receiving ciprostene stenoses diameter was reduced from 83±3 to 31±4 % by the PTCA procedure and increased to 55±9 % at 6 month. This follow up result in the ciprostene group is still significantly different to the situation before PTCA (P=0.012). The initial success of coronary artery dilatation was identical in patients receiving placebo, in which stenoses were reduced from an initial value of 81±3 % to 34±3 % after PTCA. At the 6 month follow up stenoses diameter had increased to 63±8 %. The patients in the placebo group did not exert any statistically significant difference in stenoses at the 6 month follow-up, when compared to the initial value (Fig. 1). There are no statistically significant differences in the degree of stenoses when the two groups are compared at a given time.

Figure 1

Degree of coronary artery stenoses in all patients with stable and unstable angina treated with ciprostene (n=12) or placebo (n=12).

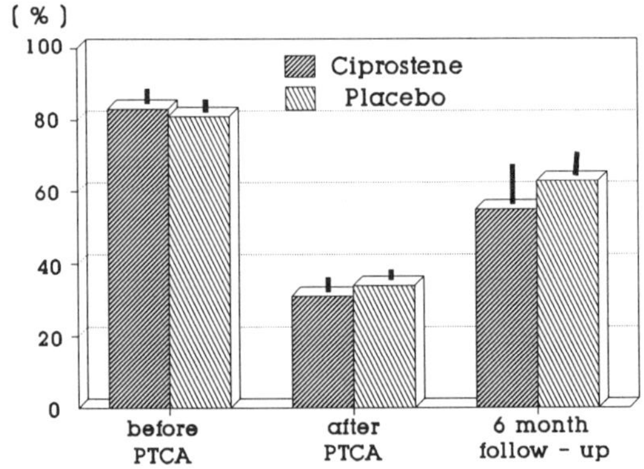

According to the clinical and electrocardiographic criteria given above 13 patients (6 ciprostene, 7 placebo) were classified as having unstable angina and 11 patients suffered from stable angina (6 ciprostene, 5 placebo). Only patients with unstable angina receiving ciprostene exerted a significant difference at the 6 month follow-up coronary angiography when compared to the percent of stenoses before PTCA (Fig. 2). There is no hint, that infusion of ciprostene in patients with stable angina improves the angiographic outcome at 6 month.

Figure 2

Degree of coronary artery stenoses in patients with unstable angina treated with ciprostene (n=6) or placebo (n=7).

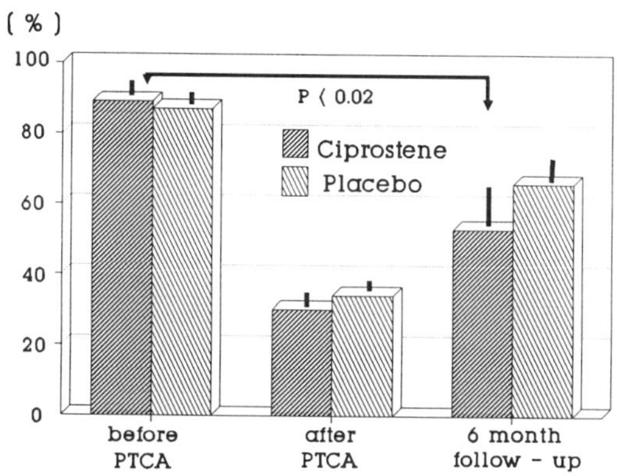

Hemodynamic drug effects

When patients receiving ciprostene were compared to the placebo group there were no statistically significant alterations in systolic or diastolic arterial blood pressure or heart rate during the infusion period.

Unwanted drug effects during the infusion period

The unwanted effects possibly related to the study medication are depicted in table 1. The number of puncture site hematomas was significantly higher in the ciprostene group (n=4) when compared to placebo (n=0). One ciprostene patient developed a bleeding from the groin after removal of the pressure cuff at a time, when ciprostene infusion had been terminated already. This patient received one unit of washed red blood cells and the further course was without any other complications. It is remarkable, that no non-catheter associated bleedings occurred.

Table 1
Unwanted events possibly related to the study medication

	Placebo (n=12)	Ciprostene(n=12)
Puncture site hematoma	0	4
Bleedings requiring transfusion	0	1
Facial flush	3	6
Headache	4	2
Nausea	2	2
Vomiting	2	1
Restlessness	1	1

Discussion

A number of studies were performed to identify alterations in medical therapy after PTCA in order to decrease the rate of restenoses. These studies included the use of platelet inhibitors (Schwartz etal, 1988), calcium antagonists (Corcos etal, 1985) or nitrovasodilators with platelet inhibitory effects like molsidomine (Darius etal, 1987). In 1990 Gershlick etal reported of a study on intravenous prostacyclin which did not show major beneficial effects. Despite of the multitude of trials undertaken to decrease restenosis significantly, no major breakthroughs were reported yet. The therapeutic approach tested in this study was the use of intracoronary and intravenous infusion of the prostacyclin analog ciprostene. In addition to inhibiting platelet aggregation PGI_2 reduces the release of mitogens like platelet derived growth factor (PDGF) from activated platelets (Stürzebecher etal, 1989). Thus, the administration of ciprostene during the PTCA procedure was performed in order to reduce the initial platelet deposition and platelet activation during angioplasty and thereby diminishing the risk of early thrombosis and late restenosis.

The angiographic analyses of the coronary artery stenoses in the two groups of patients studied did not show statistically significant differences between the two groups before PTCA and immediately thereafter. Thus, PTCA resulted in a comparable reduction in percent stenoses (Fig. 1). However, in patients receiving ciprostene stenoses at the 6 month follow up angiography was significantly lower when compared to the situation before PTCA (55 ± 9 vs 83 ± 3 %; $P=0.012$). This prolonged beneficial effect of the angioplasty procedure is due to the ciprostene infusion in patients with unstable angina. In patients with stable angina ciprostene had no detectable effect (Fig. 2).

The number of catheter associated hematomas at the puncture site was higher in the ciprostene group. Thus, during the infusion of prostacyclin analogs special attention should be paid to the concomitant medication with antiplatelet and anticoagulatory drugs.

In conclusion, in this study recruiting a limited number of 32 patients, angiographic analyses of the coronary artery stenoses hints to a possible beneficial effect of ciprostene in patients with unstable angina. Thus, further studies involving a larger cohort of patients are needed.

REFERENCES

Corcos, T., David, P.R., Val, P.G. etal (1985) Failure of diltiazem to prevent restenosis after percutaneous transluminal coronary angioplasty. Am. Heart J. 109, 926-931.

Darius, H., Rupprecht, H.J., Erbel, R., Pop, T., Brennecke, R., Meyer, J. (1987) A randomized study of pharmacologic prevention of coronary reocclusion after therapeutic PTCA.
Europ.Heart J. 8 (Suppl.2), 224.

Gershlick, A.H., Timmis, A.D., Rothman M.T., Layton C.A., Balcon, R. (1990) Post angioplasty prostacyclin infusion does not reduce the incidence of restenosis. Circulation 82 (Suppl.III), 1974.

Linet, O.I., Nishizawa, E.E., Schaub, R.G., van der Lugt, J.T., Greenwald, C.A. (1986) Tolerance and pharmacology of ciprostene, a stable epoprostenol (prostacyclin) analogue in humans. J.Clin.Pharmacol. 26, 131-140.

Meyer, J., Merx, W., Schmitz, H., et al (1982) Percutaneous transluminal coronary angioplasty immediately after intracoronary streptolysis of transmural myocardial infarction. Circulation 66, 905-913.

Schwartz, L., Bourassa, M.G., Lesperance, J. et al (1988) Aspirin and dipyridamole in the prevention of restenosis after percutaneous transluminal coronary angioplasty. N.Engl.J.Med. 318, 1714-1719.

Stürzebecher, S., Nieuweboer, B., Matthes, S., Schillinger, E. (1989) Effects of PGD_2, PGE_1, and PGI_2-analogues on PDGF release and aggregation of human gel-filtered platelets. In: Prostaglandins in Clinical Research. Cardiovascular System (K. Schrör and H. Sinzinger, Eds) Alan R.Liss, New York, pp 365-370.

AAS 37
Prostaglandins in the
Cardiovascular System

ENDOGENOUS PROSTACYCLIN PRESERVES MYOCARDIAL FUNCTION AND ENDOTHELIUM-DERIVED NITRIC OXIDE FORMATION IN MYOCARDIAL ISCHEMIA

K. Schrör, and I. Woditsch

Institut für Pharmakologie, Heinrich-Heine-Universität Düsseldorf, Moorenstraße 5, D-4000 Düsseldorf 1, FRG

SUMMARY: Nitric oxide (NO) and prostacyclin (PGI_2) release was determined in effluents of Langendorff-perfused rabbit hearts under control conditions and during reperfusion subsequent to 2 h of global, low-flow ischemia. PGI_2 release (6-oxo-$PGF_{1\alpha}$) was significantly enhanced during early reperfusion and remained enhanced during a total time of 70 min of reperfusion. NO formation was reduced during ischemia but was substantially enhanced during reperfusion. Inhibition of endogenous PGI_2 production by indomethacin resulted in severe disturbance of myocardial function and NO release. Inhibition of NO generation by L-N-nitroarginine did not affect myocardial contractility. These data suggest a cardioprotective and endothelium-protective role of PGI_2 in myocardial ischemia which also involves protection of NO generation.

INTRODUCTION

Myocardial ischemia is associated with initial stimulation and subsequent injury of vascular endothelium. This, in turn should also have consequences for endothelium-derived mediator release. Two important vasodilators with a similar profile of biological activities and putative significance for ischemic tissue perfusion are prostacyclin (PGI_2) and nitric oxide (NO) (Moncada et al, 1991). Interestingly, there appears not to be any systematic investigation addressing the question of the significance of endogenous NO and PGI_2 release for coronary and cardiac function in ischemia.

This study was designed to (i) determine PGI_2 and NO release subsequent to global low-flow ischemia in a well standardized in vitro model; (ii) study possible interactions between PGI_2 and NO release during ischemia and reperfusion by selective inhibition of PGI_2 and NO biosynthesis; (iii) evaluate the consequences of removal of PGI_2 or NO generation for cardiocoronary functions and cardiac tissue injury.

MATERIALS AND METHODS

Heart preparations and measurements. Langendorff-hearts were prepared from New Zealand White rabbits as previously described (Schrör et al, 1991). The hearts were perfused at a constant rate of 22 ml/min with Krebs-Henseleit-buffer (pH 7.4). The buffer was equilibrated with 95% oxygen + 5% CO_2 by using a membrane oxygenator (Eschweiler, Kiel, FRG). Left ventricular systolic pressure (LVSP), enddiastolic pressure (LVEDP) and coronary perfusion pressure (CPP) was measured continuously. Because of the constant volume perfusion, the CPP is a direct measure of the coronary vascular resistance. NO was determined in the coronary effluent spectrophotometrically by the oxyhemoglobin technique (Kelm and Schrader, 1988), PGI_2 by radioimmunoassay of the stable hydrolysis product 6-oxo-$PGF_{1\alpha}$.

Experimental protocol. Control readings were taken at time 0. Thereafter, oxyhemoglobin (3 µM) was added to the perfusion fluid and the perfusion continued under otherwise identical conditions. At time 60 min normothermic ischemia was induced by reduction of coronary flow to 1.2 ml/min. This low-flow ischemia was maintained for 2 h, i.e. until time 3 h. At this time, reperfusion was initiated by restoring the initial flow rate of 22 ml/min for another 0.5 h.

In experiments with blocking agents, indomethacin (3 µM) or L-N-Nitroarginine (L-NO_2-ARG, 100 µM) (Sigma, Deisenhofen, FRG) were added to the Krebs-Henseleit-buffer at time 0 to inhibit PGI_2 and NO formation, respectively.

Statistics. The data are mean ± SEM of n determinations. Statistical analysis was performed by the two-tailed t-test. P levels of $\leq$ 0.05 were considered significant.

RESULTS

NO-release in ischemia and reperfusion. There was a significant NO release under non-ischemic conditions, amounting to 0.8 ± 0.9 nmoles/min. NO generation was suppressed to values close to 0 during ischemia but rose considerably during reperfusion to 1.3 ± 0.1 nmoles/min at the end of the experiment (n = 12).

NO-release after treatment with inhibitors. Addition of L-NO_2-ARG to the perfusion buffer reduced the NO formation at the end of the experiment to 0.3 ± 0.1 nmoles/min, i.e. by 60- 70%. Treatment with indomethacin did not modify NO release under non-ischemic conditions. However, indomethacin significantly reduced NO formation during reperfusion, amounting to 0.8 ± 0.1 nmoles/min at the end of reperfusion. This was equivalent to a 35-40% inhibition as compared to untreated controls (n = 9; $P < 0.05$).

PGI_2-release in ischemia and reperfusion. Basal 6-oxo-$PGF_{1\alpha}$ release into the coronary effluent amounted to 7.5 ± 1.2 pmol/min at the beginning of the experiment. This level was significantly reduced during ischemia. Reperfusion resulted in a considerable increase of 6-oxo-$PGF_{1\alpha}$ levels, reaching a peak level of 77 ± 6

pmol/min during the second minute of reperfusion ($n = 12$; $p < 0.05$). At the end of the reperfusion period, 6-oxo-$PGF_{1\alpha}$ release remained elevated at a level, about two-fold higher than that before ischemia ($n = 12$; $P < 0.05$).

PGI_2-release after treatment with inhibitors. Treatment with indomethacin reduced 6-oxo-$PGF_{1\alpha}$ generation during non-ischemic conditions to levels close to the detection limit throughout the experiment. L-NO_2-ARG did not alter basal release of 6-oxo-$PGF_{1\alpha}$ prior to ischemia. In contrast, peak 6-oxo-$PGF_{1\alpha}$ overflow during the second minute of reperfusion was significantly reduced by this compound, from 77 ± 6 to 32 ± 3 pmol/min ($n = 8$, $P < 0.05$). There was no change in 6-oxo-$PGF_{1\alpha}$ generation at the end of the reperfusion period by L-NO_2-ARG treatment, amounting to 20 ± 3 pmoles/min in the presence and 22 ± 2 pmoles/min in absence of the inhibitor.

Cardiocoronary functions in ischemia and reperfusion. All hearts exhibited stable cardiocoronary function prior to ischemia. Reduction of flow resulted in a rapid drop to < 10 mmHg of CPP and LVSP during the first minutes. There was a time-dependent increase in LVEDP during ischemia. At the beginning of reperfusion, all functional parameters started to recover and approached constant levels at the end of the experiment.

Actions of inhibitors. Treatment with L-NO_2-ARG did not change cardiac contractility under non-ischemic conditions. There was only a modest and insignificant increase in the CPP, despite of a 70% reduction in NO release. The same treatment during ischemia and reperfusion did also not modify contractile functions of the left ventricle. In contrast, coronary perfusion pressure was considerably higher in L-NO_2-ARG-treated hearts than in untreated controls. Thus, the increase in CPP at the end of reperfusion was about twice as much as in untreated reperfused hearts ($n = 10$; $P < 0.05$) (Table I).

Treatment with indomethacin resulted in a modest increase in CPP ($P > 0.05$). However, indomethacin did severely suppress contractile functions of the myocardium during ischemia. Coronary vascular resistance was also somewhat increased (Table I).

Table I: Left ventricular enddiastolic pressure (LVEDP), actively developed systolic pressure (LVSP) and coronary perfusion pressure (CPP) in isolated rabbit hearts before ischemia and reperfusion, and its alterations by indomethacin (3 μM) and L-NO_2-ARG (100 μM) as compared to untreated controls.

Parameter	time	Control (14)	Indomethacin (12)	L-NO_2-ARG (10)
	before ischemia	63 ± 3	60 ± 4	57 ± 3
LVSP	end of ischemia	< 10	< 10	< 10
[mmHg]	end of reperfusion	58 ± 3	32 ± 5*	54 ± 4
	before ischemia	0	0	0
LVEDP	end of ischemia	28 ± 5	57 ± 4*	28 ± 7
[mmHg]	end of reperfusion	21 ± 5	58 ± 6*	25 ± 6
	before ischemia	33 ± 3	32 ± 1	29 ± 2
CPP	end of ischemia	0	0	0
[mmHg]	end of reperfusion	54 ± 4	45 ± 3	70 ± 3*

The data are x ± SEM of the number of experiments indicated in brackets.

*): $P < 0.05$ (indomethacin or L-NO_2-ARG vs. control)

Myocardial creatine phosphokinase-specific activity. Myocardial CK-specific activity amounted to about 15 IU/mg protein in non-ischemic control hearts and was reduced by 15% in reperfused ischemic hearts. L-NO_2-ARG did not modify these levels whereas indomethacin caused another 40-50% loss of CK-specific activity.

DISCUSSION

Myocardial ischemia is associated with enhanced lipid degradation, arachidonic acid accumulation and prostaglandin release during reperfusion (Engels et al, 1990). This will result in some initial overflow of 6-oxo-$PGF_{1\alpha}$ into the coronary effluent at the beginning of reperfusion which was also seen in this study.

However, this 6-oxo-$PGF_{1\alpha}$ release appears not to be a pure wash-out phenomenon of an accumulated metabolite, because 6-oxo-$PGF_{1\alpha}$ levels remained elevated for more than 1 h of reperfusion. Thus, the question arises whether enhanced PGI_2 production just indicates phospholipase activation and myocellular membrane disruption or has any biological effect by its own.

Our data and those reported previously for reperfused ischemic hearts of the rabbit (Schrör et al, 1982) and cat (Thiemermann et al, 1984) clearly suggest enhanced PGI_2 generation as an important tissue protective factor. Inhibition of PGI_2 generation by indomethacin resulted in severe depression of myocardial function, as seen from the elevation in LVEDP and decrease in myocardial contractility. Additionally, there was a considerable loss of myocellular integrity, indicated by a substantial loss of cytosolic CK in indomethacin-treated ischemic hearts as compared to untreated controls.

Our data indicate that generation and release of NO is also considerably suppressed during ischemia, confirming earlier studies of Sessa and Vane (1991) in isolated endothelial cells. With initiation of reperfusion there is a stepwise increase in NO formation that exceeds non-ischemic control levels at about 30 min of reperfusion.

Reduced endothelium-derived relaxation and/or generation of EDRF subsequent to myocardial ischemia has been described in several models, including intact hearts in vitro (Woditsch and Schrör, 1990; Tsao and Lefer, 1990). However, inhibition of NO generation in contrast to inhibition of PGI_2 formation had no major consequences for myocellular integrity or cardiac contractility. There is only some increase in coronary vascular resistance, confirming an involvement of the mediator in regulation of coronary vascular resistance of the rabbit (Amezcua et al, 1989; Humphries et al., 1991).

Indomethacin not only caused additional myocellular injury as noted above but also a reduction in NO-release. This effect was only seen in reperfusion but not prior to ischemia. This observation and the failure of L-arginine to reverse indomethacin-induced inhibition of NO formation (not shown), excludes an inhibition of the NO synthase by indomethacin or depletion of the precursor as cause of reduced NO formation. We postulate that inhibition of ischemia-induced increase in PGI_2 generation by indomethacin causes endothelial injury in a way similar to that of myocardial muscle cells.

In summary, our study demonstrates important functional interactions between PGI_2 and NO in isolated ischemic rabbit hearts which do not reflect common pathways in biosynthesis (Schröder et al, 1990). Enhanced PGI_2 generation occurs during reperfusion and appears to be necessary to maintain myocardial function and endothelium-derived NO release. There is no evidence that endothelium-derived NO at concentrations that can be formed by the heart, has any other important function than control of coronary perfusion.

REFERENCES

Amezcua, J.L., Palmer, R.M.J., de Souza, B.M., and Moncada, S. (1989) Nitric oxide synthesized from L-arginine regulates vascular tone in the coronary circulation of the rabbit, Br. J. Pharmacol. 97, 1119-1124.

Engels, W., Van Bilsen, M., De Groot, M.J.M., Lemmens, P.J.M.R., Willemsen, P.H.M., Renemann, R.S., and Van der Vusse, G.J. (1990) Ischemia and reperfusion induced formation of eicosanoids in isolated rat hearts, Am. J. Physiol. 258, H1865-H1871.

Humphries, R.G., Carr, R.D., Nicol, A.K., Tomlinson, W., and O'Connor, S.E. (1991) Coronary vasoconstriction in the conscious rabbit following intravenous infusion of L-N^G-nitro-arginine, Br. J. Pharmacol. 102, 565-566.

Kelm, M., and Schrader, J. (1988) Nitric oxide release from the isolated guinea pig heart, Eur. J. Pharmacol. 155, 317-321.

Moncada, S., Palmer, R.M.J., and Higgs, E.A. (1991) Nitric oxide - physiology, pathophysiology, and pharmacology, Pharmacol. Rev. 43, 109-142.

Schröder, H., Machunsky, Ch., Strobach, H., and Schrör, K. (1990) Nitric oxide but not prostacyclin has an autocrine function in porcine aortic endothelial cells, Adv. Prostaglandin Thrombox. Leukotriene Res. 21, 671-674.

Schrör, K., Darius, H., Addicks, K., Köster, R., and Smith III, E.F. (1982) PGI_2 prevents ischemia-induced alterations in cardiac catecholamines without influencing nerve-stimulation induced catecholamine release in non-ischemic conditions, J. Cardiovasc. Pharmacol. 4, 741-748.

Schrör, K., Förster, S., and Woditsch, I. (1991) On-line measurement of nitric oxide release from organic nitrates in the intact coronary circulation, Naunyn-Schmiedeberg's Arch. Pharmacol. 344, 240-246.

Sessa, W.C., and Vane, J.R. (1991) Ischaemic conditions inhibit the release of EDRF from cultured endothelial cells, Br. J. Pharmacol. 102, 120P.

Thiemermann, C., Steinhagen-Thiessen, E., and Schrör, K. (1984) Inhibition of oxygen-centered free radical formation by the stable prostacyclin-mimetic iloprost (ZK 36 374) in acute myocardial ischemia, J. Cardiovasc. Pharmacol. 6, 365-366.

Tsao, P.S., and Lefer, A.M. (1990) Time course and mechanism of endothelial dysfunction in isolated ischemic and hypoxic-perfused hearts, Am. J. Physiol. 259, H1660-1666.

Woditsch, I., Strobach, H., and Schrör, K. (1990) Endothelium-dependent vasodilatation in the reperfused ischemic rabbit heart, Circulation, 82, Suppl. III, III-378.

AAS 37
Prostaglandins in the
Cardiovascular System

ROLE OF PROSTACYCLIN IN NORMAL AND ARTERIOSCLEROTIC HUMAN CORONARY ARTERIES DURING HYPOXIA

G. Siegel[1], F. Schnalke[1], K. Rückborn[2], J. Müller[3] and R. Hetzer[3]

[1]Institute of Physiology, Biophysical Research Group, The Free University of Berlin, D-1000 Berlin 33; [2]Institute of Physiology, The University of Rostock, D-2500 Rostock 1; [3]German Heart Institute Berlin, D-1000 Berlin 65, Germany

SUMMARY: Human coronary arteries were taken from heart transplant patients. Arteriosclerotic arteries were more depolarized and constricted over the whole P_{O_2} range between 535 and 0 mm Hg. During oxygen deficiency, control preparations showed a maximal hyperpolarization of $\Delta V = 10.9$ mV and a maximal relaxation of $\Delta T = 0.466$ g. Arteriosclerotic arteries, however, became hyperpolarized by merely $\Delta V = 7.1$ mV and relaxed by $\Delta T = 0.258$ g. The isometric pretension was 2 g in all investigations. Two series of experiments, one with an application of indomethacin and another one with deendothelialized blood vessels, confirmed the hypothesis that the endothelium of arteriosclerotic coronary arteries may produce less prostacyclin and EDHF. In normal coronary arteries, indomethacin reduced the hypoxic hyperpolarization and dilatation at 30 mm Hg P_{O_2} by about 51%. The reduction was 26% in arteriosclerotic vessels. The complete removal of the endothelium caused a 49% (74%) restriction of dilatory vascular reactivity. The relation was quite similar for a carbogen Krebs solution (resting, control conditions). The hyperpolarizing and dilatory contribution by prostacyclin was 32% in normal and 12% in arteriosclerotic coronaries. The rest can be attributed to the basal release of the endothelial dilator EDHF. Thus, it may be concluded that, in arteriosclerotic blood vessels, PGI_2 synthesis and release are predominantly diminished or its effectivity is impaired. Finally we found the ratio PGI_2/EDHF in the voltage and tension changes strongly shifted to the PGI_2 side with a declining oxygen concentration. This is true for normal and arteriosclerotic vessels. In accordance with the activation curve for vascular smooth muscle, the hyperpolarization leads to relaxation via a closure of Ca^{2+} channels. 2.5 mV hyperpolarization reduces the tension developed by half.

Eicosanoids and cytokines play a role in regulating vascular cholesterol homeostasis and have a profound effect on cholesterol delivery and trafficking within the vessel wall. It also appears that the eicosanoid pathway is linked to the cytokine network regarding the modulation of vessel wall lipolytic activities. Furthermore, it has been suggested that endothelial cells are the early target sites in the pathogenesis of atherosclerosis. Certain dysfunctions which occur very early after the onset of hypercholesterolemia, including a marked loss of ability to produce the eicosanoid prostacyclin (PGI_2) and endothelium-derived hyperpolarizing factor (EDHF) provide evidence for this. The cellular mechanisms of these important changes, as well as the ability of agents such as prostacyclin mimetics to protect the endothelium and smooth muscle cells from such dysfunction, will be discussed.

MATERIALS AND METHODS

Experimental Preparations and Solutions

Intracellular potential recordings and measurements of isometric tension were performed on the vascular smooth muscle of the human coronary artery [15]. Coronary arteries were taken from heart transplant patients who had been suffering from a dilative cardiomyopathy or extensive atherosclerosis. There was a clear differentiation between normal and atherosclerotic vessels where the preparations had been subjected to light and electron microscopic examination. All arterial segments were equilibrated in a Krebs solution of the following composition: Na^+ 151.16, K^+ 4.69, Ca^{2+} 2.52, Mg^{2+} 1.1, Cl^- 145.4, HCO_3^- 16.31, $H_2PO_4^-$ 1.38, glucose 7.77 mmol/l (temp. 37°C, pH 7.35). The solution was usually aerated with a 95% O_2 - 5% CO_2 gas mixture (carbogen). Blood substitute solutions were equilibrated with $O_2/CO_2/N_2$ mixtures containing different oxygen concentrations, but a constant concentration of carbon dioxide (5 ml/dl) to vary the oxygen tension. Microelectrodes consisting of platinum cathodes were used for continuous oxygen tension measurements in the Krebs solution close to the blood vessel strip [4]. Indomethacin (Vonum, Econerica, Germany) was applied in a concentration of 10^{-5} mol/l. Each solution was freshly prepared. Endothelium-denuded preparations were obtained by gently scraping off the endothelial layer. Whether the procedure was successful was verified using light and electron microscopy.

Mechanical and Electrical Recording

Cylinders from the coronary arteries, 4-5 mm long, were cut lengthwise. Since muscle cells of the arteries are arranged circularly, the folded-out vessel ring, 5-10 mm long, was attached at the cut ends to an isometrically measuring tension device (KWS 522.C, K 52 C; Hottinger-Baldwin, Darmstadt, Germany) [15]. The specimens were superfused with a carbogen Krebs solution at 50-60 ml/min for 15 min at an initial tension of 2 g. This high flow rate was used in order to bring about quick changes in P_{O_2} and reach low pressures. After this time, the tension was steady and amounted to 0.995 ± 0.156 g (n=10). Then, solutions with first decreasing, then increasing oxygen partial pressures (reversibility) were applied for 15 min each. After these periods, the mechanical tension had reached a steady state value at each concentration step [13]. All values are the means ± SEM of the indicated number of preparations. Statistical significance (error probability P) was calculated according to the one-tailed t-test for dependent or independent samples.

Intracellular recordings of membrane potential were made with glass capillary microelectrodes, filled with 3 mol/l KCl, simultaneously with the mechanical tension registration. The electrode resistances ranged from 60-100 MΩ and the tip potentials from -40 to -80 mV [13,15]. Electrode resistances and tip potentials were measured before and after impalement. Only when these values were unchanged was the recorded membrane potential included in the evaluation. The electrodes were shielded to just below the tips; otherwise conventional recording techniques were used [11]. The microelectrode was inserted into the arterial muscle cell from the intimal surface. Arteries in a normal Krebs solution with membrane potentials between -50 and -80 mV were selected for the final averaging. Membrane potentials more positive than -50 mV (20% of all impalements) had to be discarded because, according to our own measurements and those of other authors [9,15], they stem from endothelial cells.

At each oxygen concentration step, the membrane potential had attained a steady state value after 3 min and the tension after 7 min at the most. In principle, intracellular recordings were carried out after the fifth minute. In all preparations at least ten impalements per oxygen concentration were averaged. The mean values of the membrane potential of all the canine carotids and human coronaries at each oxygen tension were averaged and are represented in the figures.

RESULTS

Fig. 1 illustrates the effect of hypoxia on membrane potential and tension of normal and arteriosclerotic human coronary arteries which were taken from heart transplant patients. Voltage and tension, as a function of P_{O_2}, showed similar courses to those already described for the canine carotis [11,13,15]. There was a continuous hyperpolarization and relaxation with a reduction of P_{O_2} from 535 to 30 mm Hg, and a depolarization and contraction between 30 and 0 mm Hg. It is striking that, in the case of atherosclerosis, vascular smooth muscle cells were more depolarized and had more tone. This was true for all O_2 tensions. In normal carbogen Krebs solution, the membrane potential amounted to -60.4 ± 0.3 mV (n=5) and the initial force to 0.985 ± 0.096 g (n=5). Arteriosclerotic coronaries were depolarized to -59.8 ± 1.0 mV (n=5) and contracted to 1.316 ± 0.061 g (n=5; $P < 0.02$). During oxygen deficiency, control preparations showed a maximal hyperpolarization of 10.9 mV and a maximal relaxation of 0.466 g. Arteriosclerotic arteries, however, became hyperpolarized by merely 7.1 mV and relaxed by 0.258 g.

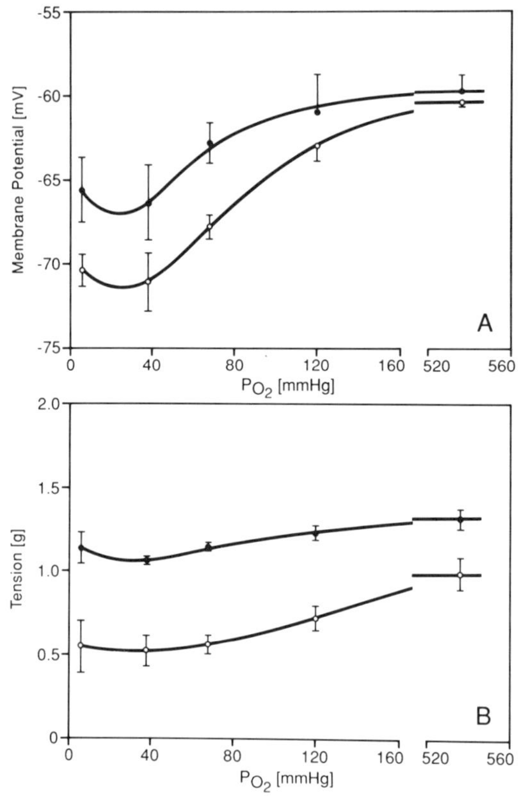

Fig. 1. Membrane potential (A) and mechanical force development (B) of isolated human coronary arteries in response to changes in the oxygen tension of the Krebs solution. Mean values from five experiments each. (○) Normal coronary arteries, (●) arteriosclerotic coronary arteries.

Two series of experiments, one with an application of indomethacin (Figs. 2,3b) and another one with deendothelialized blood vessels (Figs. 2,3c), confirmed the hypothesis that the endothelium of arteriosclerotic coronary arteries may produce less prostacyclin (PGI_2) and endothelium-derived hyperpolarizing factor (EDHF). For reasons of clearness, the points measured and their deviations were omitted. In normal coronary arteries, indomethacin reduced the hypoxic hyperpolarization and dilatation at 30 mm Hg P_{O_2} by about 51% (Fig. 2). The hyperpolarizing and

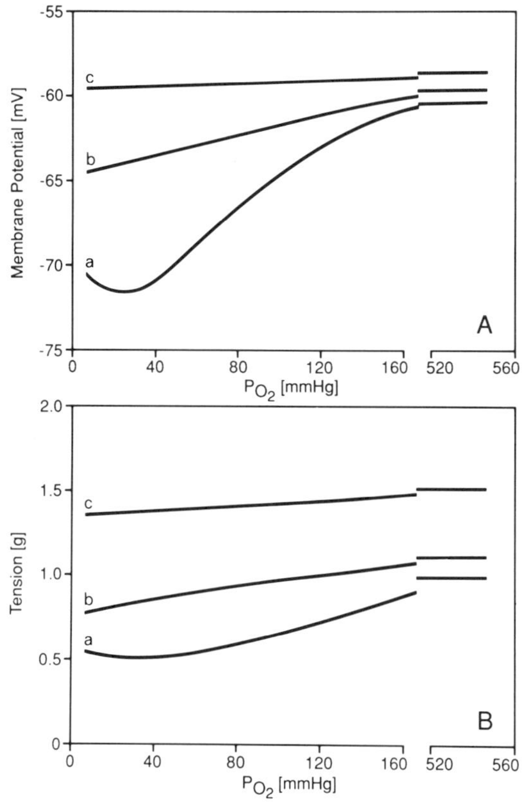

Fig. 2. Membrane potential (A) and tension (B) in isolated vascular strips of human coronary arteries in dependency on the oxygen partial pressure of the Krebs solution. Mean values from 15 experiments. *a:* Normal Krebs solution; *b:* Krebs solution with indomethacin (10^{-5} mol/l); *c:* Normal Krebs solution, endothelial layer of the coronary segments removed.

dilatory contribution by PGI_2 was only about 32% for a carbogen Krebs solution (resting, control conditions). Without mentioning that arteriosclerotic coronary arteries were more depolarized and contracted, they became less hyperpolarized and relaxed by a fall in oxygen partial pressure (Fig. 3). With indomethacin, the hypoxic hyperpolarization and vasorelaxation was attenuated by merely 26%. The share of prostacyclin in dilatory vascular reactivity was restricted to 12% in normal Krebs solution. These

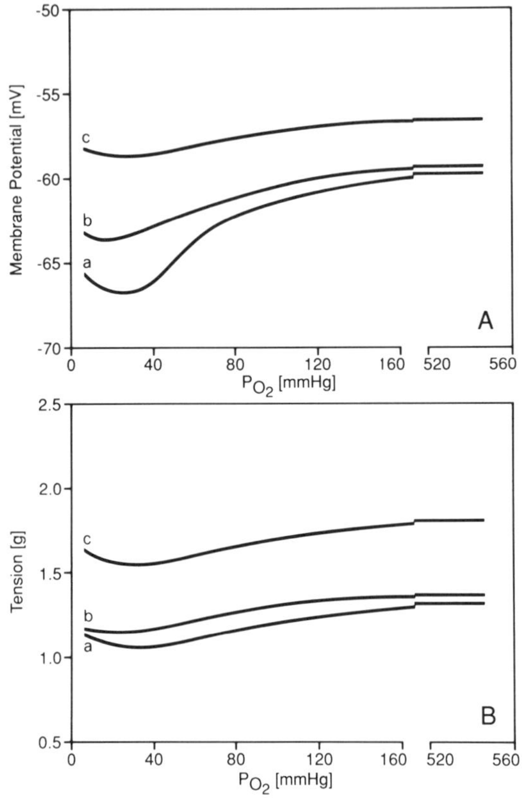

Fig. 3. Membrane potential (A) and tension (B) in isolated vascular strips of arteriosclerotic human coronary arteries in response to the oxygen partial pressure of the Krebs solution. Mean values from 15 experiments. *a:* Normal Krebs solution; *b:* Krebs solution with indomethacin (10^{-5} mol/l); *c:* Normal Krebs solution, endothelial layer of the coronary segments removed.

results can be qualitatively realized by the closed up curves a and b for arteriosclerotic blood vessels (cf. Fig. 3) as compared with the normal ones (cf. Fig. 2). Thus, it may be concluded that in arteriosclerotic blood vessels PGI_2 synthesis and release are predominantly diminished.

The beneficial effect of a compensation of the PGI_2 lacking is demonstrated in Fig. 4. As natural prostacyclin is unstable we used iloprost, a stable carbacyclin analogue. Iloprost, in a

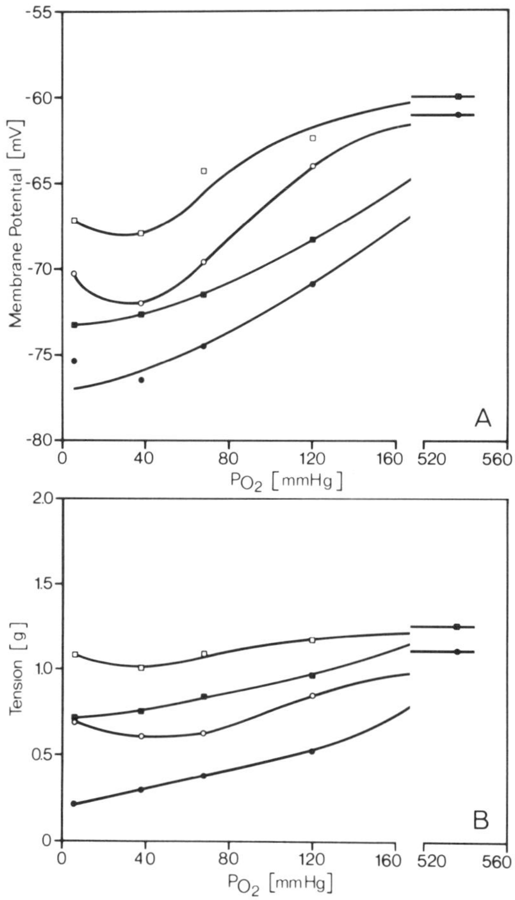

Fig. 4. Membrane potential (A) and tension (B) in isolated vascular strips of human coronary arteries dependent on the oxygen partial pressure of the Krebs solution. Mean values from five experiments each. (○) Normal coronary arteries with intact endothelium, (●) plus iloprost 10^{-7} mol/l; (□) arteriosclerotic coronary arteries, (■) plus iloprost 10^{-7} mol/l.

concentration of 10^{-7} mol/l, was able to induce hyperpolarization and relaxation at all O_2 partial pressures, even with maximal hyperpolarization and dilatation at about 30 mm Hg P_{O_2}. In normal and in atherosclerotic blood vessels, the hypoxic depolarization and contraction with oxygen pressures below 30 mm Hg was prevented by iloprost [12,15]. These results emphasize that also with an oxygen deficiency, additional hyperpolarization and vasodilatation can be attained by the intervention of a K^+ channel opener.

DISCUSSION

The response of vascular smooth musculature to a decline in oxygen tension presents itself as a balanced interplay between hyperpolarizing-vasodilatory (PGI_2, EDHF) and depolarizing-vasoconstrictory factors (noradrenaline, 20-HETE, endothelin). The same holds true for the adjustment of muscle tone under stationary resting conditions because all these compounds have a basal release [11,15]. This balance between relaxing and constricting factors seems to be disturbed and shifted to the constriction side in arteriosclerosis. Since atheromatous plaques contain high concentrations of lipid peroxides, which are known to inhibit prostacyclin synthetase [5,7], it was suggested that the prostacyclin production might be severely impaired in this disease [6]. Human arteriosclerotic iliac and femoral arteries form less 6-keto-prostaglandin $F_{1\alpha}$ than arteries obtained from healthy controls [16]. Endothelium-dependent relaxations to acetylcholine were reduced or absent in isolated atherosclerotic human coronary arteries [3]. These findings are fully confirmed by our observations. Arteriosclerotic human coronary arteries were more depolarized by 0.6 mV and more contracted by 0.331 g as compared to normal ones in a carbogen Krebs solution [12]. This difference was even greater with a P_{O_2} of 30 mm Hg: $\Delta V = 4.5$ mV; $\Delta T = 0.539$ g. The endothelial function is possibly limited in this tissue. Apparently, less PGI_2 and/or EDHF are produced by arteriosclerotic vessels. The distribution of both substances has changed as well. Under resting conditions, prostacyclin takes part in the basal release of hyperpolarizing and relaxing factors by 32% in normal coronaries, but only by 12% in arteriosclerotic coronaries. The rest can be attributed to the basal release of the endothelial dilator EDHF. In principle, a decline in O_2 tension shifts this ratio to the side of PGI_2. In normal coronary arteries, PGI_2 contributed by 51% at 30 mm Hg P_{O_2} to the hypoxic hyperpolarization and relaxation, however, to the minor changes in arteriosclerosis, only by 26%. Therefore, in arteriosclerotic blood vessels, PGI_2 synthesis and release may be restricted. An alternative explanation could be that impairment of PGI_2-dependent hyperpolarization and relaxation in the circulation of arteriosclerotic coronaries is not due to diminished PGI_2 formation but, in spite of an unchanged or even enhanced synthesis and release, due to a reduced action (increased inactivation, reduced sensitivity of the vasculature) of liberated PGI_2 [18]. Finally, we were able to analyze the portion of the hyperpolarizing and relaxing factors in a normal blood vessel at an oxygen partial pressure of 30 mm Hg: 20.6% smooth muscle prostacyclin, 30.2% endothelial prostacyclin [cf. 2], and 49.2% endothelium-derived hyperpolarizing factor.

The lack in prostacyclin of arteriosclerotic vessels could be compensated by externally applied PGI_2 [12,15]. The prostacyclin analogue iloprost 'transformed' arteriosclerotic coronaries into normal ones as far as their membrane potential and tone response to a reduction in O_2 partial pressure is concerned. Above all, membrane depolarization and vasoconstriction failed to appear with O_2 pressures below 30 mm Hg even in arteriosclerotic vessels. This is a very important result because such low P_{O_2} values were found during coronary angiography in the large coronary blood vessels of man with extensive arteriosclerosis. Therefore, even lower values may be expected in peripheral arteries and arterioles. An application of iloprost may be beneficial for the following reasons: P_{O_2} values can be expected where hypoxic depolarization and vasoconstriction appear in peripheral vascular disease, especially with pronounced atherosclerosis. Moreover, a low P_{O_2} causes the ratio of PGI_2/EDHF action to shift towards PGI_2. Conversely, not as much PGI_2 is produced in arteriosclerotic tissue, or else it loses its efficacy. Thus, the exogenous supply of prostacyclin mimetics prevents hypoxic depolarization and vasoconstriction.

Within the context of an explanation for the hypoxic membrane hyperpolarization we would like to say a few words about K^+ channel opening. The cause of hypoxic hyperpolarization is probably an increase in K^+ conductance for both compounds, PGI_2 and EDHF [1,11,12,14,15]. The central starting point of the physiological mode of action of K^+ channel openers is the hyperpolarization of the smooth muscle cells which leads to relaxation by closing T- and/or L-type Ca^{2+} channels without, in the classical sense, the participation of cAMP or cGMP [14]. In the case of prostacyclin, cAMP plays a part in the increase of the Ca^{2+}-activated K^+ outward current [14,15,17]. As suggested by Sadoshima et al. [10], the cAMP-dependent protein kinase seems to increase the Ca^{2+} sensitivity of the Ca^{2+}-activated K^+ channel. Obviously, one or two types of K^+ channels (perhaps the Ca^{2+}-activated K^+ channel and the delayed rectifier K^+ channel) are stimulated by phosphorylation with cA-PK. Therefore, the hyperpolarizing and relaxing effect of PGI_2 may be explained by interventions of cA-PK at the Ca^{2+}-activated K^+ channel, the sarcolemmal Ca^{2+} pump, and the $I_{Ca(s)}$ [17]. In principle, the effect of EDHF seems to be the same, but its effector chain proceeds via cG-PK. We presume that an ATP-sensitive channel, especially with respect to the effect of prostacyclin, is not responsible for the K^+ channel opening resulting in the hypoxic hyperpolarization, but the Ca^{2+}-activated K^+ channel [14,15]. The effect of the vasodilator EDHF, however, might be mediated by an ATP-sensitive K^+ channel [8].

Acknowledgements: The authors thank Mrs. Ch. Fuhrmann for her excellent technical assistance and Mr. H. Ewald from the mechanical workshop for his constant help. We are grateful to Mrs. M. Krawczynski for her outstanding work in preparing the illustrations and Mr. P. Holzner for the photographs. We are indebted to Mrs. A. Scheuermann for the translation and editorial elaboration of the manuscript.

REFERENCES

1. Bonnet, P., Gebremedhin, D., Rusch, N., Lombard, J.H., and Harder, D.R. (1991) Hypoxia increases K^+ conductance in cerebral arterial muscle cells. Circ. Res. (submitted).
2. Domae, M., and Kuriyama, H. (1986) Effects of prostaglandin I_2 synthesized in the endothelium and in the smooth muscle on mechanical properties of the canine thoracic aorta. Naunyn-Schmiedeberg's Arch. Pharmacol. **333**, 294-302.
3. Ginsburg, R., and Zera, P.H. (1984) Endothelial relaxant factor in the human epicardial coronary artery. Circulation **70** (Suppl. II), 122.
4. Grote, J., Siegel, G., Zimmer, K., and Adler, A. (1988) The influence of oxygen tension on membrane potential and tone of canine carotid artery smooth muscle. Adv. Exp. Med. Biol. **222**, 481-487.
5. Gryglewski, R.J., Bunting, S., Moncada, S., Flower, R.J., and Vane, J.R. (1976) Arterial walls are protected against deposition of platelet thrombi by a substance (prostaglandin X) which they make from prostaglandin endoperoxides. Prostaglandins **12**, 685-713.
6. Lüscher, T.F. (1988) Endothelial vasoactive substances and cardiovascular disease. Basel, München, Paris, London, New York, New Delhi, Singapore, Tokyo, Sydney: S. Karger.
7. Moncada, S., Gryglewski, R.J., Bunting, S., and Vane, J.R. (1976) A lipid peroxide inhibits the enzyme in blood vessel microsomes that generates from prostaglandin endoperoxides the substance (prostaglandin X) which prevents platelet aggregation. Prostaglandins **12**, 715-737.
8. Nelson, M.T., Patlak, J.B., Worley, J.F., and Standen, N.B. (1990) Calcium channels, potassium channels, and voltage dependence of arterial smooth muscle tone. Am. J. Physiol. **259**, C3-C18.
9. Northover, B.J. (1980) The membrane potential of vascular endothelial cells. Adv. Microcirc. **9**, 135-160.
10. Sadoshima, J.-I., Akaike, N., Kanaide, H., and Nakamura, M. (1988) Cyclic AMP modulates Ca-activated K channel in cultured smooth muscle cells of rat aortas. Am. J. Physiol. **255**, H754-H759.
11. Siegel, G., Grote, J., Schnalke, F., and Zimmer, K. (1989) The significance of the endothelium for hypoxic vasodilatation. Z. Kardiol. **78** (Suppl. 6), 124-131.
12. Siegel, G., Rückborn, K., Schnalke, F., Müller, J., and Warnecke, H. (1991) Hypoxische Vasodilatation und Vasokonstriktion an normalen und arteriosklerotischen Koronargefäßen des Menschen. In: Koronare Herzkrankheit: Molekulargenetische Aspekte und zelluläre Mechanismen, Risikoprofile vor und nach invasiven Therapieverfahren (G. Assmann, E. Betz, H. Heinle and H. Schulte, Eds), Verlag Vieweg, Braunschweig, pp. 98-108
13. Siegel, G., Walter, A., Bostanjoglo, M., Jans, A.W.H., Kinne, R., Piculell, L., and Lindman, B. (1989) Ion transport and cation-polyanion interactions in vascular biomembranes. J. Membrane Sci. **41**, 353-375.

14. Siegel, G., Walter, A., Schnalke, F., Schmidt, A., Buddecke, E., Loirand, G., and Stock, G. (1991) Potassium channel activation, hyperpolarization and vascular relaxation. Z. Kardiol. **80** (in press).
15. Siegel, G., Wenzel, K., Schnalke, F., Mironneau, J., Schultz, G., Schröder, G., Schillinger, E., Grauhan, O., and Hetzer, R. (1990) Prostacyclin analogues as K^+ channel openers. Clin. Pharmacol. **7**, 72-96.
16. Sinzinger, H., Feigl, W., and Silberbauer, K. (1979) Prostacyclin generation in atherosclerotic arteries. Lancet **II**, 469.
17. Sperelakis, N., and Ohya, Y. (1990) Cyclic nucleotide regulation of Ca^{2+} slow channels and neurotransmitter release in vascular muscle. Prog. Clin. Biol. Res. **327**, 277-298.
18. Woditsch, I., Hohlfeld, Th., and Schrör, K. (1991) Reduced endothelium-dependent relaxation in hypercholesterolaemic rabbits is not due to diminished NO formation. Portland Press (in press).

AAS 37
Prostaglandins in the
Cardiovascular System

INVOLVEMENT OF PAF IN ATHEROGENESIS

Brief Review

Matyas Koltai and Pierre G. Braquet

Institut Henri Beaufour, 17, avenue Descartes, 92350 Le Plessis Robinson, France

ABSTRACT: Crucial points have been recently explored between formation, release and breakdown of PAF and atherosclerotic plaque formation. Experimental and clinical studies suggest that an autocatalytic feedback network among PAF, cytokines and growth factors contributes to atherogenesis. This novel approach to atherogenesis deserves future therapeutical importance.

Abbreviations: ACh, acetylcholine; ADP, adenosine-5'-diphosphate; β-TG, β-thromboglobulin; cAMP, cyclic adenosine-5'-monophosphate; EDRF, endothelium-derived relaxing factor; FMLP, formyl-methionyl-leucyl-phenylalanine; GM-CSF, granulocyte-monocyte colony-stimulating factor; IL, interleukin; LDL, low density lipoproteins; LT, leukotriene; PAF, pletelet-activating factor; PG, prostaglandin; PLA_2, phospholipase A_2; PMNL, polymorphonuclear leukocytes; TNF, tumor necrosis factor; TX, thromboxane; VLDL, very low density lipoproteins.

INTRODUCTION

Cardiovascular ischemic disease, developing as a consequence of atherosclerosis, is the main cause of mortality. The 'response to injury' hypothesis by Ross and Glomset (1976) emphasizes the similarity of the inflammatory response to atherosclerotic lesions, implicating the endothelial injury as a primary determinant for the disease. PAF is mediator in inflammation, anaphylaxis, immune disorders and ischemic diseases (see for reviews Braquet et al., 1987; Koltai et al., 1991). Inflammatory cells, such as macrophages, PMNL and platelets as well as endothelial cells synthesize, release and metabolize PAF which may be involved in atherogenesis in several ways: (i) its synthesis, metabolism and breakdown is related to lipid metabolism which profoundly changes in atherogenesis; (ii) as a mediator of inflammation and immune response; and (iii) as a potent vasoactive mediator inducing abnormal vascular reactions during atherosclerosis. PAF is, therefore, likely involved in atherogensis. This review is an attempt to summarize evidence for this concept.

PAF IN THE PATHOMECHANISM OF ATHEROGENESIS

.PAF in atherosclerotic plaque formation and dyslipidemias: Primary vascular injury may result from hyperlipidemia and endothelial cell activation. The earliest consequence of denuding endothelial injury is platelet adhesion. PAF infusion to the mesenteric artery induces pathological alterations similar to that found in early atherogenesis (Bourgain et al., 1985). PAF released from activated platelets and endothelial cells attracts monocytes/macrophages to the site of injury. Hypercholesterolemia induces direct adhesion of monocytes to intact endothelium. Free radical formation in PMNL induced by PAF modulates lipoprotein uptake by subendothelial tissue. Free radicals oxidize LDL, modified LDL is recognized by specific receptors on macrophages and increases intracellular cholesterol accumulation. These "scavenger cell" receptors play a role in the formation of macrophage-derived foam cells (Henriksen et al., 1981). *In vivo* PAF is rapidly transformed to inactive lyso-PAF by a specific acetylhydrolase (see for review Braquet et al., 1987) which is associated with lipoproteins (Stafforini et al., 1987), mainly LDL and VLDL. While good correlation has been recognized between plasma LDL levels and atherosclerosis (Ross, 1986), a recent work has shown that plasma from patients with atherosclerosis, hypertension and ischemic cerebrovascular disorders exhibits a markedly increased capacity for PAF degradation *via* LDL associated PAF-acetylhydrolase (Östermann et al., 1988, Satoh et al., 1988).

FMLP did not alter resistance of large arteries in normal monkeys, but produced marked constriction in atherosclerotic animals (Lopez et al., 1989). In parallel, LTD_4 and PAF had minimal effects, while atherosclerosis potentiated the constrictor effect of TXA_2. Patients with obliterative arteriosclerosis of the lower limbs showed increased sensitivity of platelets to ADP and PAF, increased levels of β-TG and TXB_2 as well as decreased levels of 6-keto-$PGF_{1\alpha}$ and cAMP. Basal levels of PAF in patients with essential hypertension were not different from healthy individuals, however, changes in circulating PAF levels positively correlated with arterial blood pressure and creatinine clearance, but not with plasma Na^+ and Cl^- concentrations or plasma volume in response to dietary salt restriction, indicating that PAF plays a compensatory role in essential hypertension (Masugi et al., 1989). Whole blood aggregation induced by ADP and collagen in cigarette smokers with or without major symptomatic peripheral vascular disease was higher than in non-smokers, but no difference in TXB_2 and lyso-PAF production was found (Sturm et al., 1989). However, Taylor et al. (1989) reported a correlation of plasma lyso-PAF levels to cigarette smoking and atherosclerosis.

Marked shape change induced by LDL in human platelets was accompanied by increased phosphatidylinositol turnover, free intracellular Ca^{2+} and TXB_2 levels. High concentrations of LDL exerted increased platelet aggregation (Aviram et al., 1983). Evidence has been presented that LDL isolated from human plasma, contain PAF, and the shape change induced by LDL might be due to or modified by the presence of PAF. However, preincubation of human platelets with PAF antagonists did not affect shape change reaction induced by LDL (Pletscher et al., 1989), but completely suppressed shape change due to PAF. Alternatively, preincubation of platelets with PLA_2 abolished PAF-induced shape change, but did not influence the shape change due to LDL.

We have recently presented evidence for the involvement of PAF in the atherosclerotic process by examining the effect of BN 52021, a specific PAF receptor antagonist, on cholesterol accumulation in the rabbit aorta induced by an atherogenic diet (Feliste et al., 1989). Hypercholesterolic diet resulted in a rapid, 50-fold increase in plasma cholesterol levels, Treatment with BN 52021 for two months did not affect hypercholesterolemia, however it markedly reduced free and esterified cholesterol accumulation in the aortic wall of animals fed atherogenic diet. BN 52021 showed no effect on the cellular cholesterol esterification and liver acyl-CoA cholesterol acyl-transferase activity remained unchanged. These findings suggest that BN 52021 exerts its protective effect on atherosclerotic plaque formation by inhibiting PAF-induced endothelial damage and cell infiltration.

PAF and endothelium-dependent relaxation: PAF produced a concentration-dependent vasodilatory effect in rabbit mesenteric artery which was significantly inhibited by CV-6209, a PAF receptor antagonist, while ACh-induced vasodilation remained uneffected (Kamata et al., 1989). These data suggest that PAF produces dilation of resistance vessels through EDRF release which might account for the its strong hypotensive effect produced *in vivo*. In rat aortic rings precontracted with $PGF_{2\alpha}$, addition of unstimulated canine PMNL or PMNL stimulated with FMLP in the presence of cytochalasin B moderately decreased ACh-induced vasorelaxation (Pieper & Gross, 1989). Preincubation of stimulated PMNL with PAF suppressed endothelium-dependent relaxation by ACh, but not that induced by nitroglycerin. CV-3988 or catalase blocked the response to PAF. Thus, PAF-primed PMNL impairs EDRF production *via* oxygen-derived free radicals. This finding provides additional evidence for the interaction of PMNL with PAF and other lipid mediators which may contribute to the regulation of vascular tone.

PAF/cytokine interaction in atherogenesis: Like PAF, cytokines, such as TNF and various interleukins can interact with endothelial cells, resulting in injury characterized by bleb formation, vacuolization and plasma leakage (Bevilacqua et al., 1986). PAF is a potent chemotactic agent for PMNL, inducing superoxide release, aggregation, degranulation (Braquet et al., 1989a), and stimulates TNF production from peripheral blood derived monocytes (Bussolino et al., 1988). These effects are inhibited by PAF antagonists (Bonavida et al., 1989). TNF also enhances PMNL superoxide production and adherence (Berkow et al., 1987). We have shown that TNF primes PAF-induced superoxide generation in human PMNL, and this effect is completely abolished by PAF antagonists, being also able to decrease superoxide anion production elicited solely by TNF. This indicates that TNF-induced superoxide generation is partially mediated by PAF (Paubert-Braquet et al., 1990).

PAF, IL-1 and TNF also exert direct effects on the vascular system (Braquet et al., 1989a). TNF, IL-1 and lymphotoxin, but not IL-2, IL-3, IL-6, γ-IFN and colony- stimulating factors, induce cultured endothelial cells to synthesize PAF (Bussolino et al., 1988). GM-CSF, another cytokine produced by activated T cells, also primes PAF-induced production of superoxide and LTs (McColl et al., 1990). This suggests that GM-CSF interacts with PAF during various inflammatory reactions and atherogenesis.

CONCLUSION

In conclusion, complex interactions between PAF and cytokines, amplifying the inflammatory response, appear to contribute to atherosclerotic plaque formation. PAF may increase atherogenesis by increasing hypercholesterolemia, while elevation of plasma lipid levels may delay the breakdown of PAF. The beneficial effect of BN 52021 in hypercholesterolemia supports the assumption that PAF antagonists protect primarily endothelial cells (Feliste et al., 1989). Atherogenesis induces microcirculatory failure leading to ischemia. PAF antagonists provide protection against myocardial and cerebral ischemia (Braquet et al., 1989b), known as major consequences of atherogenesis

The complex multicomponent nature of degenerative processes at the vascular wall suggests that combination of drugs, such as protease inhibitors, calcium antagonists, PGI_2 analogues, inhibitors of cytokines and growth factors, anti-TNF antibodies, with PAF antagonists may represent a successful therapeutic regimen in atherosclerotic patients or for the prevention of the disease.

REFERENCES

Aviram, M. and Brook, J.G. (1983) Platelet interaction with high and low density lipoproteins. Atherosclerosis 46, 259-268.

Berkow, R.L., Wang, D., Larrich, J.W. (1987) Enhancement of neutrophil superoxide production by preincubation with recombinant human tumor necrosis factor. J. Immunol. 139, 378-379.

Bevilacqua, M.P., Pober, J.S., Majeau, G.R., Fiers, W., Cotran, R.S.S. and Gimbrone, M.A. Jr. (1986) Recombinant tumor necrosis factor induces procoagulant activity in cultured human vascular endothelium: Characterization and comparison with the actions of interleukin 1. Proc. Natl. Acad. Sci. USA 83, 4533-4537.

Bonavida, B., Mencia-Huerta, J.M. and Braquet, P. (1989) Effect of platelet-activating factor (PAF) on monocyte activation and production of tumour necrosis factor. Int. Archs Allergy Appl. Immun. 88, 157-160.

Bourgain, R.H., Maes, L., Braquet, P. and Deby, C. (1985) The effect of 1-0-alkyl-2-acetyl-sn-glycero-3-phosphocholine (PAF-acether) on the arterial wall. Prostaglandins 30, 185-197.

Braquet, P., Paubert-Braquet, M., Bourgain, R., Bussolino, F. and Hosford, D. (1989a) PAF/cytokine autogenerated feedback networks in microvascular immune injury: consequences in shock, ischemia and graft rejection. J. Lipid Med. 1, 75-112.

Braquet, P., Paubert-Braquet, M., Koltai, M., Bourgain, R., Bussolino, F. and Hosford, D. (1989b) Is there a case for PAF antagonists in the treatment of ischemic states? Trends Pharmacol. Sci. 10, 23-30.

Braquet, P., Touqui, L., Shen, T.S. and Vargaftig, B.B. (1987) Perspectives in platelet-activating factor research. Pharmacol. Rev. 39, 97-145.

Bussolino, F., Camussi, G. and Baglioni, C. (1988) Synthesis and release of platelet-activating factor by human vascular endothelial cells treated with tumor necrosis factor or interleukin 1α. J. Biol. Chem. 263, 11856-11861.

Feliste, R., Perret, B., Braquet, P. and Chap, H. (1989) Protective effect of BN 52021, a specific antagonist of platelet-activating factor (PAF-acether) against diet-induced cholesteryl ester deposition in rabbir arta. Atherosclerosis 78, 151-158.

Friedman, R.J., Moore, S. and Singal, D.P. (1975) Repeated endothelial injury and induction of atherosclerosis in normolipemic rabbits by human serum. Labor. Invest. 32, 404-412.

Frieman, R.C., Mitchell, G.G., Heistad, D.D., Armstrong, M.L. and Harrison, D.G. (1986) Atherosclerosis impairs endothelium-dependent vascular relaxation to acetylcholine and thrombin in primates. Circ. Res. 58, 783-789.

Henriksen, T., Mahoyen, E.M. and Steinberg, D. (1981) Enhanced macrophage degradation of low density lipoproteins previously incubated with cultured endothelial cells: recognition by receptors for acetylated low density lipoproteins. Proc. Natl. Acad. Sci. USA 78, 6499-6513.

Kamata, K., Mori, T., Shigenobu, K. and Kasuya, Y. (1989) Endothelium-dependent vasodilator effects of platelet-activating factor on rat resistance vessels. Br. J. Pharmacol. 98, 1360-1364.

Koltai, M., Hosford, D., Guinot, P., Esanu, A. and Braquet, P. (1991) Platelet activating factor (PAF): a review of its effects, antagonists and possible future clinical implications. Drugs 42, Part I, 9-29, Part II, 174-204.

Lopez, J.A., Armstrong, M.L., Harrison, D.G., Piegors, D.J. and Heistad, D.D. (1989) Vascular responses to leukocyte products in atherosclerotic primates. Circ. Res. 65, 1078-1086.

Löbel, P. and Schrör, K. (1989) Stimulation of vascular prostacyclin and inhibition of platelet function by oral defibrotide in cholesterol-fed rabbits. Atherosclerosis 80, 69-79

Ludmer, P.L., Selwyn, A.P., Shook, T.L., Wayne, R.R., Mudge, G.H., Alexander, R.W. and Ganz, P. (1986) Paradoxical vasoconstriction induced by acetylcholine in atherosclerotic coronary arteries. N. Engl. J. Med. 315, 1046-1050.

Masugi, F., Sakaguchi, K., Saeki, S., Imaoka, M. and Ogihara, T. (1989) Dietary salt, blood pressure and circulating levels of 1-0-hexadecyl-2-sn-glycero-3-phospho-choline in patients with essential hypertension. J. Lipid Med. 1, 341-348.

McColl, S.H., Krump, E., McDonald, P. and Naccache, P. (1990) Granulocyte-macrophage colony-stimulating factor enhances the synthesis of leukotriene B_4 by human neutrophils in response to PAF-acether. J. Lipid Med. 2, 119-128.

Östermann, G., Lang, A., Holtz, H., Ruhlino, K., Winkler, L. and Till, U. (1988) The degradation of platelet-activating factor in serum and its discriminative value in atherosclerotic patients. Thrombos. Res. 52, 529-540.

Paubert-Braquet, M., Hosford, D., Koltz, P., Guilbaud, J. and Braquet, P. (1990) TNF primes PAF-induced superoxide release by human neutrophils: possible involvement of G protein. J. Lipid Med. 2, 1-14.

Pieper, G.M. and Gross, G.J. (1989) Selective impairment of endothelium-dependent relaxation by oxygen-derived free radicals: Distinction between receptor versus non-receptor mediators. Blood Vessels 26, 44-47.

Pletscher, A., Ferracin, F. and Gurari-Rotman, D. (1989) LDL induced shape change reaction of platelets is not due to PAF. Thrombos. Res. 56, 571-572.

Ross, R. (1986) The pathogenesis of atherosclerosis - an update. N. Engl. J. Med. 314: 488-500.

Ross, R. and Glomset, J.A. (1976) The pathogenesis of atherosclerosis. N. Engl. J. Med. 295, 369-377.

Satoh, K., Imaizumi, T.A., Kawamura, Y., Hoshida, H., Takamatsu, S., Mizono, S., Shojo, B.I. and Takamatsu, M. (1988) Activity of platelet-activating factor (PAF) acetylhydrolase in plasma from patients with ischemic cerebrovascular disease. Prostaglandins 35, 685-698.

Stafforini, D.M., McIntyre, T.M., Carter, M.E. and Prescott, S.M. (1987) Human plasma platelet-activating factor acetylhydrolase. Association with lipoprotein particles and role in the degradation of platelet-activating factor. J. Biol. Chem. 262, 4215-4222.

Sturm, M.J., Strophair, J.M., Kendrew, P.J., Vandongen, R., Beilin, L.J. and Taylor, R.R. (1989) Whole blood aggregation and plasma lyso-PAF related to smoking and atherosclerosis. Clin. Exp. Pharmacol. Physiol. 16, 597-605.

Taylor, R.R., Sturm, M., Kendrew, P.J., Vandongen, R. and Beilin, L.J. (1989) Plasma levels of the lyso-derivative of platelet-activating factor are related to age. Clin. Sci. 76, 195-198.

AAS 37
Prostaglandins in the
Cardiovascular System

ILOPROST PRESERVES ENDOTHELIAL FUNCTION AGAINST CYCLOSPORIN A AND SENSITISES MICROVESSELS TOWARDS ENDOTHELIUM-DEPENDENT AND -INDEPENDENT VASODILATATION

G.A. Burton, B. Müller and M. Schmidtke

Research Laboratories of Schering AG, Department of Cardiovascular Pharmacology, Müllerstr. 170-178, W-1000 Berlin 65, Germany

SUMMARY: The effects of iloprost have been investigated on the endothelial damage produced by cyclosporin-A (Cy-A) and on the microvascular reactivity to sodium nitroprusside (SNP), acetylcholine (ACh) and isoprenaline (ISO) following iloprost treatment i.e. in the absence of effective plasma levels, using the hamster cheek pouch. It has been shown that iloprost protects the microvascular arteriolar endothelium from functional damage by Cy-A and that iloprost infusion for 12 - 14 hr sensitizes the arterioles to ACh, SNP and ISO, an effect which is evident 5 hr but not 24 hr following treatment and in the case of ACh is abolished by indomethacin.

INTRODUCTION

The prostacyclin analogue, iloprost has previously been shown to protect the endothelium under various conditions such as, reperfusion following ischaemia, exposure to inflammatory agents (Müller et al., 1987) and loss of endothelial function under hypoxia (Türker and Demirel, 1988). As such it was of interest to examine whether iloprost could protect vascular endothelial function in a clinically relevant situation in vivo.

Cy-A is a potent immunosupressant which is highly effective in prolonging allograft survival. However, clinical use of Cy-A is complicated by 2 prominent adverse effects i.e. hypertension and vasculogenic nephrotoxicity. Short term administration of Cy-A seems to result in functional damage to the endothelium while long term administration would appear also to affect vascular smooth muscle function (Bossaller et al., 1989).

In addition, despite the short half life of iloprost in man (< 30 min), infusion of iloprost for 6 hr per day for 28 days has been shown to result in sustained and significant clinical improvement in 85 % of patients suffering from severe peripheral vascular occlusive disease (PVOD; Flessinger and Schäfer, 1990).

The present study comprises essentially two separate experiments. The first, in order to determine whether a prostacyclin mimetic can protect the microvascular endothelium against the damaging effects of Cy-A and the second to investigate whether iloprost can influence microvascular reactivity in the absence of effective plasma levels (i.e. following iloprost treatment).

MATERIALS AND METHODS

Hamster cheek pouch: Male Syrian Hamsters (100 - 120 g; BGA, Berlin) previously allowed free access to food and water were anaesthetised with pentobarbital sodium (60 mg/kg, i.p.). Exteriorisation of the cheek pouch and preparation for intravital microscopy were as previously described (Duling, 1973). The hamster cheek pouch was continuously superfused (5 ml/min) with warm (37 °C) physiological salt solution (composition in mM: NaCl 131, KCl 4.7, $CaCl_2$ 2, $MgSO_4$ 1.2, $NaHCO_3$ 18) gassed with 95% N_2/5% CO_2.

Microscopic observation and videosampling using a Leitz intravital microscope amd modified Sony video system were carried out at a final magnification (videomonitor) of x120. Arterioles were contrasted from the surrounding tissue by fluoresene isothiocyanate labelled dextran (FITC-dextran 70 KD Sigma; 500 mg/kg, i.v.). Intravascular fluorescence was observed using filtered incident light at 425 nm. Diameters of pre-selected 1st - 3rd branching order arterioles were measured from videotape using an electronic, adjustable square.

Experimental design 1: 26 animals were randomly assigned to 1 of 4 experimental groups: Group 1: control (no treatment, n=6); Group 2: Cy-A (Sandimmun®, 30 mg/kg/day, i.p. for 7 days, n=7); Group 3: iloprost (0,3 mg/kg/min s.c. for 7 days, n=6); Group 4: iloprost (as above) + Cy-A (as above, for 7 days, n=7).

Iloprost (dissolved in 0.9% NaCl + 1.25 mg/ml $NaHCO_3$) was administered s.c. by means of minipumps (Alzet®) implanted on day 1. On day 8 the minipumps were removed at least 1.5 hr prior to experimentation. Due to its short half-life in rodents (15 min) it was considered that iloprost was not present at relevant plasma concentrations during the microscopy studies. After surgical preparation of the cheek pouch an equilibration period of 30 min was allowed prior to measurement of control vascular diameters. Following control measurements the superfusion solution was replaced for a period of 5 min with solutions containing ACh ($1x10^{-7}$ M, Sigma), SNP ($5x10^{-8}$ M, Riedel de Haen) or U46619 ($1x10^{-7}$ M, UpJohn). A 10 minute washout period with normal superfusion solution was allowed following administration of each vasoactive agent. Vascular diameters of 1st - 3rd branching order arterioles were measured immediately prior to, at 2 and 5 min during, and at 5 and 10 min following administration of each vasoactive agent.

Experimental design 2: Iloprost (0.3 μg/kg/min s.c.) was administered by minipumps for a period of 12 - 14 hr following which the minipumps were removed. At 5 and 24 hr following removal of the minipumps the microvascular reactivity of 1st - 3rd branching order arterioles was examined following topically applied ACh (10^{-7} M), SNP ($5x10^{-8}$ M) and ISO (10^{-7} M, EGA-Chemie, n=6). Vascular diameters were measured at the same time intervals as described above. Vasodilatation to ACh and SNP was investigated both in the presence and absence of indomethacin (10 mg/kg i.p.) administered 1 hr prior to the vasoactive agents.

A descriptive statistical evaluation using the Mann-Whitney U test was performed where $P < 0.05$ was taken as a significant difference.

RESULTS

Experiment 1: Topical application of ACh produced an increase in resting diameters of 1st - 3rd branching order arterioles of 10 - 13 % in control animals. Following pretreatment with Cy-A, ACh produced a vasoconstriction with arteriolar diameters decreasing by 19 - 24 %. Pretreatment with iloprost alone produced a significant potentiation of ACh-induced vasodilatation when compared to control responses ($P < 0.05$). Vasodilatation to ACh was further potentiated following pretreatment with Cy-A and iloprost combined (Fig. 1).

U46619 produced a marked vasoconstriction in all arterioles studied i.e. 55 %, 42 % and 29 % in 1st, 2nd and 3rd order arterioles respectively. The vasoconstriction induced by U46619 was unaffected by any of the pretreatments studied (data not shown).

Application of SNP increased arteriolar diameters in control animals by 20 - 27 %. Pretreatment with Cy-A had no significant effect on SNP-induced vasodilatation, however, pretreatment with iloprost alone and in combination with Cy-A increased the vasodilatation response to SNP when compared to control animals. This vasodilatation was only significant in the case of second order arterioles (Fig. 1).

Experiment 2: Topical application of ACh, 5 hr following the cessation of iloprost infusion, produced a significant ($P < 0.05$) potentiation of vasodilatation in all arterioles studied when compared to controls, however, this potentiation was no longer evident at 24 hr (Fig. 2).

Application of SNP following iloprost also produced a potentiation of the vasodilatation response which was significant in both 1st and 3rd order arterioles ($P < 0.05$, Fig. 2). At 24 hr vasodilatation was still evident in all arterioles studied and was significantly different from controls in 1st ($P < 0.05$) and 3rd ($P < 0.1$) order arterioles (data not shown).

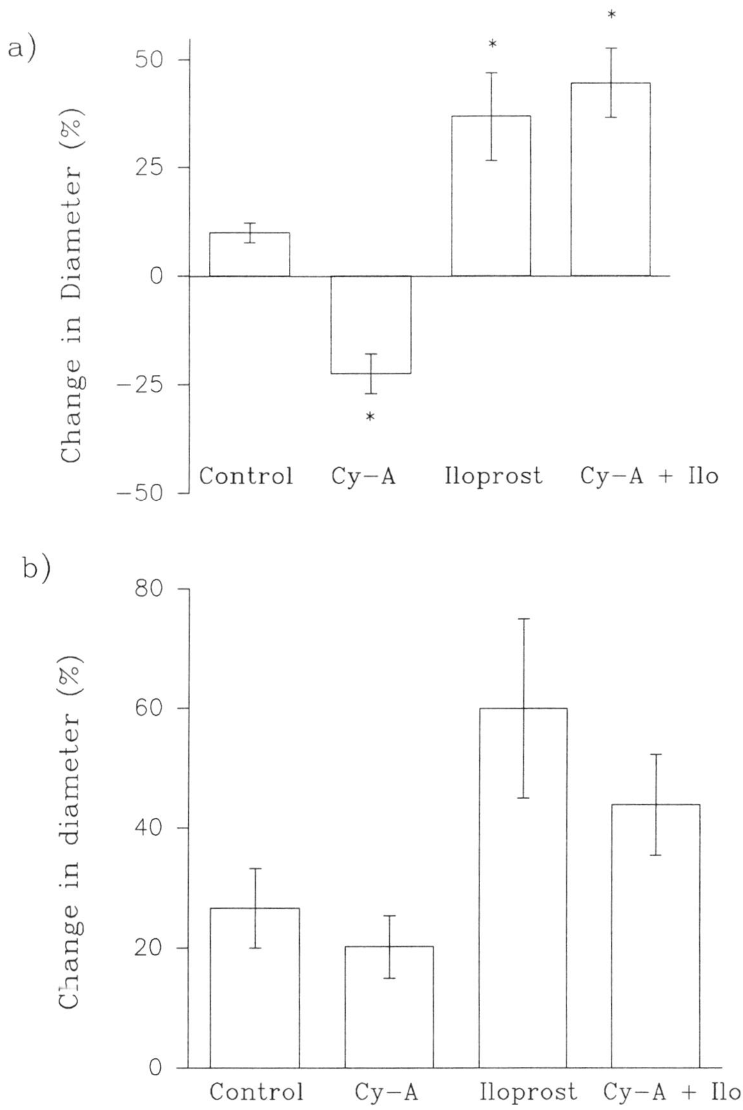

Fig. 1. Effects of Cy-A (30 mg/kg/day), iloprost (0.3 μg/kg/min) and Cy-A + iloprost on a) ACh-induced and b) SNP-induced diameter changes of 1st branching order arterioles (resting diameter 53.7 ± 10.3 μm). Data are expressed as means ± SEM, n ≥ 6, * $P < 0.05$.

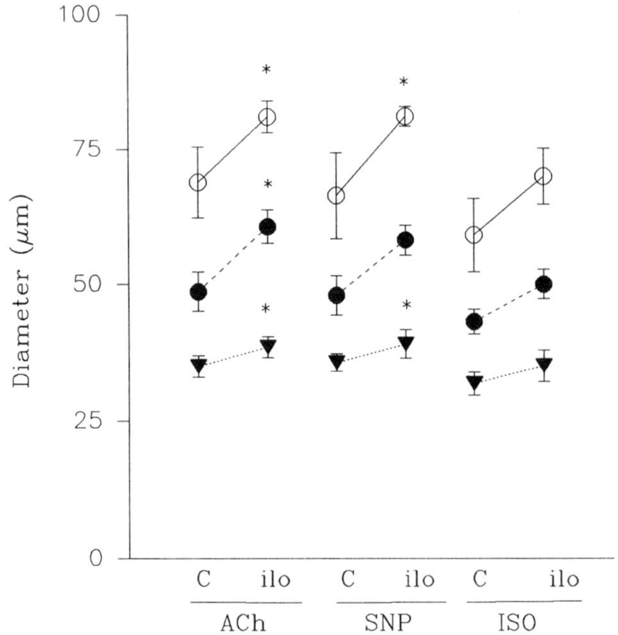

Fig. 2. Diameter changes in 1st (○—○), 2nd (●—●) and 3rd (▼—▼) order arterioles induced by ACh, SNP and ISO, 5 hr following cessation of iloprost infusion. C = control, ilo = 5 hr after iloprost. Data are expressed as means ± SEM, $n \geq 6$. * $P < 0.05$.

ISO failed to produce vasodilatation in control vessels studied at 5 and 24 hr. However, in animals pretreated with iloprost, ISO produced vasodilatation at 5 hr in all vessels studied although this failed to reach statistical significance (Fig. 2). At 24 hr vasodilatation was only evident in 1st order vessels (data not shown).

Administration of indomethacin 1 hr prior to application of ACh and SNP abolished the potentiation of vasodilatation observed previously following ACh and reduced that following SNP (data not shown).

DISCUSSION

ACh-induced vasodilatation has been shown to be dependent on an intact endothelium and to be mediated by endothelium-derived relaxing factor (EDRF; Furchgott and Zawadski, 1981). In the present study it has been shown that in the hamster cheek pouch Cy-A treatment for 7 days converts the vasodilatory response to ACh to vasoconstriction, an effect known to occur in the absence of an intact endothelium. Pretreatment with Cy-A did not however influence the response to the endothelium independent vasodilator, SNP, indicating that Cy-A has damaged the vascular endothelium. Iloprost prevented the loss of ACh-induced vasodilatation following Cy-A suggesting that iloprost may be capable of protecting the microvasculature from Cy-A induced endothelial damage.

Iloprost pretreatment alone, resulted in potentiation of both endothelium-dependent and -independent vasodilatation although the mechanism by which this occurs requires further investigation. U46619-induced vasoconstriction was unaffected by any of the pretreatments studied, indicating that in this study Cy-A did not induce changes in vascular smooth muscle. These effects occured at least 1.5 hr after termination of iloprost administration i.e. in the absence of effective plasma levels, suggesting that the effects of iloprost are not receptor-mediated From the results of the second part of the study, obtained with ACh, SNP and ISO following iloprost pretreatment, vasodilatation induced by SNP and ACh were potentiated and ISO-induced vasodilatation became evident indicating a sensitizing effect of iloprost on the microvasculature. Evidence to suggest that more than one mechanism is involved in this sensitization was provided by the abolishment of ACh-induced vasodilatation by indomethacin while responses to SNP were unaffected. It can be speculated that these mechanisms may include stimulation of prostacyclin release by EDRF, regulation of membrane receptors, G proteins or second messengers.

CONCLUSION: Iloprost protects the microvascular endothelium from functional damage induced by Cy-A. Modulation of vasodilatory effects persisting beyond the presence of effective plasma levels may explain the therapeutic effects on PVOD which are achieved with prostacyclin mimetics infused daily for only a few hours.

REFERENCES

Bossaller, C., Förstermann, U., Hertel, R., Olbricht, C., Reschke, V., Fleck, E. (1989) Eur. J. Pharmacol. 165 (1), 165-169
Duling, B.R. (1973) Microvasc. Res. 5, 423-429
Flessinger, J.N., Schäfer, M. (1990) Lancet 335, 555-557
Furchgott, R.F., Zawadski, J.V. (1980) Nature 288, 373-376
Müller, B., Schmidtke, M., Witt, W. (1987) Prost. Leuk. Med. 29, 187-198
Türker, R.K., Demirel, E. (1988) Pharmacology 36, 151-155

AAS 37
Prostaglandins in the
Cardiovascular System

ILOPROST IN CARDIOPULMONARY BYPASS PROCEDURES

H.R.Watson[1],G.Belcher[1],J.K.Brierley[2] & W.P.Dole[3].

[1]Cardiovascular Clinical Research Unit, Schering Health Care, Burgess Hill, West Sussex, England, [2]Department of Cardiothoracic Anaesthesia, Freeman Hospital, Newcastle-upon-Tyne, England, [3]Berlex Laboratories Inc., Wayne, N.J., U.S.A.

SUMMARY: The inhibition of platelet aggregation during cardiopulmonary bypass and effects on post-operative cerebral deficits were investigated in a placebo-controlled study of 145 patients. Significant preservation of platelet numbers and function were shown without significant haemodynamic problems, but no effect on cerebral deficits could be found. The use of iloprost in patients with severe thrombocytopenia seems justified, but the clinical benefits from its use in routine cardiopulmonary bypass remain to be shown.

INTRODUCTION

Cardiopulmonary bypass surgery is associated with the problems of platelet consumption and post-operative organ dysfunction. It is hypothesised that the reported organ dysfunction, notably cerebral, pulmonary and renal, may be a consequence of platelet activation and microaggregate formation in the extracorporeal circuit. Strategies to reduce the complications of bypass have included the use of membrane instead of bubble oxygenators, arterial line filters to remove microaggregates from the circulation and the inhibition of platelet aggregation.

Iloprost is a chemically stable prostacyclin analogue with a short half-life in man. Like prostacyclin it is a very potent inhibitor of platelet aggregation and vasodilator. The platelet inhibitory property encouraged the use of iloprost in cardiopulmonary bypass procedures. The results of the three earlier studies in routine cardiopulmonary bypass are summarised below (Table I). Two of these three placebo-controlled studies showed a significant prevention of platelet loss and aggregation by iloprost (10-12 ng/kg/min). All of the studies also showed a reduction in blood pressure with iloprost, but differed in the extent to which this unwanted effect could be controlled.

TABLE I: Studies of iloprost in routine cardiopulmonary bypass procedures

Investigator	n	Platelet Effects	Haemodynamic Effects
Addonizio (unpublished)	50	↓ platelet loss preservation of platelet function	↓ blood pressure controlled with pressor agent + fluids
Blauth et al (1987)	20	No significant effect	↓ blood pressure (not controlled)
Spyt et al (1988)	50	↓ platelet loss preservation of platelet function ↓ platelet sequestration in bypass circuit	↓ blood pressure controlled with fluids

Two further publications on the use of iloprost in cardiac surgery have addressed the particular problems of cardiopulmonary bypass in patients suffering from clinically severe thrombocytopenia associated with the use of heparin (Addonizio et al 1987, Kraenzler et al 1988). In these cases higher doses of iloprost (up to 36 ng/kg/min) were used in order to ensure reduced loss of platelets and platelet function. By this means it was possible to successfully perform cardiac surgery which would not otherwise have been feasible without large transfusions of platelet concentrates.

With these results in mind it was decided to conduct a further study in cardiopulmonary bypass surgery to confirm the reduction of platelet aggregation with iloprost, to confirm that the haemodynamic problems are not insurmountable and to investigate whether an inhibition of platelet aggregation results in a reduction in post-operative cerebral deficits.

METHODS

One hundred and forty-five patients admitted to hospital for elective coronary artery bypass graft surgery were entered into the study and randomised to either iloprost or placebo. Treatment consisted of an intravenous infusion of iloprost (10 ng/kg/min) or placebo from induction of anaesthesia until reversal of heparinisation after the completion of bypass.

Platelet effects were studied by recording platelet count before, during and after bypass, and by investigating the aggregation of platelets in platelet-rich plasma to collagen. Haemodynamic parameters were recorded during the operation and in the early post-operative period.

Screening for cerebral deficits was performed pre-operatively and repeated seven days and six months after surgery. This consisted of a comprehensive neurological examination, all seven subtests of the Wechsler Memory Scale, two components of the Wechsler Adult Intelligence Scale (block design test and vocabulary test) and the Halstead-Reitan Trail-making test part B.

RESULTS

The 145 patients entered were randomised, 75 to receive iloprost and 70 to receive placebo. There were no significant differences between the two groups with respect to demographic data or preoperative factors which might have influenced the clinical outcome.

Figure 1. Platelet Count.

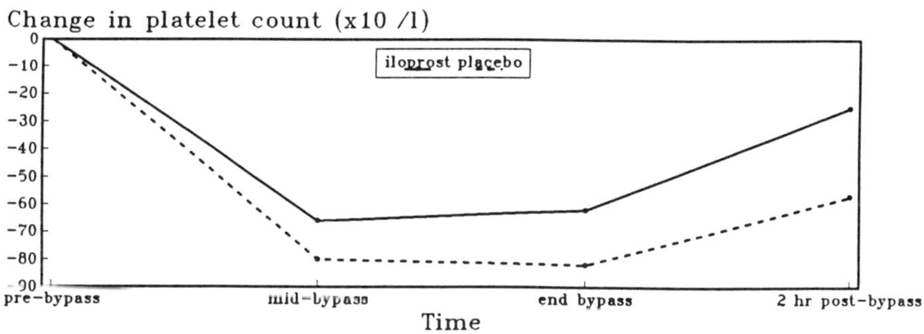

Figure 2. Platelet aggregation to collagen.

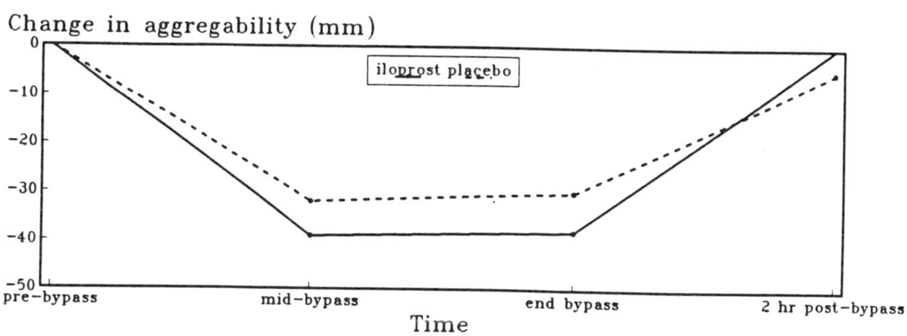

Loss of circulating platelets occurred during cardiopulmonary bypass in both treatment groups, but was significantly reduced in the iloprost group when compared to the control group at the end of bypass (p=0.009) and 2 hours post-operatively (p=0.0002) (figure 1). Platelet aggregability to collagen was reduced during bypass in both treatment groups compared to preoperative values, but 2 hours post-operatively platelet function was significantly better in the iloprost group (p=0.045) (figure 2).

The mean blood loss was numerically less in the iloprost group, and there was a significant reduction in blood transfusion requirements with iloprost (p=0.012) (table II). Haemodynamic parameters showed no significant differences intra-operatively. The highest pump flow rate, the lowest perfusion pressure recorded, duration of perfusion < 50 mmHg and the use of pressor agents to maintain blood pressure were all similar in the two groups. In the early post-operative period, however, a lower incidence of hypertensive episodes and a slightly higher use of inotropes were recorded in the iloprost group.

New neurological deficits were observed in 59% of cases on assessment before discharge from hospital, but only two of these were major strokes (one in each treatment group) and over half of these were primitive reflexes. There was no significant difference between the two treatment groups. By the 6 month assessment many of these deficits had resolved with only 33% of patients confirmed to have new deficits compared to pre-operative examination. Again there was no difference between the two treatment groups.

The sensitivity of the neuropsychological tests used was confirmed by the finding of significant deterioration in the mean scores in 4 of the 10 tests used at discharge with respect to pre-operative tests. After 6 months the mean scores showed that the patient groups as a whole had improved considerably with none of the 10 tests showing a deterioration compared to preoperative scores and 6 out of 10 showing a significant improvement. However, in all of these neuropsychological tests there were no statistically significant differences between the two treatments in terms of either the changes in mean scores recorded in each test or in terms of the number of patients showing a significant change in their individual score.

TABLE II: Blood loss and transfusion requirements

		Iloprost n = 75	Placebo n = 70	p value
Blood loss (ml)	mean	406	473	n.s.
	s.d.	223	306	
Blood transfused (ml)	mean	246	457	0.012
	s.d.	398	523	

DISCUSSION

The platelet parameters studied in this latest series of patients showed that the circulating platelets were protected from damage in the extracorporeal circuit to a significant extent by iloprost, but nevertheless some reduction in post-operative aggregability and loss of platelets did occur. A reduction in blood transfusion requirements was also observed in the iloprost group. In contrast to earlier studies no significant haemodynamic problems in the use of iloprost were encountered.

The incidence of neurological and neuropsychological deficits recorded were in line with previous reports and confirm the sensitivity of the methods used (Shaw et al 1985). However, there was no indication in the results of neurological screening, or in the neuropsychological scores that the patients were in any way protected from cerebral injury by the use of iloprost. There are two possible explanations for the lack of influence of iloprost in this respect. Firstly, the inhibition of platelet aggregation achieved may have been too weak to prevent microaggregates forming in the face of the strong stimulus from the artificial surfaces. Secondly, platelet microaggregates may not be responsible for the cerebral injury occuring in cardiopulmonary bypass. It is possible that both are true, but the finding that there was no effect on cerebral deficits despite a degree of platelet inhibition, suggests that the second explanation is probably the correct one.

The platelet preservation and lack of haemodynamic problems in this study support the use of iloprost in cases where thrombocytopenia is a clinical problem such as those patients suffering from heparin-associated thrombocytopenia. However, the clinical benefits of iloprost use in routine cardiopulmonary bypass procedures beyond the reduction in platelet loss and blood transfusion requirements remain to be shown.

REFERENCES

Addonizio V.P., Fisher C.A., Kappa J.R., Ellison N., (1987). Prevention of heparin-induced thrombocytopenia during open-heart surgery with iloprost (ZK36374). Surgery 102 796-807.

Blauth C., Brady A., Arnold J., Brannan J., Schulenburg W.E., Frackowiak R and Taylor K.M., (1987). A double-blind clinical trial of iloprost during cardiopulmonary bypass.
Perfusion 2 271-76.

Kraenzler E.J., Starr N.J., (1988). Heparin-associated thrombocytopenia: Management of patients for open heart surgery.
Anesthesiology 69 964-967.

Shaw P.J., Bates D., Cartlidge N.E.F., Heaviside D., Julian D.G., Shaw D.A., (1985). Early neurological complications of coronary artery bypass surgery.
Br. Med. J. 291 1384-1387.

Spyt T.J., Wheatley D.J., Walker I.D., Davidson J.F., MacArthur K.J.D., Martin W., (1988). Placebo-controlled study of iloprost (ZK36374) in cardiopulmonary bypass surgery.
Perfusion 3 179-186.

AAS 37
Prostaglandins in the
Cardiovascular System

EFFECTS OF ILOPROST AND FACTORS AFFECTING OUTCOME IN PATIENTS WITH SEVERE INOPERABLE LOWER LIMB ISCHAEMIA

G. Belcher for U.K. Severe Limb Ischaemia Study Group

Cardiovascular Clinical Research Unit, Schering Health Care, Burgess Hill, West Sussex, U.K.

SUMMARY: The effects of i.v. iloprost given for 14-28 days on six month outcome in patients with severe inoperable lower limb ischaemia were investigated in a double-blind placebo controlled study. More iloprost patients (64%) survived with a viable limb than placebo patients (42%). Iloprost improved prognosis in all subgroups of patients, but patients with lower presenting ankle Doppler pressures had a worse outcome than patients with higher pressures.

INTRODUCTION

The prognosis for patients with severe lower limb ischaemia with rest pain and/or ulcers remains poor. The U.K. Vascular Surgery Group reported only 56% of such patients were alive with a viable limb one year after presentation (Wolfe 1988). The treatment of choice remains vascular surgery or angioplasty, but for patients where this is not possible the prognosis is even worse. Further, although several studies report long-term outcome in patients with severe ischaemia few describe the outcome and the factors affecting outcome in this subgroup of inoperable patients. There is, therefore, a need for further investigation of these patients and for effective medical treatment. Several groups have reported that the prostacyclin analogue iloprost (Schering AG) can reduce rest pain and improve the healing rate of ulcers in inoperable patients. (Diehm et al., 1989, Balzer et al., 1987) and that there was a tendency for reduced amputation rates at 5 months after treatment (Norgren et al., 1990). This current study further investigated the effects of iloprost particularly emphasising long term outcome in terms of the number of patients alive with a viable limb, probably the most important end-point from the patients points of view. An analysis to investigate factors affecting long term outcome to assess whether iloprost might be particularly effective in subgroups of patients has also been performed.

METHODS

The study was randomised multicentre, double blind and placebo controlled. Hospitalised patients with severe limb ischaemia who were deemed inoperable at entry were randomised to receive i.v. iloprost or placebo. Treatment consisted of infusions of drug for 6 hours each day at a maximum tolerated dose up to 2.0 ng/kg/min. Patients with rest pain only received up to 14 days treatment and patients with trophic lesions up to 28 days treatment. At the end of treatment patients were assessed for relief of symptoms and 6 months later were reviewed to assess the number of patients surviving without a major amputation. Demographic factors (age, sex, diabetes, previous operation, presence of distal disease, presenting symptom and presenting ankle Doppler pressure) were then investigated in univariate analyses to assess whether any of these factors was predictive of long term outcome in the iloprost and placebo groups and whether iloprost might be particularly effective in any subgroups of the population.

RESULTS

The patients were reasonably well matched at entry to the study and demonstrated the expected characteristics of severe lower limb ischaemia (table I). There were rather more diabetics in the placebo group and more patients with rest pain in the iloprost group. A high proportion of patients had previously had vascular surgery, which then failed.

	ILOPROST (80)	PLACEBO (71)
Age	73 ± 10	73 ± 10
Males	52 (65%)	36 (51%)
Diabetics	25 (31%)	35 (49%)
Previous operation	36 (45%)	31 (44%)
Distal disease	87%	79%
AB index	0.48 ± 0.04	0.47 ± 0.04
Presenting Symptoms		
Rest pain	37 (46%)	27 (38%)
Painless ulcers	14 (18%)	9 (13%)
Painful ulcers	29 (36%)	35 (49%)

TABLE I: Patient Characteristics

At six months significantly more iloprost patients (64%) were alive with a viable limb than placebo patients (42%) (table II). More placebo patients (47%) than iloprost patients (31%) underwent major amputation.

	ILOPROST (76)	PLACEBO (71)
Major amputation	23 (31%)	33 (47%)
Death	4 (5%)	8 (11%)
Alive with viable limb	49 (64%)	30 (42%)*

* sig. $p<0.05$

TABLE II: Patient outcome at six months following treatment

In all the subgroups analysed iloprost patients had a better prognosis than placebo patients. Age, sex, previous vascular surgery, diabetes, presence of calf vessel disease and presenting symptoms were not found statistically significantly to affect outcome (table III).

		ILOPROST		PLACEBO	
		n	Survival	n	Survival
Age:	<60	5	100%	5	60%
	60-69	16	50%	15	60%
	70-79	36	61%	32	31%
	>80	20	70%	19	42%
Sex:	Male	50	70%	34	50%
	Female	26	56%	37	35%
Diabetic:	Yes	25	56%	34	41%
	No	48	73%	35	46%
Distal Disease:	Yes	52	60%	46	41%
	No	14	71%	12	33%
Previous Operation:	Yes	34	65%	31	45%
	No	42	67%	40	40%
Symptoms:	Rest Pain	36	58%	27	33%
	Painful Ulcers	27	63%	35	43%
	Painless Ulcers	13	85%	9	66%

TABLE III: Factors affecting outcome (survival with a viable limb) at six months.

The best predictor of outcome was presenting ankle Doppler pressure (Mantel-Haenszel test sig. $p<0.01$). The lower the absolute pressure or ABPI the more likely patients were to die or undergo major amputation (Fig. I). Iloprost improved prognosis at all levels of ankle pressure, but the greatest difference between iloprost and placebo responses were in the middle ranges of Doppler pressures.

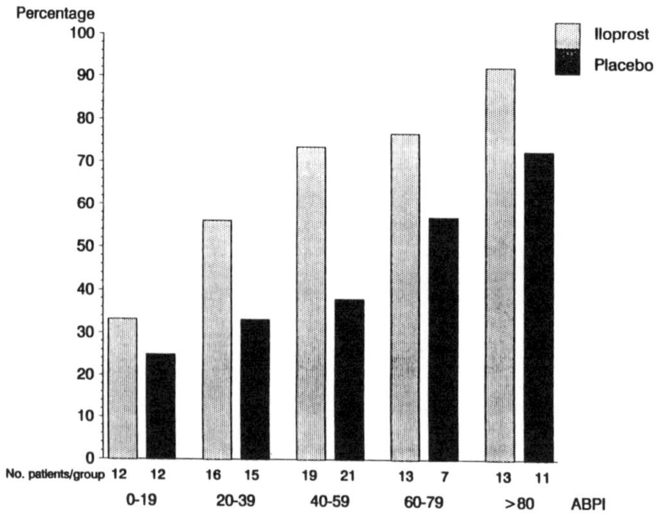

Fig I: Percentage of patients alive with a viable limb at 6 months divided by presenting ankle brachial pressure indices (ABPI).

DISCUSSION

The results show iloprost treatment can improve outcome at 6 months in patients with severe inoperable lower limb ischaemia and are similar to those reported previously (Norgren et al 1990). Iloprost improved prognosis in all subgroups of patients studied. The only factor found to significantly predict outcome was presenting ankle doppler pressure. Patients with low pressures had a poorer prognosis than patients with higher pressures. Despite this no particular pressure below which all patients were amputated or above which all patients survived could be demonstrated making a definition of critical ischaemia using Doppler pressures difficult. Iloprost improved outcome at all doppler pressure levels, but the potential to improve prognosis of patients with very low pressures was limited.

CONCLUSIONS: Iloprost treatment compared with placebo increases the number of patients alive with a viable limb at 6 months following treatment. Patients in all subgroups benefited from iloprost treatment, but the lower the presenting ankle doppler pressure the worse the prognosis in both treatment and control groups.

REFERENCES

Balzer K., Bechara G., Bisler H., Cleverth D., Diehm C., Heistg G., Held K., Mahfoud Y., Moerl H, et al. Placebo controlled double-blind multicentre study on the efficacy of iloprost in the treatment of ischaemic rest pain in patients with peripheral arterial ciculatory disease. Vasa Suppl 1987; 20: 379-381.

Diehm C., Abri O., Baitch G., Bechara G., Beck K., Breddin H.K., Brock F.E., Clevert H.D., Gorovic D., Marshall M., Rahmel B., Scheffler P., Schmidt W., Oberender H.A. Iloprost, ein stabiles Prostacyclinderivat, bei arterieller Verschlusskrankheit in Stadium IV D.M.W. 1989; 114: 783-788.

Norgren L., Alwmark A., Angqvist K.A., Hedberg B., Bergqvist D., Takolander R., Claes G., Lundell A., Holm J., Jivegard L., Risberg B., Ortengren T., Ortenwall P., Salenius J.P., Kaukinen S., Shtonen O., Huttunen M., Ylitalo P., Nizankowski R., Szczeklik A., Krolidowski W., Oberender H.A. A stable prostacyclin analogue (iloprost) in the treatment of ischaemic ulcers of the lower limb. A Scandinavian-Polish placebo-controlled, randomised multicentre study. Eur. J. Vasc. Surg. 1990; 4: 463-467.

Wolfe J.N.H. The definition of critical ischaemia - is this a concept of value? In Greenhalgh R.M., Jamieson C.W., Nicolaides A.N., eds. Limb Salvage and Amputation for Vascular Disease. London: W.B. Saunder Co., 1988; 3-10.

AAS 37
Prostaglandins in the
Cardiovascular System

ANY PHYSIOLOGICAL ROLE FOR PROSTACYCLIN IN REGULATION OF FETAL VESSEL TONE?

W. Klockenbusch*, H. Strobach, and K. Schrör

Institut für Pharmakologie und *Frauenklinik der Heinrich-Heine-Universität Düsseldorf, Moorenstraße 5, D-4000 Düsseldorf 1, FRG

SUMMARY: This study investigates the contribution of endogenous prostacyclin and nitric oxide (NO) for maintenance of umbilical artery tone in vitro. Treatment with indomethacin as well as removal of the endothelium was followed by contractions of umbilical arteries and a reduced formation of prostacyclin. In contrast, vessel tone was not affected by inhibition of NO synthesis, using nitro-L-arginine. Thus, prostacyclin rather than nitric oxide appears to be the endogenous endothelium-derived factor in the umbilical circulation that is involved in regulation of vessel tone.

INTRODUCTION

Generation of endothelium-derived vasoactive mediators is of key importance for control of vessel tone (Vane & Botting, 1991). There is evidence that endothelial formation of prostacyclin (PGI_2) in fetal vessels is much greater than in vessels of the adult (Remuzzi et al., 1979; Kawano & Mori, 1983). However, its contribution to low vascular resistance in the fetal circulation is still unsettled. In contrast to PGI_2, NO appears to play a crucial role in the regulation of blood pressure in the adult circulation (Rees et al., 1989).

To evaluate the physiological significance of PGI_2 in the fetus, we compared its vasodilator activities with those of endothelium-derived nitric oxide (NO).

In addition, we determined the generation of these endogenous mediators by umbilical arteries. The contribution of PGI_2 and NO to vessel tone was examined by selective inhibitors, i.e. indomethacin and nitro-L-arginine, respectively.

MATERIALS AND METHODS

Umbilical artery rings of normal pregnancies were prepared and suspended in organ baths containing low-oxygenated (2% O_2, 5% CO_2, 93% N_2) Krebs-Henseleit solution (37°C) of the following composition [mM]: Na^+ 143, K^+ 5.8, Ca^{2+} 2.5, Mg^{2+} 1.2, Cl^- 128, HCO_3^- 25, $H_2PO_4^-$ 1.2, SO_4^{2-} 1.2, glucose 5.1. After an equilibration period of about 5 h, a resting tone of 10 mN was applied. Submaximal standard contractions were induced by equieffective concentrations of serotonin (0.1 µM) or bradykinin (1 µM) and are expressed in percent of maximal response, elicited by serotonin at a concentration of 10 µM.

Changes in tension were measured isometrically under control conditions, in the presence of the cyclooxygenase inhibitor indomethacin (3 µM) or the inhibitor of NO formation nitro-L-arginine (100 µM). Alternatively, the endothelium was removed by gentle rubbing.

Generation of PGI_2 by the vessel segments was determined by measuring the accumulation of its stable hydrolysis product 6-oxo-$PGF_{1\alpha}$ in the incubation medium using a previously described radioimmunoassay technique (Schrör & Seidel, 1988). NO formation was quantified in terms of its second messenger cyclic GMP. Vessel segments were deep-frozen in liquid nitrogen and later homogenized, extracted and radioimmunoassayed for cyclic GMP as previously described (Steiner et al., 1972).

The data are mean and standard errors ($\bar{x} \pm$ SEM) of n experiments. Statistical analysis was performed by the two-tailed t-test. P values of ≤ 0.05 were considered significantly.

RESULTS

There was a significant accumulation of 6-oxo-$PGF_{1\alpha}$ by the vessel segments during the incubation period. Neither serotonin nor bradykinin did affect this basal release. Generation of 6-oxo-$PGF_{1\alpha}$ was decreased after treatment with indomethacin or removal of the endothelium (Table I).

Table I: PGI_2-generation by umbilical artery segments during 50 min incubation in Krebs-Henseleit solution

Treatment	n	6-oxo-$PGF_{1\alpha}$ [pmol/g ww]
none (Control)	10	154 ± 32
Serotonin [0.1 μM]	6	154 ± 16
Bradykinin [1 μM]	7	167 ± 30
Indomethacin [3 μM]	5	38 ± 13 *)
Endothelium removal	6	30 ± 11 *)

*): $p < 0.05$ (treatment vs. control)

Isolated artery segments also exhibited a marked cyclic GMP accumulation. This basal formation was not significantly altered by serotonin or bradykinin. Treatment with nitro-L-arginine or removal of the endothelium, however, considerably reduced the generation of cyclic GMP (Table II).

Table II: Cyclic GMP generation in umbilical artery segments during 15 min incubation in Krebs-Henseleit solution at 37°C

Treatment	n	cyclic GMP [pmol/g ww]
none (Control)	4	249 ± 41
Serotonin [0.1 µM]	3	490 ± 149
Bradykinin [1 µM]	4	278 ± 18
Nitro-L-Arginine [100 µM]	4	97 ± 27 *)
Endothelium removal	4	103 ± 13 *)

*): $p < 0.05$ (treatment vs. control)

Endothelium removal as well as treatment with indomethacin increased contractile tension induced by serotonin or bradykinin. In contrast, contractile actions remained unaltered in the presence of nitro-L-arginine (Table III).

Table III: Effects of indomethacin (IND), nitro-L-arginine (NLA) and endothelium revomal (- ENDO) on serotonin (5-HT) or bradykinin (BK)-induced contraction of umbilical arteries

Treatment	n	Tension (% max. response)
5-HT (0.1 µM)	12	67 ± 4
+ IND (3 µM)	9	74 ± 6
+ NLA (100 µM)	8	66 ± 6
- ENDO	10	90 ± 6 *)
BK (1 µM)	10	71 ± 4
+ IND (3 µM)	8	82 ± 3 *)
+ NLA (100 µM)	7	72 ± 6
- ENDO	10	89 ± 7 *)

*): $p < 0.05$

Constrictor effects of endothelium removal and indomethacin are exemplified in Fig. 1. In comparison to maximum contraction, elicited by serotonin, the peak contraction induced by bradykinin in a control artery segment was markedly reducedr. This difference in peak contraction disappeared after removal of the endothelium or treatment with indomethacin. Furthermore, the decrease in tension after peak contraction was substantially reduced both by indomethacin and endothelium removal (Fig. 1).

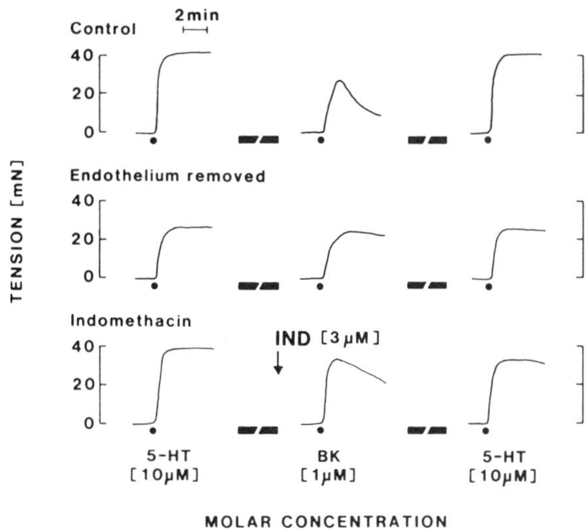

<u>Figure 1:</u> Original tracing of bradykinin (BK)-induced contractile tension after endothelium removal or treatment with indomethacin (IND) in comparison to maximal response induced by 5-HT (10 µM)

Fig. 2 shows that indomethacin as well as endothelium removal significantly reduced the time-dependent decrease of bradykinin-induced contractile peak. In contrast, inhibition of NO formation by nitro-L-arginine did not affect changes in tension (Fig. 2).

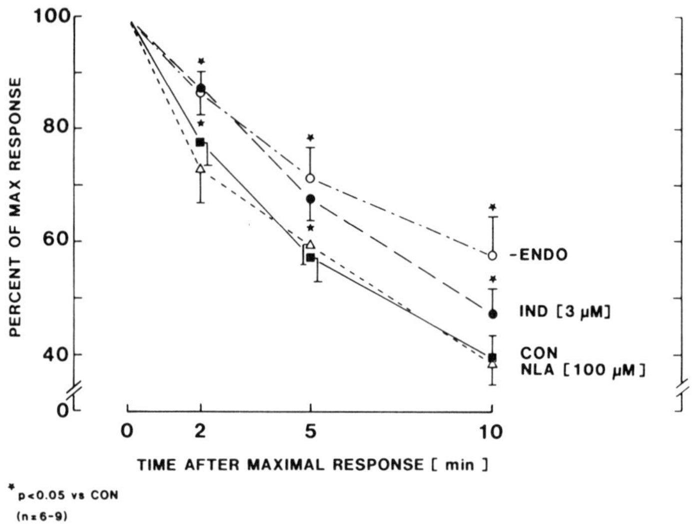

<u>Figure 2:</u> Time-dependent decrease of bradykinin-induced contractile peak in the presence of indomethacin (IND), nitro-L-arginine (NLA) or after removal of the endothelium (- ENDO)

DISCUSSION

This study demonstrates enhanced umbilical vessel tone and decreased formation of PGI_2 and NO after removal of the endothelium, indicating that endothelium-dependent relaxation takes place also in the vessel under the conditions of our study. In agreement with this, others have shown endothelial damage in pregnancy-induced hypertension (Dadak et al., 1984; Roberts et al., 1989), often associated with intrauterine growth retardation and reduced umbilical blood flow. These clinical symptomes could be explained at least partially by a diminished formation and/or action of endothelium-derived PGI_2 and NO. It is, however, unclear whether these mediators really act as relaxant agents in the fetus under physiological conditions.

Previously, a positive correlation between PGI_2 formation and blood flow in umbilical arteries has been shown (Mäkilä et al., 1983). However, the generation of PGI_2 could be the result of increasing blood flow during pregnancy rather than the immediate cause of low vascular resistance. Here we report that endogenous

PGI_2 generation reduces vascular tension of umbilical artery segments. Inhibition of endogenous PGI_2 production by indomethacin results in a significantly elevated tone of isolated artery segments. This suggests a role for endogenous PGI_2 in lowering vessel tension in the umbilical circulation.

In addition to PGI_2, a significant NO synthesis by umbilical arteries was also found in these experiments. In adult subjects, the basal release of NO keeps the vasculature in a dilated state (Vane & Botting, 1991). Concerning the fetal circulation, an increased perfusion pressure of placental vessels has been observed after inhibition of NO formation by methylene blue. This led to the conclusion that NO acts as a vasodilator in the fetal-placental circulation (Myatt et al., 1991). However, methylene blue is rathe nonspecific and may also prevent endogenous PGI_2 formation. In the present study, treatment with the selective inhibitor of NO synthesis, nitro-L-arginine, did not alter umbilical vessel tone. This suggests that NO has no or only minor functions for the maintenance of low vascular resistance in the umbilical circulation.

We conclude that in the umbilical circulation PGI_2 rather than NO appears to be the endogenous endothelium-derived relaxing factor. With respect to the available literature, this suggests a fundamental difference between fetal and adult circulation since in adult subjects NO rather than PGI_2 appears to be the key-endogenous vasodilating factor.

REFERENCES

Dadak, C., Ulrich, W., and Sinzinger, H. (1984) Morphological changes in the umbilical arteries of babies born to pre-eclamptic mothers: an ultrastructural study. Placenta 5, 419-426.

Kawano, M., and Mori, N. (1983) Prostacyclin producing activity of human umbilical, placental and uterine vessels. Prostaglandins 26, 645-662.

Mäkilä, U.M., Jouppila, P., Kirkinen, P., Viinikka, L., and Ylikorkala, O. (1983) Relation between umbilical prostacyclin production and blood-flow in the fetus. Lancet I, 728-729.

Myatt, L., Brewer, A., and Brockman, D.E. (1991) The action of nitric oxide in the perfused human fetal-placental circulation. Am. J. Obstet. Gynecol. 164, 687-692.

Rees, D.D., Palmer, R.M.J., and Moncada, S. (1989) Role of endothelium-derived nitric oxide in the regulation of blood pressure. Proc. Natl. Acad. Sci. (USA) 58, 531-538.

Remuzzi, G., Misiani, R., Muratore, D., Marchesi, D., Livio, M., Schiepatti, A., Mecca, G., de Gaetano, G., and Donati, M.B. (1979). Prostacyclin and human foetal circulation. Prostaglandins 18, 341-348.

Roberts, J.M., Taylor, R.N., Musci, T.J., Rodgers, G.M., Hubel, C.A., and McLaughlin, M.K. (1989) Preeclampsia: an endothelial disorder. Am. J. Obstet. Gynecol. 161, 1200-1204.

Schrör, K., and Seidel, H. (1988) Blood-vessel wall arachidonate metabolism and its pharmacological modification in a new in vitro assay system. Naunyn-Schmiedeberg's Arch. Pharmacol. 337, 177-182.

Steiner, A.L., Parker, C.W., and Kipnis, D.M. (1972) Radioimmunoassay for cyclic nucleotides. J. Biol. Chem. 247, 1106-1113.

Vane, J.R., and Botting, R.M. (1991) Endothelium-derived vasoactive factors and the control of the circulation. Semin. Perinatol. 15, 4-10.

AAS 37
Prostaglandins in the
Cardiovascular System

SEXUAL DIMORPHISM IN BLOOD PRESSURE RESPONSE TO THROMBOXANE AGONIST U 46619 AND TO ENDOTHELIN

Chr. Taube and M. Schirner

Institut für Pharmakologie und Toxikologie der Martin-Luther-Universität Halle, Leninallee 4, D-O-4020 Halle/Saale, FRG

SUMMARY: The blood pressure rising effect of two vasconstrictoryacting substances (the thromboxan agonist U 46619 and the endothelium-derived peptide endothelin-1) differs in male and in female rats and this fact depends on normotensive or hypertensive levels of blood pressure. Whereas in male rats the the drug effect was changed by pretreatment with aspirin, in female rats aspirin was uneffective in changing the blood pressure response to the agents.It could be suggested that the mechanism(s) for blood pressure regulation, especially the vasoconstrictor system, is different in males and females.

INTRODUCTION

From clinical and experimental data it is known, that incidence and complications of hypertension occur in a sex different manner. In former studies (Taube et al, 1988) we could show a sexual dimorphism in the formation of prostanoids in various organs of normotensive and especially of hypertensive rats. Now we looked for a sexual dimorphism in the blood pressure response curve to the thromboxane agonist U 46619 and to the endothelium-derived peptide endothelin-1. The blood pressure increasing potency of these substances depends on normotensive or hypertensive state of the animals (Tomobe et al., 1988). Therefore in our experiments we used male as well as female rats with normotensive and hypertensive blood pressure levels and looked for any difference in the blood pressure response to the vasoconstrictors.

MATERIAL AND METHODS

Animals: Normotensive Wistar rats (NTR) and spontaneously hypertensive Okamoto rats (SHR) of both sexes, 6 month old, wheighing 200-400 g were used.
Pretreatment: Aspirin (100 mg/kg) or saline (1 ml/kg) were injected intraperitoneally 24 h and 1 h before the experiment was started.
Blood pressure measurement: The animals were anesthetized with pentobarbital (50 mg/kg). A catheter was inserted into the carotid artery for measuring blood pressure and heart rate.
Drug application: U 46619 (5 µg/kg or endothelin-1 (1nM/kg) were injected into the jugular vein. Control animals were given saline (1 ml/kg) for preatreatment and treatment.
Experimental design: On each day the equivalent number of male and female rats (NTR and SHR) pretreated with aspirin and with saline, resp., and control animals was investigated.
Statistical analysis: Results are expressed as means ± s.e.m. Statistical analysis of data was conducted by students t-test. $p < 0.05$ indicated statistical significance.

RESULTS

As shown in Figure 1, the thromboxane agoist U 46619 increased the mean arterial blood pressure of male SHR at + 9.8 % in the 15th min., and + 13,1 % in the first min. ($p < 0.05$, $n = 10$). Pretreatment with aspirin attenuated this effect of U 46619 to approximately + 20 % ($p < 0.05$). The blood pressure in the control group was unchanged by the experimental procedure. In contrast to the results in male SHR in female ones there was no significant change in bloo d pressure after application of U 46619, independently of a pretreatment with or without aspirin. The blood pressure in the control group was unchanged, too, (Figure 2).
The results in SHR are shhown in Figure 3 and 4. In NTR, in contrast to SHR, the application of U 46619 caused a

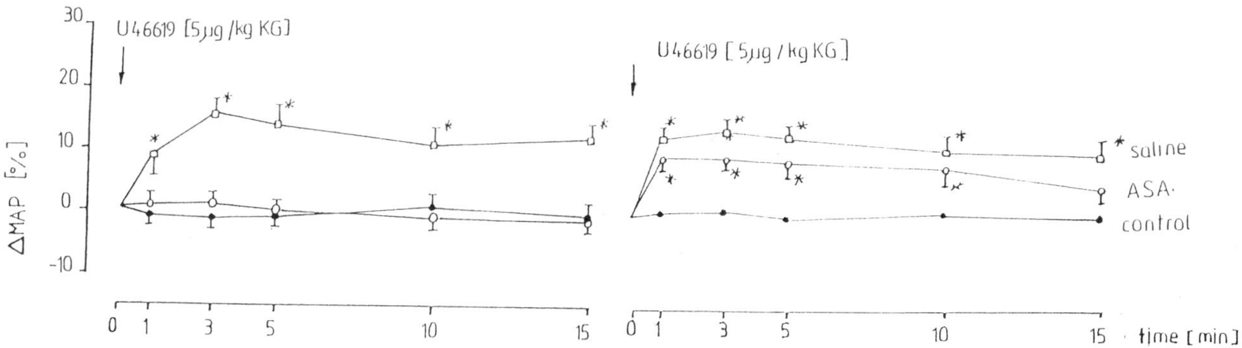

Fig. 1 and 2: Changes (% from baseline) of mean arterial blood pressure (MAP) by i. v. injection of U 46619 to male (left fig.) and to female (right fig.) SHR pretreated with aspirin (O - O) or saline (-) and in comparison to control animals (-)

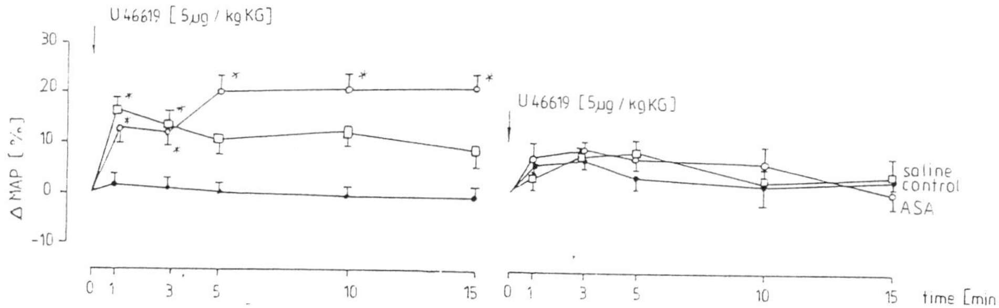

Fig. 3 and 4: Changes (% from baseline) of mean arterial blood pressure (MAP) by i. v. injection of U 46619 to male (left fig.) and to female (right fig.) NTR pretreated with aspirin (O - O) or saline (-) and in comparison to control animals (-)

significant increase in blood pressure in male as well as in female animals pretreated with saline. However, aspirin pretreated NTR showed significant differences between males and females: in male NTR aspirin abolished the blood pressure increasing potency of U 46619 to the value of control animals. The results in NTR are shown in Figure 3 and 4. In NTR, in contrast to SHR, the application of U 46619 caused a significant increase in blood pressure in male as well as in female animals pretretet with saline. However, aspirin pretreated NTR showed significant differences between males and females: in male NTR aspirin abolished the blood pressure increasing potency of U 46619 to the values of the control animals. In contrast to males in female rats pretreated with aspirin the increase in blood pressure by U 46619 was only slightly diminished, and the response curve was significantly different from the controls (Figure 4) As shown in Figure 5 in male SHR endothelin-1 caused initially a short lasting fall and after them a long lasting increase in blood pressure reaching + 36 % from baseline 15 minutes after application. Pretreatment with aspirin abolished the vasoconstrictor action of endothelin-1, whereas the depression in blood pressure during the first minutes was attentuated by aspirin. The blood pressure changes in female SHR, following the application of endothelin-1, however, differed from the results obtained in male ones (Fig. 6). There was no vasoconstrictor effect in female SHR independently of the pretreatment with or without aspirin. The blood pressure was depressed immidiately after application of endothelin-1 and this effect was more pronounced in aspirin pretreated SHR in comparison to controls. Calculating the correlation coeffizient r between the values of blood pressure 15 min. after injecting endothelin-1 and the blood pressure level of the animal measured before the endothelin was given we could show a significant correlation only for male SHR ($r = -0.9167$, $p < 0.01$), whereas for female rats the correlation coeffizient was insignificant ($r=0.087$, $p > 0.05$).

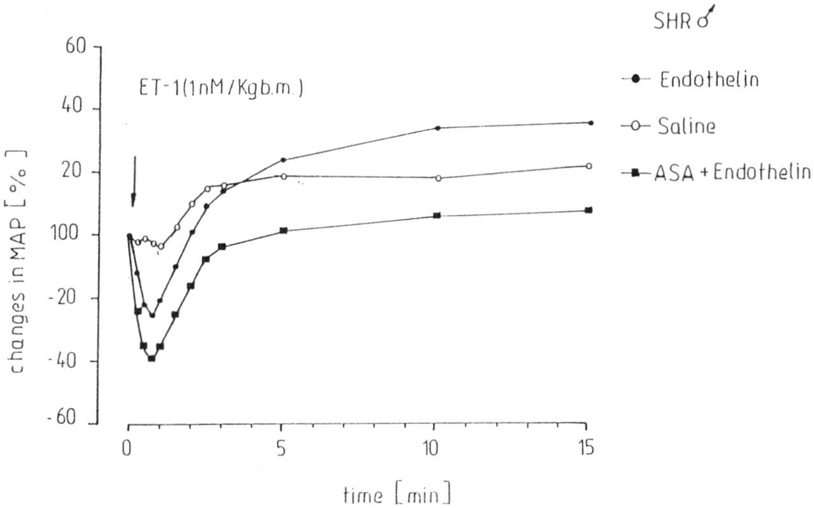

Fig. 5: Changes (% from baseline) of mean arterial blood pressure by i. v. application of endothelin-1 male SHR pretreated with aspirin (-) or saline (-) and in comparison to control animals (O -O)

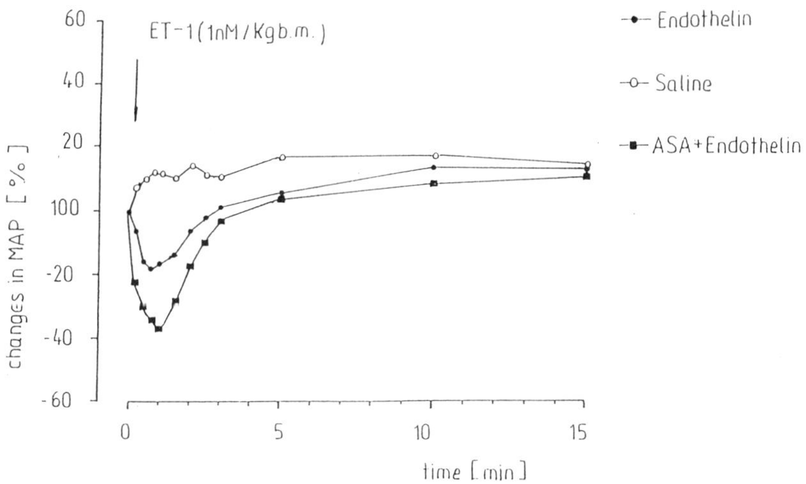

Fig. 6: Changes (% from baseline) of mean arterial blood pressure by i. v. injection of endothelin-1 to male SHR pretreated with aspirin (-) or saline (-) and in comparison to control animals

DISCUSSION

The present study demonstrates a significant sexual dimorphism in the vasoconstrictor effect of U 46619 as thromboxane agonist and of endothelin-1 as vasoconstrictive peptide . However, the relaxing effect of endothelin-1 immediately after performing the injection was similar in males and in females. Pretreatment with aspirin caused potentiating effects of U 46619 in male SHR and diminishing effects of U 46619 in male NTR and on endothelin-1 in male SHR. In contrast aspirin did not change the action of both agents in female rats. The initial and transient fall in blood pressure after bolus injection of endothelin-1 is possibly caused by a release of endothelin-derived relaxing factor (EDRF) and of prostacyclin (de Nucci et al., 1988). Inhibition of cyclooxygenase by indomethacin in rats did not change the depressor response to endothelin-1 (Winquist et al., (1988). This is in agreement with our studies: pretreatment with aspirin pronounced the depressor response in male as well as in female SHR, but the pressor response to endothelin-1 was completely diminished in male SHR. This lack in the pressor response to endothelin after aspirin pretreatment could possibly be explained by the inhibition of cyclopxygenase and therefore an inhibited formation of thromboxane A 2, which is the mediator for the pressor effect of endothelin. The missed effect of the vasocoonstrictor activity of endothelin-1 in female SHR suggests a difference in the mechanism of vasoconstriction in males and females. This hypothesis could be underlined by the fact that the thromboxane agonist U 46619 as potent vasoconstrictor acts different in male and in female SHR and that in normotensive rats a complete inhibition of soconstrictor effect of U 46619 by pretreatment with aspirin occured only in males. Cunard et al. (1987) also described a sexual dimorphism in the formation of endothelium-derived contracting substances in the rat pulmonal artery. Summarizing the results we suggest a sexual dimorphism in the vasoconstrictory mechanism(s) of blood pressure regulation, which is more pronounced in hypertensive rats than in normotensive ones. Prostanoids could be involved in this process.

REFERENCES

Cunard, C., Y. Maddox, M. Falcon: Eicosanoid expression of vascular sexual dimorphism. In: Prostacyclin and its stable analogue Iloprost, eds. by R. J. Gryglevski, G. Stock (1987) Springer Berlin, pp. 115-121

de Nucci, G., Thomas, R., d'Orlean-Juste, P., Antunes, E., Walder, C., Warner, T. D., Vane, J.R.(1988), Pressor effects of circulating endothelin are limited by its removal in the pulmonary circulation and by the release of prostacyclin and endothelium-derived relaxing factor. Proc. natn. Acad. Sci. USA 85: 9797-9800

Taube, Ch., S. Martin, A. H. Köhler, A. R. Köhler, H.-J. Mest: (1988) Influence of acetylsalicylic acid and BM 13177 on blood pressure and efficacy of antihypertensive drugs inspontaneously hypertensive rats, Biomed. Biochim. Acta 47, 94-99

Tomobe, Y., Miyauchi, T., Saito, A., Yanagisawa, M., Kimura, S., Goto, K., Masaki, T. (1988) Effects of endothelin on the renal artery from spontaneously hypertensive and Wistar-Kyoto rats. Eur. J. Pharmacol. 152: 373-374

Winquist, R. J., Bunting, P. B., Garsky, V. M., Lumma, P. K., Schofield, T. L. (1989) Prominent depressor response to endothelin in spontaneously hypertensive rats. Eur. J. Pharmacol. 163: 199-203

Subject index